VETERINARY NURSING OF EXOTIC PETS

Simon Girling
BVMS (Hons) DZooMed CBiol MIBiol MRCVS

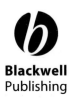

Blackwell
Publishing

© 2003 by Blackwell Publishing Ltd
Editorial Offices:
9600 Garsington Road, Oxford OX4 2DQ, UK
  Tel: +44 (0)1865 776868
108 Cowley Road, Oxford OX4 1JF, UK
  Tel: +44 (0)1865 791100
Blackwell Publishing USA, 350 Main Street, Malden, MA
02148-5018, USA
  Tel: +1 781 388 8250
Iowa State Press, a Blackwell Publishing Company, 2121
State Avenue, Ames, Iowa 50014-8300, USA
  Tel: +1 515 292 0140
Blackwell Munksgaard, Nørre Søgade 35, PO Box 2148,
Copenhagen, DK-1016, Denmark
  Tel: +45 77 33 33 33
Blackwell Publishing Asia, 550 Swanston Street, Carlton
South, Victoria 3053, Australia
  Tel: +61 (0)3 9347 0300
Blackwell Verlag, Kurfürstendamm 57, 10707 Berlin,
Germany
  Tel: +49 (0)30 32 79 060
Blackwell Publishing, 10 rue Casimir Delavigne, 75006
Paris, France
  Tel: +33 1 53 10 33 10

First published 2003

A catalogue record for this title is
available from the British Library

ISBN 1-4051-0747-2

Library of Congress
Cataloging-in-Publication Data
Girling, Simon.
    Veterinary nursing of exotic pets/Simon Girling.
        p. cm.
    Includes bibliographical references and index.
    ISBN 1-40510-747-2 (softcover)
    1. Exotic animals–Diseases.   2. Wildlife diseases.
    3. Pet medicine.   4. Veterinary nursing.   I. Title.

    SF997.5.E95 G57 2003
    636.089′073–dc21   2002038565

Set in 9.5 on 12 pt Times
by SNP Best-set Typesetter Ltd., Hong Kong
Printed and bound in Great Britain by
Ashford Colour Press, Gosport

For further information on
Blackwell Publishing, visit our website:
www.blackwellpublishing.com

Contents

The colour plate section may be found following page 154.

Preface

Veterinary nurse and veterinary student training in exotic species has come a long way in the last four or five years. Previously often consigned to the category of 'alsorans', exotic species are increasingly seen in general veterinary practice, to the point where the house rabbit has officially become the UK's third most commonly kept pet, after the cat and dog. Even more telling is the fact that numbers of cats and dogs in the UK are on the decline, yet the number of small mammals, reptiles and birds kept by the public continues to rise.

With this increase in these species kept as household pets, improved training in their care has thankfully started to become more important. Many veterinary schools and veterinary nurse training providers are devoting more time to teaching the husbandry and medicine of exotic species. Indeed, 2001 saw the start of the first course in Veterinary Nursing of Exotic Species, run through Edinburgh's Telford College and leading to a City and Guilds recognised qualification.

There is no turning the clock back. Exotic pet species are here to stay. It is therefore our duty as veterinary surgeons and veterinary nurses to ensure that we are up-to-date with the latest husbandry and medical details so that we may offer as good, if not better, levels of care as that provided for more traditional domestic pets.

I hope that this book will help in that quest and may be of use to veterinary nurse, technician and veterinary student alike.

Simon J. Girling

Avian Species

Chapter 1
Basic Avian Anatomy and Physiology

Classification

Birds are classified into many different family groups, according to a number of physical, anatomical and evolutionary factors. It is useful to know to which group a bird belongs as this gives an indication of the other birds it is related to. This is of some help when faced with a species that you have not seen before.

Table 1.1 contains some of the more commonly encountered family groups of birds seen in general and avian orientated practices.

The Psittaciformes are among the most colourful of birds kept as pets.

Nervous system

The avian brain is extremely smooth, lacking the many *gyri* (the ridges in the brain) seen in mammals (Fig. 1.1). Sight appears to be the dominant sense in birds. Two large optic lobes lie between the cerebral hemispheres and the cerebellum, and it is here where the optic nerves communicate and disseminate information.

The avian nervous system is not dissimilar to that seen in its mammalian counterpart. Birds possess 12 cranial nerves, the same number as the cat and dog. In the bird, the optic nerve is the largest.

Each of the wings has a nervous supply from a brachial plexus derived from the spinal nerves in the caudal cervical area. A lumbar plexus in the cranial kidney area supplies the body wall and upper leg muscles. Unlike dogs and cats, birds have an ischiatic plexus which is derived from spinal nerves in the sacral area and which is situated in the mid-kidney structure. It gives rise to the principal nervous supply for the hind

limbs – the ischiadic nerve. Finally, a pudendal plexus forms in the caudal kidney area from the spinal nerves and innervates the tail and cloacal area.

Musculoskeletal system

Most birds have the power of flight. The dense, cumbersome bones of the earthbound mammal would require too much effort to lift into the air. Birds have therefore adapted their skeletal structure, simplifying the number of bones by fusing some together, and generally lightening the whole structure by creating air spaces within many of the bones.

To further lighten the skeleton several of the larger bones, and even some of the vertebrae in the spine, are connected directly or indirectly to the airways, and are said to be *pneumonised*. This replaces the thick medullary cavity or bone marrow present in the center of mammalian bones, and produces a light, trabecular structure. While light, the structure is nevertheless extremely strong.

Figure 1.2 shows a generalised avian skeleton.

Skull

Beak

The beak, or bill, is the principle feature of the avian skull. It has been modified into a bewildering number of shapes and sizes, depending mainly on the diet to which the bird has become adapted. In all cases it is composed of an upper (maxillary) and lower (mandibular) beak which are covered in a layer of keratin, a tough protein compound similar to that which forms the exoskeleton of

Table 1.1 Avian family groups commonly encountered in veterinary practice.

Psittaciformes	This is the order of birds which includes those we know as 'parrots'. This includes the budgerigar, the amazons, the macaws, cockatiels, African grey parrots (Plate 1.1), cockatoos (Plate 1.2), parakeets and others.
Passeriformes	This is the largest order of birds and includes the canary, the finch family, birds of paradise, the mynah birds, ornamental starlings, sparrows and others.
Anseriformes	This order includes: • the duck family, for example the mallard, shovellor and shelduck; • the goose family, for example the barnacle, and greylag; • the sea duck family, for example the eider and smew; • the swan family, for example the mute, Whooper's and Bewick's swans.
Rhamphastidae	This order includes the toucan, toucanette and hornbill families.
Strigiformes	This covers the owl families.
Falconiformes	This order covers: • the Falconidae family, for example the peregrine falcon, the saker, the llanner, the gyrfalcon; • the Accipitridae family such as the buzzards (common, rough-legged and honey), the sparrowhawk, goshawk, golden eagle. } These are known as raptors

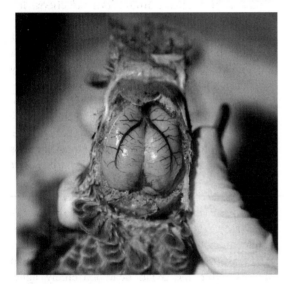

Fig. 1.1 Dorsal aspect of avain cerebral hemispheres showing lack of gyri.

insects. This keratin layer is known as the *rhamphotheca*. It is further classified so that the maxillary layer is referred to as the *rhinotheca*, and the mandibular layer as the *gnatotheca*. The rhinotheca and gnatotheca grow from a plate at the base of the respective sides of the beak, the rate of replacement depending upon the type of food eaten and the abrasion the beak receives.

In Psittaciformes (Table 1.1), the upper beak is powerfully developed and ends in a sharp point overhanging the broader, stouter lower beak (Plate 1.3). The tremendous power in a parrot's beak is due to a synovial joint or hinge mechanism, known as the *kinetic joint*, which joins the beak to the skull. The parrot's lower beak has a series of pressure sensors at its tip, which allow it to test the consistency and structure of objects grasped.

In raptors, the upper beak is extremely sharp and pointed, but lacks the kinetic joint attachment so it cannot produce such powerful downward force. Instead, it is used as a ripping instrument.

In Anseriformes (the duck family), the beak is flattened and may have fine serrations at the edges that allow the bird to filter fine particles from the water. Ducks such as mallards and shovellors have this type of beak. These serrations may be further developed to a jagged edge (for example, in the aptly named sawbill family) which allows the bird to grip slippery food, such as fish. Anseriformes also have nerve endings in a plate at the tips of their beaks (known as the 'nail') that allows them to find food hidden in mud.

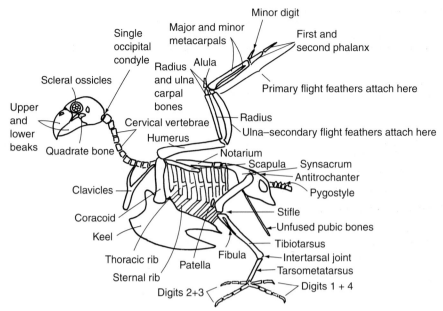

Fig. 1.2 Avian skeleton.

In all birds there is a series of smaller bones behind the lower and upper beaks which allows them to move the beak independently of the skull. These include the palatine, quadrate and pterygoid bones and the jugal arches. Their exact movements are beyond this text to describe, but many of the references at the end of this chapter give good accounts of their function.

Nostrils

The nostrils, or nares, lie at the base of the upper beak in most birds and are often surrounded by an area of featherless skin known as the *cere*. This may be highly coloured in some species, such as the budgerigar, where they may be used to identify the sex of the bird. In many Anseriformes the nares lie more towards the tip of the beak. The nares themselves are merely openings into the sinus chambers, which in turn connect with a branching network of bony chambers throughout the bird's head. These sinuses vary according to the species, but the majority of avian patients have an infraorbital sinus. This sits below the eyes, and is often involved in sinus and ocular infections. These sinuses also communicate with head and neck air-sacs. The function of these air sacs is not clear, but they may help with voice resonance.

When a bird suffers from sinus infections, the narrow inlets to these sinuses may become partially blocked and act as one-way valves, allowing air into the sacs but not out. The sacs may then overinflate and soft swellings are then commonly seen over the back or nape of the bird's head.

The sinuses and external nares communicate with the oropharynx via the choanal slit. This is a narrow opening in the midline of the hard palate. It is often the area chosen for taking samples when trying to isolate infectious agents for upper airway disease in birds.

The skull of the avian patient connects to the *atlas* (or first spinal vertebra) via only one occipital condyle at the base of the skull, unlike the mammalian two. There are also a large number of highly mobile cervical vertebrae. These two factors make the avian head extremely agile. However, the atlanto-occipital joint is also a weak point, making dislocation at that site very easy.

Vertebral column

Cervical vertebrae

The cervical vertebrae (Fig. 1.2) are independently mobile in the avian patient, as they are in the mammalian patient, and vary in number depending on the species between 11–25. They are generally box-like in form.

Thoracic vertebrae

The thoracic vertebrae (Fig. 1.2) are fused in raptors, pigeons and many other species to form a single bone known as the *notarium*. In other species they have some limited mobility. There are then two intervertebral joints between the notarium and the fused lumbar and sacral vertebrae. These fused vertebrae are known as the *synsacrum*.

Coccygeal vertebrae

The majority of the caudal coccygeal vertebrae (Fig. 1.2) are usually fused into a single structure known as the *pygostyle* – which forms the 'parsons nose' part of the chicken!

Pelvis

The roof of the pelvis is formed by the synsacrum (Fig. 1.2). The two 'sides' of the pelvis are reduced in size compared with mammals but consist of the ilial and ischial bones, with the *acetabulum* being created where they meet. The acetabulum in birds is not a complete bony socket as it is in mammals, but a fibrous sheet. There is a ridge on the lateral pelvis known as the *antitrochanter*, which articulates with the greater trochanter of the femur. The function of this ridge is to prevent the limb from being abducted when perching. The pubic bones of the pelvis do not fuse in the ventral midline as in mammals. Instead they form fine long bones which extend caudally towards the vent. They provide support for the skin covering the caudal abdomen and enough space for the passage of eggs in the female bird.

Ribcage

Psittaciformes have eight pairs of ribs (Fig. 1.2). Each rib has a dorsal segment known as the thoracic rib, and a ventral segment, or sternal rib. These ribs point backwards and rigidly connect the thoracic vertebrae dorsally and the keel, or sternum, ventrally.

Sternum

The sternal vertebrae are fused in birds to form the keel. The keel has a midline ridge which divides the pectoral muscles into right and left sides. The ridge may be a deep structure, as is seen in pigeons, raptors and Psittaciformes, allowing large pectoral muscles to attach for strong flight. Alternatively the keel may be flattened, as with Anseriformes, to provide a boat-like structure more suited to floating.

Wings

The shoulder joint is formed by the meeting of three bones, the humerus, the scapula (which is more tubular than the flattened mammalian one) and a third bone, known as the *coracoid* (Fig. 1.2). This latter bone forms a strut propping the shoulder joint against the sternum. The supracoracoid muscle attaches to the keel, then passes through the *foramen*, or opening, formed at the meeting point of these bones, and so reaches the dorsal aspect of the humerus where it attaches. Contraction of this muscle, along with some elastic tissues which are also present, helps to raise the wing. The pectoral muscles attach from the keel onto the humerus to pull the wing downwards. The fused clavicles, or wishbone (often referred to as the *furcula*), articulate with the coracoid bone and provides a degree of spring to the flapping of the wings. The humerus is pneumonised, which means that it cannot be used for intraosseous fluid therapy. This is also an important point to consider when repairing fractures.

The humerus articulates with the radius and ulna at the elbow joint. The radius is the smaller of these two bones, and lies cranially. The ulna provides the source of attachment for the secondary flight feathers, which insert directly into the periosteum of this bone (Fig. 1.3). The ulna is often used for intraosseous fluid administration in birds.

The radius and ulna articulate with one radial carpal bone and one ulnar carpal bone respectively. These in turn articulate with three metacarpal bones. The first metacarpal bone is the equivalent of the avian 'thumb'. It is known as the *alula*, or 'bastard wing', and forms a feathery pro-

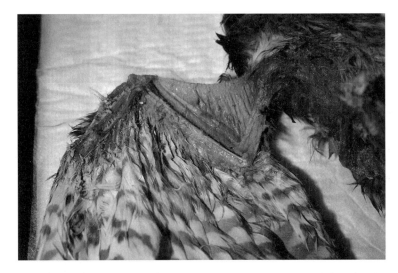

Fig. 1.3 Ventral aspect of a kestrel's (*Falco tinnunculus*) wing with covert feathers removed showing the attachment of the primaries to the manus and the secondaries to the ulna.

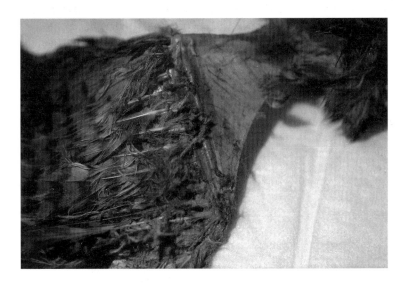

Fig. 1.4 Dorsal aspect of a kestrel's (*Falco tinnunculus*) wing with covert feathers removed showing the elastic sheet of the propatagium bridging the elbow joint.

jection from the cranial aspect of the carpometacarpal joint. The remaining two metacarpal bones are known as the major and minor metacarpal bones, and articulate with the first phalanx cranially and the minor digit caudally. The first phalanx then articulates with the second phalanx, forming the wing tip. The primary feathers attach to the periosteum of the phalanges and minor metacarpal bones (Fig. 1.3).

The area of the wing is enlarged by thin sheets of elastic tissue which span from one joint surface to another. The largest extends from the shoulder to the carpal joint cranially and is known as the *propatagium*, or 'wing web' (Fig. 1.4). This can be used in some species, such as pigeons, for vaccine administration.

Pelvic limb

The acetabulum of the pelvis holds the femoral head (Fig. 1.2). The limb may be locked, and prevented from being abducted, by the greater trochanter of the femur engaging with the antitrochanteric ridge on the pelvis. The femur is pneumonised in many birds. At the stifle joint the femur articulates with the patella and the tibiotarsal bone. The tibiotarsal bone is so called because it is formed from the fusion of the tibia and the proximal row of tarsal bones, and may also be used for intraosseous fluid administration. On the lateral aspect of the proximal tibiotarsus is the much reduced fibula.

Distally, the tibiotarsal bone articulates with the tarsometatarsal bone. This bone is formed by the fusion of the distal row of tarsal bones with the solitary metatarsal bone. The joint between the tibiotarsus and the tarsometatarsus is known as the intertarsal, or *suffrago*, joint. The tarsometatarsus then articulates with the phalanges.

In Psittaciformes, two digits point forwards (the second and third) and two backwards (the first and fourth), creating a *zygodactyl* limb. The first digit has two phalanges, the second digit has three phalanges, the third has four phalanges and the fourth has five phalanges. In perching birds (Passeriformes) and raptors, the second, third and fourth digits point forwards and the first points backwards creating an *anisodactyl* limb. Some species, such as the osprey (*Pandion haliaetus*), may move the fourth digit to face forwards or backwards to aid capturing its prey, creating a *semi-zygodactyl* limb.

Special senses

Eye

The avian eye is unique in that it contains a series of small bones. These are known as the *scleral ossicles* (Fig. 1.2). They form a ring-shaped structure which supports the front of the eye. The avian eye also differs from the mammalian eye in that it is not a globe, but pear-shaped, with the narrower end outermost.

The avian eye is large in proportion to the overall size of the skull, with only a paper-thin bony septum separating the right and left orbits. Birds have a mobile, translucent third eyelid, and upper and lower eyelids, the lower of which is more mobile than the upper. Two tear-producing glands commonly exist: the third eyelid, or *Harderian* gland, which is located at the base of the third eyelid, and the lacrimal gland situated caudo-laterally, as in mammals.

The colour of the iris may change with age in some parrots, for example the African grey parrot has a dark grey iris until 4–5 months of age, when it turns yellow/grey, and then silver as it continues to age. In others the iris may be used as an indicator of the sex of the bird: in large cockatoos, for example, the female has a bright, red-brown iris, whereas the male's is a dark, brown-black.

The avian retina is thick and possesses no visible surface blood vessels, unlike that of mammals. To provide nutrition to the retina, birds possess a pleated and folded vascular structure called the *pecten oculi*, which is found at the point where the optic nerve enters the eye. It contracts intermittently, expelling nutrients into the vitreous humour.

Finally, the avian iris has skeletal-muscle fibres within it, unlike mammals, which possess only smooth-muscle fibres. This means the avian patient can constrict and dilate its pupil at will, so reducing the value of the pupillary light reflex as a tool in determining ocular function. Because the two optic nerves are completely separated from each other, the consensual light reflex is also a poor indicator of cerebral function.

Ear

There is no pinna in birds, although some species, such as the long and short eared owls, have feathers in this area. There is a short, horizontal external canal, covered by feathers, which is located caudo-lateral to the ocular orbit. The tympanic membrane may be clearly seen. The middle ear connects to the oropharynx via the Eustachian canal. The mammalian aural ossicles are replaced in the bird by a lateral, extra columella cartilage and a medial columella bone which transmit sound waves to the inner ear.

The inner ear contains the cochlea and the semicircular canals, which fulfil the same functions as in mammals.

Respiratory anatomy

Upper respiratory system

The nares open into the nasal passages, which in turn communicate with the glottis of the larynx via a midline aperture in the hard palate which forms the roof of the caudal mouth. This aperture is called the *choanal* slit. The sinus system and cervicocephalic air sacs have been previously mentioned.

Larynx

Birds have a reduced laryngeal structure, lacking an epiglottis, the thyroid cartilage, and the vocal folds seen in cats and dogs. The main structure is the glottis, which protects the entrance to the trachea. External muscles pull the glottis and trachea forwards so that it communicates directly with the choanal slit, allowing the bird to breathe through its nostrils. The glottis is held closed when at rest, only opening on inspiration and expiration.

Trachea

The trachea of avian species differs from the mammalian trachea in that its cartilage rings are complete, signet-ring-shaped circles, interlocking one on top of the other, rather than the C-shaped rings of the mammalian trachea. In Psittaciformes and diurnal raptors the shape of these cartilage rings is slightly flattened in a dorso-ventral direction, whereas in most Passeriformes they are round.

In some species, such as the Whooper's swan and the guinea fowl, the trachea forms a series of loops and coils at the thoracic inlet. Other species, such as the emu, have a midline ventral split in the trachea three quarters of the distance between the head and the thoracic inlet. The tracheal lining mucosa projects through this slit to form a tracheal sac. This improves vocal resonance. In male ducks such as mallards, there is a swelling in the last portion of the trachea, often just inside the thorax, known as the *tracheal bulla*.

Syrinx

Before the trachea divides into the two main bronchi, there is a structure known as the *syrinx* (Fig. 1.7). This is where the bird produces most of its voice. It is composed of a series of muscles and two membranes which can be vibrated, independently of inspiration or expiration.

Lower respiratory system

Lungs

The lungs of avian species are rigid in structure and do not inflate or deflate significantly. They are flattened in shape and firmly attached to the ventral aspect of the thoracic vertebrae and vertebral ribs. There is no diaphragm in birds and the common body cavity is referred to as the *coelom*.

The paired bronchi are supported by C-shaped rings of cartilage, unlike the trachea. The primary bronchi supply each of the two lungs, and rapidly divide into secondary and tertiary bronchi, or *parabronchi*. There are four main groups of secondary bronchi supplying the lung but their role in gas exchange is minimal. The tertiary bronchi however do play a role in gas exchange, as their walls are filled with membranes capable of gaseous exchange. These areas appear as small pits, or *atria*, to which are connected even finer tubes known as *air capillaries*. These intertwine with each other to form a three-dimensional mesh interwoven with the blood capillary beds. These air capillaries vary in size but average around 3–5 µm in diameter. This extremely small diameter produces very high forces of attraction between their walls when fluid secretions are present, resulting in rapid blocking of the respiratory surfaces. To stop this from occurring, there are cells within the parabronchi which secrete surfactant, to ensure the airways stay open.

The lung structure may be further classified by the direction of airflow within it into the *neopulmonic* lung and the *paleopulmonic* lung. These will be mentioned later on when discussing respiratory physiology.

Air sacs

The final part of the avian lower respiratory system is composed of the air sacs. These are balloon-like sacs which act as bellows, pumping the air into and out of the rigid avian lungs. The air-sac walls are very thin and composed of simple squamous epithelium which covers a layer of poorly-vascularised elastic connective tissue.

In the majority of birds there are nine air sacs. One of these is the separate air sac already mentioned, the cervicocephalic air sac, which does not communicate with the lungs at all. The other eight all communicate with the lungs via a secondary bronchus (except the abdominal air sacs which connect to the primary bronchus on each side). Figure 1.5 shows the air sac system of a duck.

In addition to the separate cervicocephalic air sac, the other standard eight air sacs are:

(1) A single cervical air sac which lies between the lungs and the dorsal oesophagus, and communicates with air spaces within the cervical vertebrae.
(2) A single clavicular air sac which has two diverticuli, one of which involves the heart and, cranial to this, the thorax. The other extends around the bones and muscles of the pectoral girdle and crop. This air sac communicates with the air spaces within the medullary cavity of the humeri, scapulae and sternum.
(3) The paired cranial thoracic air sacs lie dorso-laterally in the chest, ventral to the lung field and immediately caudal to the heart.
(4) The paired caudal thoracic air sacs lie immediately caudal to the cranial air sacs. These are again positioned dorso-laterally within the chest and tend to be slightly smaller than the cranial ones.
(5) The paired abdominal air sacs lie caudal to the caudal thoracic air sacs. They touch the

caudal aspect of each lung field before spreading caudally into and around the gut. This communicates with the air spaces in the medullary cavities of the notarium, synsacrum, pelvis and femurs.

Respiratory physiology

Respiratory cycle

The downward movement of the sternum and the cranial and lateral movement of the ribs inflate the air sacs and draw air into the lungs. There are two portions to the avian lung, known as the *neopulmonic* and *paleopulmonic* sections. The neopulmonic part of the lung is caudolateral and is absent in certain species, such as penguins. It differs from the paleopulmonic lung in that air passes through the paleopulmonic section of the lung in one direction only, whereas the neopulmonic lung receives air on inspiration and expiration. The avian cycle of inspiration and expiration is given in Fig. 1.6.

It can be seen that the avian respiratory system is extremely efficient at extracting oxygen from the air. For one thing, the whole cycle occurs over two inspirations and expirations, allowing oxygen to be extracted on both inspiration *and* expiration. In addition, the air flow through the parabronchial tubes is at right angles to the accompanying blood flow. This creates a cross current system, wherein oxygen in the airway is always at a higher concentration than its accompanying blood vessel, so encouraging the movement of oxygen from airway to bloodstream.

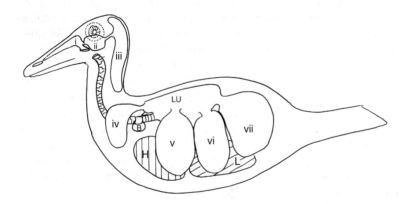

Fig. 1.5 Avian air-sac system in a duck. (i) nasal passages; (ii) infra-orbital sinus; (iii) cervicocephalic air-sac (single); (iv) clavicular air-sacs; (v) cranial thoracic air-sacs; (vi) Caudal thoracic air-sacs; (vii) Abdominal air-sacs; H = heart; L = liver; Lu = lungs; B = syringeal bulla (male ducks).

Inspiration	Fresh air and the air in the dead space of the trachea and the primary bronchi move into the secondary and tertiary bronchi, where gas exchange can begin. In addition some of this air travels through the neopulmonic tertiary bronchi into the caudal thoracic and abdominal air sacs where it takes no part in respiration.
Expiration	The caudal thoracic and abdominal air sacs contract and expel their air back through the neopulmonic part of the lung and into part of the paleopulmonic lung where gas exchange occurs.
Second Inspiration	The air expelled during expiration through the neopulmonic and paleopulmonic lung continues to move cranially into the cervical, clavicular and cranial thoracic air sacs.
Second Expiration	The air in the clavicular, cervical and cranial thoracic air sacs is expelled through secondary bronchi to the primary bronchi and so out of the body.

Fig. 1.6 Avian respiratory cycle.

Physiological control of respiration

This is in many ways similar to mammalian respiratory control. Carotid body chemoreceptors in the carotid arteries monitor the partial pressure of oxygen in the blood, while carbon dioxide sensitive receptors in the paleopulmonic parabronchi of the airways stimulate respiration once the airway partial pressure of carbon dioxide reaches a critical threshold. Some anaesthetic gases, such as halothane, can depress the function of these carbon dioxide receptors, creating apnoea in the patient.

Digestive system

Oral cavity

The functions of this part of the digestive system are prehension, mastication and manipulation of food into the oesophagus, just as other mammals use their teeth, lips and tongue. The avian oral cavity differs from the mammalian, in that it possesses relatively few taste buds, and produces little saliva during the mastication process.

Tongue

The avian tongue may be relatively immobile and strap-like, as in Passeriformes (perching birds such as the canary, finch and songbird families), or it may be highly muscular and mobile as in the Psittaciforme family. Alternatively, it may be extensible and specialised as is found in the hummingbirds, and, to a lesser extent, in the nectar-eating parrots, the lories and lorikeets.

Oesophagus and crop (Fig. 1.7)

The oesophagus is a muscular tube connecting the oral cavity to the first stomach. As in the lower digestive system, a series of peristaltic waves pass along the oesophagus when food is present, pushing the bolus of food towards the stomach. The oesophagus runs to the right of the trachea in the neck, and is lined with many salivary glands. Some fish-eating species of bird have a series of hooks and papillae, directed caudally to force slippery food items to travel in one direction only.

Along its route, usually at the thoracic inlet, some species have a diverticulum of the oesophagus, known as the *crop*. This is an expansible sac acting as a storage chamber for food. It has no digestive-enzyme secreting properties, although in some species, such as pigeons, a form of lipid 'milk' is produced from the lining of the crop, which acts as a source of nutrition for the young.

Some species, such as a few grain-eating finches, penguins, gulls, toucans, ducks and geese, do not have a specific crop, but instead have a much more distensible oesophagus, which can be used in the same way. The crop empties into the thoracic portion of the oesophagus, which passes dorsally over the heart before entering the proventriculus or true stomach.

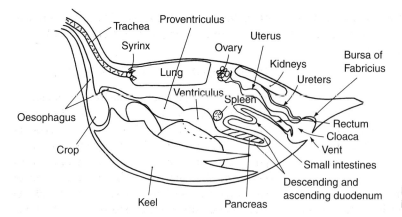

Fig. 1.7 Generalised view of the internal organs of a female bird.

Avian 'stomachs'

Birds have two stomachs (Fig. 1.7). The first of these is the 'true' stomach, known as the *proventriculus*. This organ is responsible for the secretion of the digestive enzyme pepsin and hydrochloric acid. Unlike mammals, the secretion of these two substances occurs from the same compound gland, rather than two separate ones. Other glands are present which secrete a protective mucus. The sac-like proventriculus empties in to the more circular ventriculus, also known as the *gizzard*, or grinding stomach. There is often movement of food backwards and forwards between proventriculus and gizzard to mix and digest food thoroughly before passing it on to the rest of the gut.

In seed-eating species, the gizzard is larger than the proventriculus and very muscular. In nectar-eating species, such as the lories and lorikeet family of parrots and other species, such as hummingbirds and raptors, the gizzard is much smaller. The mucosa of the gizzard is lined with deep tubular glands. These glands secrete a protein substance which, in conjunction with cells shed from the inside of the gizzard, forms a tough sheet-like layer known as the *koilin*, or cuticle. This layer becomes heavily stained with bile refluxing into the gizzard from the duodenum (Plate 1.4). Its function appears protective and it is periodically replaced. Some species of raptor will regurgitate the koilin as a neat package when expelling waste fur and bones from prey which has been consumed.

The gizzard itself is constructed of two pairs of muscles, one pair of smaller muscles and one larger pair, forming an asymmetric structure. Each muscle bundle is separated from its neighbour by a sheet of tendinous tissue. The gizzard lies on the left side of the avian coelomic cavity, caudally, and empties into the duodenum. Food outflow from the gizzard is regulated by a fold-like sphincter.

Grit particles may be consumed by the bird and lodge in the gizzard, and act as an abrasive source for food grinding. This is important for seed eating, or granivorous, birds which do not remove the outer husks with their beaks, for example pigeons and gamebirds.

Small intestine

The first part of the small intestine is the duodenum. It forms a descending and then an ascending limb which are adherent to each other, but separated by the pancreas (Fig. 1.7). The duodenum has separate openings into it from the liver biliary system and the pancreatic ducts.

The proximal duodenum contains many mucus secreting goblet cells which serve to protect its lining from the acidic food mixture leaving the gizzard. As in the mammalian duodenum, the avian duodenum is covered with a thick carpet of villi, which increases its absorptive area. The small intestinal brush border cells secrete some disaccharidase and monosaccharidase enzymes to further digest food. There is no evidence of the enzyme lactase in birds, so the feeding of milk-sugar or lactose containing foods is not recommended. The jejunum and ileum are very small in avian patients, and difficult to define.

Large intestine

The large intestine is frequently referred to as the 'rectum' in birds, because of its small size. It is smaller in diameter than the small intestine (Fig. 1.7). The rectum is responsible for the absorption of water and some electrolytes.

At the junction of the ileum and rectum are the caeca. These may be absent in most Psittaciformes or reduced in many Passeriformes to one or two lymphoid deposits. In some other species such as the duck family or the domestic fowl the caeca may be relatively large. Other examples of species with large caeca are ratites, such as the ostrich or emu, willow grouse and red grouse which live off twigs and shoots such as heather. The caeca in these species often act as fermenting chambers for the microbial digestion of cellulose and hemicellulose present in these tougher vegetable foods. The rectum empties directly into the most cranial part of the cloaca known as the coprodeum.

Cloaca

This is the communal chamber into which the digestive, urinary and reproductive systems empty (Fig. 1.7). The most cranial segment is the *coprodeum* which receives faeces from the rectum.

The coprodeum is separated by a mucosal fold from the next chamber of the cloaca, known as the *urodeum*. The urodeum receives the urinary waste from the ureters, and the reproductive tract opens into it as well. The mucosal fold may be everted, or pushed out through the vent, so ensuring that the faeces do not contaminate the urodeum and therefore the reproductive system. This fold can also close off the coprodeum from the urodeum completely when the male ejaculates, or when the female is egg laying, so as to prevent faecal contamination of semen or egg.

The last chamber of the cloaca before the vent is the *proctodeum*. The proctodeum is connected to the bursa of Fabricius which is the germinal centre for the B lymphocyte line of the immune system (see the Lymphatic System section).

Gastrointestinal tract innervation

The intestines and avian stomachs are supplied by branches of the tenth cranial nerve, the *vagus*, which also carries branches of the parasympathetic nervous system. The sympathetic nervous system also contributes to gut innervation, mainly via the intestinal nerve, which is a large plexus of sympathetic nerves that is close to the cranial and caudal mesenteric arteries and supplies the small and large intestines.

Liver

The liver is bilobed and lies caudal to the heart, ventral to the proventriculus and cranial to the gizzard (Fig. 1.7). The liver produces bile salts and bile acids, which are excreted into the duodenum via bile canaliculi and bile ducts, and aid in the emulsification of fats in the small intestine.

Some species have a gall bladder, but many parrots and pigeons do not possess one. In those species with a gall bladder, it tends to receive bile only from the right lobe of the liver, the left lobe draining directly into the duodenum.

The main bile pigment in birds is biliverdin. This means that measurement of total bilirubin levels is of no clinical use in birds for assessing liver disease. It does mean that liver inflammation may often be indicated by the presence of biliverdin pigments in the urate portion of the droppings. These pigments turn the urates mustard yellow or lime green. Starved blood bile acid levels are therefore preferred as indicators of liver function.

Pancreas

The pancreas lies between the descending and ascending loops of the duodenum (Fig. 1.7). It has three lobes: dorsal, ventral and splenic. The gland is tubuloacinar in structure, similar to that of mammals, and is responsible for the secretion of the enzymes amylase, lipase, trypsin, chymotrypsin, carboxypeptidases, ribonucleases, deoxyribonucleases and elastases. As in mammals, it is also responsible for the production of bicarbonate ions which help neutralise the hydrochloric acid from the stomachs. The pancreas also produces the endocrine chemicals insulin and glucagon.

Urinary anatomy

Kidney

The kidneys are paired structures found within the pelvis. They are tightly adhered to the backbone in the lumbosacral area (Fig. 1.7). Each kidney is divided into cranial, middle and caudal lobes (Fig. 1.8).

Nephron

The nephron is the functional unit of the kidney, as it is in mammals, however there are two types in birds. One is the *cortical* form of nephron which lacks a loop of Henle. It makes up 70–90% of the nephrons, depending on the species, and is found only in the outer cortex of the kidney. The other is known as the *medullary* nephron, which accounts for the other 10–30%. This *has* a loop of Henle, which, like its mammalian counterpart, dips into the inner medullary region of the kidney.

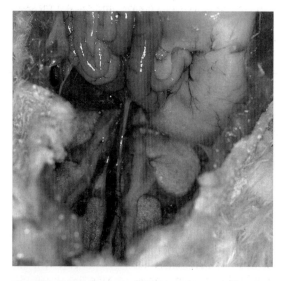

Fig. 1.8 Ventral aspect of African grey parrot (*Psittacus erithacus erithacus*) kidneys (bottom of picture) showing vascular supply and 3 lobed appearance.

Irrespective of the type of nephron, they both start with a Bowman's capsule and a glomerulus. Both types of nephron empty into the collecting ducts, the duct tubes becoming fewer and fewer and their diameter becoming larger and larger until they empty into the ureter.

Ureters

Each kidney has a ureter which arises from its cranial lobe. The ureter then passes caudally, on the ventral surface of the middle and caudal renal lobes, receiving branches from the amalgamation of the collecting ducts. Each ureter continues caudally and finally empties into the urodeum segment of the cloaca, on its dorsal surface. Birds do not have a urinary bladder or urethra.

Renal blood supply

Each kidney in the avian patient is supplied by three renal arteries, the cranial, middle and caudal renal arteries, which supply the cranial, middle and caudal renal lobes respectively.

In addition to this arrangement, the avian kidney also receives blood from the renal portal system. The renal portal veins form a ring of vessels surrounding the kidneys and connect with the vertebral sinus cranially and the caudal mesenteric vein caudally. Within the common iliac vein, draining the hindlimb and anastomosing with the renal portal veins, is a valve. This renal portal valve can divert blood in a number of directions. For instance:

- It can allow blood through from the leg and so on into the caudal vena cava, bypassing the kidneys altogether.
- It could shut and so divert blood from the hind limb into the kidney tissues. (This is of importance theoretically when administering potentially nephrotoxic drugs or drugs which are excreted by the kidneys, into the hind-limbs of birds.)
- The blood could equally be shunted towards the liver via the caudal mesenteric vein or into the internal vertebral venous sinus within the spinal canal. The blood flow is therefore complex and may alter almost at will.

Renal physiology

The anatomy of the cortical nephrons is significant because they do not have a loop of Henle, and so there is no counter-current multiplier system by which the urine may be made more concentrated than the plasma. Therefore most of the urine produced by birds is isosmotic, that is it is of the same concentration as the extracellular fluid.

The rennin–angiotensin system present in mammals is also present in birds and functions primarily to control sodium balance. It does this by causing the release of aldosterone from the adrenal glands or by altering the resistance of the afferent and efferent glomerular arterioles. This causes an alteration of the volume of the filtrate produced.

In *mammals*, when an animal becomes dehydrated, antidiuretic hormone (also known as *arginine vasopressin*) is released from the posterior pituitary. This causes the opening of channels in the renal collecting ducts for further absorption of water. In *birds* the chemical released is *arginine vasotocin* (AVT). This chemical works on several areas of the bird's body as, unlike mammals, birds do not rely solely on the kidneys for water conservation. This is because of their poor ability to produce concentrated, hypertonic urine. AVT therefore has more of an effect on the blood flow through the glomeruli rather than on the glomeruli themselves. By reducing this, it reduces the amount of filtrate produced and so conserves water.

To remove the salts which build up during dehydration, many species of bird have salt glands which excrete concentrated sodium chloride from the body. They are present in their nostrils and are also influenced, positively this time, by AVT.

Finally, some fluid is reabsorbed in the avian rectum, as urine enters the urodeum of the cloaca and may then be refluxed back through the coprodeum and into the rectum.

Cardiovascular system

Heart

The avian heart has four chambers and is larger in proportion to the rest of its body than its mammalian counterpart, averaging 1–1.5% body weight as compared to 0.5% body weight on average in mammals (Fig. 1.9).

The sinus venosus, which forms part of the wall of the mammalian right atrium, is actually a separate chamber in the bird, into which the caudal vena cava and the right cranial vena cava empty. The left vena cava empties nearby but is separated from the other two vessels by a septum. There are also sinoatrial valves separating the caudal vena cava entrance and the right cranial vena cava from the rest of the right atrium.

The two atria are separated from the ventricles by atrioventricular (AV) valves. The right AV valve has only one muscular flap with no chordae tendinae. The left AV valve is much the same as in the cat and dog as it has two valves. In some birds there may be three.

There are two coronary arteries supplying blood to the myocardium, and four major coronary veins as opposed to the single mammalian coronary vein.

Blood vessels (Fig. 1.9)

The avian patient differs from the mammalian in that the aorta curves to the right side of the chest rather than the left.

The avian 'abdominal' contents are supplied with the same coeliac, cranial and caudal mesenteric arteries as the mammalian. The main difference is that three arteries supply the kidneys. In the case of the reproductive organs, the testes are supplied by arteries arising from the cranial renal arteries, while the left ovary is supplied by an artery branching off from the left cranial renal artery. (There is often only one ovary – see the Reproductive System section.)

The legs are supplied by a femoral artery arising from the external iliac artery. However the leg is also supplied by a larger vessel than the femoral artery, known as the *ischiadic artery*. This arises from a common vessel offshoot of the aorta which also creates the middle and caudal renal arteries, and so passes through and over the kidney structure. It continues down the leg, changing into the popliteal and cranial tibial arteries.

The head is supplied with blood chiefly by the left and right carotid arteries which arise from the

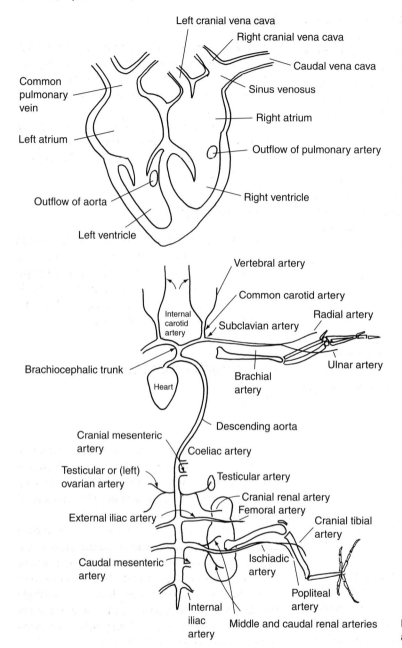

Left cranial vena cava

Right cranial vena cava

Caudal vena cava

Common pulmonary vein

Sinus venosus

Right atrium

Left atrium

Outflow of pulmonary artery

Outflow of aorta

Right ventricle

Left ventricle

Vertebral artery

Common carotid artery

Radial artery

Internal carotid artery

Subclavian artery

Brachiocephalic trunk

Heart

Ulnar artery

Brachial artery

Descending aorta

Cranial mesenteric artery

Coeliac artery

Testicular or (left) ovarian artery

Testicular artery

Cranial renal artery

Femoral artery

External iliac artery

Cranial tibial artery

Caudal mesenteric artery

Ischiadic artery

Popliteal artery

Internal iliac artery

Middle and caudal renal arteries

Fig. 1.9 Dorsal view of Avian heart and circulation.

left and right brachiocephalic arteries. The wings are supplied from the subclavian arteries which also supply the pectoral muscles forming the breast. The subclavian artery gives rise to the brachial artery which supplies the humeral region. The brachial artery then gives rise to the radial and ulnar arteries to supply the rest of the more distal wing.

The head is drained chiefly by the right and left external jugular veins. In the majority of avian species the right jugular vein is much larger than the left.

The abdominal contents of the bird are drained through a series of vessels. The main vessel returning to the heart is the caudal vena cava which is supplied by two large hepatic veins and many minor ones. The liver is supplied by two hepatic portal veins from the intestines as opposed to the one vessel in the mammal system. The caudal vena cava also receives blood from the common iliac vein and the two testicular or one ovarian vein depending on the sex of the bird.

The common iliac vein receives supplies from the caudal and cranial renal veins and from the structure known as the renal portal circulation.

The majority of the blood from the legs is drained by first the tibial vein, then into the popliteal vein, then femoral vein and finally the external iliac vein which itself empties into the common iliac vein.

The wing is drained by the radial and ulnar veins which converge to form the brachial vein. This runs alongside the humerus on its caudoventral aspect and can be used for intravenous injections in many species. The brachial vein runs into the subclavian vein and so on into the left or right cranial vena cava.

Lymphatic system

Spleen

The avian spleen is spherical in many species of Psittaciformes, but may be more strap-like in other species, and sits adjacent to the proventriculus. It has white and red pulp areas, as in mammals, and acts to remove old red blood cells, as well as functioning as part of the immune system and in cell production. It is particularly important in systemic infectious diseases, such as psittacosis, where due to antigenic stimulation it may increase ten fold in size.

Thymus

This is a series of islands of lymphoid tissue strung out along the neck and thoracic inlet. It is responsible for the production of T-lymphocytes which are necessary for cellular immunity. As with mammals the thymus decreases in size with age.

Lymph nodes

These do not occur as recognisable organs in birds except in some waterfowl such as ducks and geese. These waterfowl have two main nodes, one near to the gonads and kidneys and one near to the thoracic inlet.

In other species lymphatic tissue is present in accumulated areas within the internal body organs such as the kidneys, liver, digestive system, pancreas and lungs.

Bursa of Fabricius

This is a structure unique to birds. It is situated in the dorsal wall of the proctadeum segment of the cloaca. It is where the avian B-lymphocyte population, responsible for humoral/antibody immunity, is produced. The bursa, as does the thymus, decreases in size with age.

Reproductive anatomy

Male

Testes

There are two testes, both of which, unlike in mammals, sit entirely within the abdominal/ coloemic cavity. They are positioned cranial to the kidneys and are tightly adherent to the dorsum of the body wall either side of the midline.

The testes often enlarge during the reproductive season, most noticeably in species such as the pigeon and dove family (Columbiformes), where the testes may enlarge by up to twenty times their out-of-season size. From each testis runs a single vas deferens or spermatic cord which traverses the ventral surface of the kidney before entering the urodeum section of the cloaca.

Phallus

There is no phallus in many species of bird. Instead the semen is transferred by the apposition of the male cloacal vent to female cloacal vent.

Some species do have a phallus, including the Anseriformes, or duck, goose and swan family, as well as the ratite (ostrich, cassowary, emu and rhea) family and the domestic chicken.

The phallus lies in its dormant state on the ventral aspect of the cloaca. When aroused it engorges with blood and everts through the vent to curve in a ventral and cranial direction. Along the dorsal surface of the erect phallus runs the seminal groove. The semen drops from the vas deferens openings in the cloaca into the groove, which then guides the sperm into the female cloaca. The phallus therefore plays no part in the process of urination, unlike its mammalian counterpart.

Female (Fig. 1.10)

Ovary

There is only one ovary, the left, in most species. One or two species have two ovaries, the kiwi and many hawks for example. The ovary is cranial to the left kidney, suspended from the dorsal body wall by a mesentery containing numerous short ovarian arteries. For this reason, when speying an avian patient, only the uterus is removed, leaving the ovary intact.

Infundibulum

From this one ovary arises a one-sided reproductive system. Adjacent to the ovary is the *fimbria* or funnel part of the infundibulum. This 'catches' the oocyst when it is shed into the reproductive tract. Attached immediately to the funnel is the tubular part of the infundibulum, which is also known as the *chalaziferous* region.

Magnum

Joining onto the infundibulum is the magnum portion of the reproductive system. This is highly coiled and much larger in diameter than the infundibulum, with many folds to its lining. There are multiple ducts leading to the lumen of the magnum, with the most caudal portion containing mucus glands as well.

Attached to the caudal portion of the magnum is the isthmus which is narrower in diameter and less coiled, but with more prominent longitudinal folds.

Uterus

Attached to the caudal portion of the isthmus is the shell-gland or uterus. This is a short portion of the tract with many leaf-like folds. It empties into the S-shaped vagina, from which it is separated by a muscular sphincter.

Reproductive physiology

Male

The male avian testes are primarily composed of seminiferous tubules. In between these are the interstitial, or *Leydig*, cells which are the main source of androgens, such as testosterone, in the male bird. The seminiferous tubules are similar to their mammalian counterparts and contain the Sertoli cells in which the spermatozoa are nourished and develop.

In perching birds (Passeriformes) each *vas deferens* forms an enlarged area just before entering

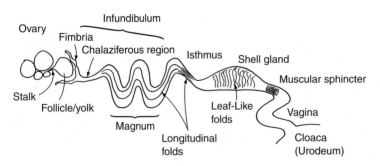

Fig. 1.10 Avian female reproductive tract.

the urodeum, known as the *seminal glomus*. The two glomi become so swollen during the breeding season as to form one mass, known as the *cloacal promontory*, which acts as the storage chamber for sperm. These can be used to sex many species of Passeriformes.

In general, the testes will enlarge during the reproductive season, with sperm production ceasing during the winter months. In many birds the left testis is larger than the right, following a pattern similar to that of the female gonad. The colour of the testes may also change during the breeding season, going from a yellow, or in some instances blackened, colour to a grey or white as they enlarge with spermatozoa.

Female

In the ovary, *folliculogenesis* (production of the oocyte and its yolk) is similar to that seen in mammals. The cycle is as follows:

(1) Each follicle starts with the oocyte. The oocyte obtains its 'yolk' of lipids and proteins from the liver via the bloodstream in response to follicle stimulating hormone (FSH) which is secreted by the anterior pituitary.
(2) Over the surface of the follicle lies a white band known as the stigma which splits, shedding the oocyst from the follicle into the infundibulum. This occurs as a result of a release of luteinising hormone (LH) from the anterior pituitary.
(3) The corpus haemorrhagicum and corpus luteum that are seen in mammals are absent in birds, although some progesterone hormone production may occur from remaining cells.
(4) The ovum is fertilised in the infundibulum (assuming a successful mating) 15–20 minutes after ovulation. The fertilised ovum moves through the tubular portion of the infundibulum (the chalaziferous portion). Here the chalazion, or egg yolk supporting membrane, is deposited around the egg yolk. This is a dense layer of albumen, or inner egg white. The ovum moves on into the magnum where the bulk of the egg white (albumen) is deposited. After this the egg moves into the isthmus gaining the tough shell membranes. Finally it moves into the uterus or shell gland where the mineralised shell is deposited. It is here also that 'plumping' occurs. This is when the bulk of the water content is added, mainly to the albumen portion of the egg. When the egg is ready, the uterine/vaginal sphincter opens, allowing the egg to move into the vagina.
(5) The vagina acts as the main storage site for spermatozoa immediately after copulation, and is where the sperm mature. It also is responsible for the deposition of the outer egg surface (cuticle) providing a microporous, protective breathing membrane on the egg's surface. When the egg is ready, the vagina expels it by muscular contractions.

Sex determination and identification

In the majority of species of birds sexual identity is chromosomally (i.e. genetically) determined.

Sex identification may be performed in three main ways:

(1) Some species show sexual dimorphism. That is the two sexes appear physically different. For example:
  — When sexually mature, the male budgerigar (in 95% of cases) has a blue cere, and the female a brown one.
  — Male cockatiels have a solid-coloured underside to their tails and a vivid orange cheek patch, whereas females have horizontal light and dark bars to the underside of the tail and a paler cheek patch. (Problems do arise in these two species when dilute colour variants (known as lutinos) and albino birds appear as there is often no pigmentation in the cere in these species.)
  — In some species the two sexes have totally different body feather colours. For example, the male eclectus parrot is a vivid green with a yellow beak, yet the female is red and deep blue with a black beak.
  — Male large species cockatoos have a dark brown iris and the females a red/brown one.

— Male canaries will sing during the breeding season.
— Many male songbirds are more highly coloured than the female. This is also true of many waterfowl, for example the ducks.
— In raptors there may be a wide variation in colours and size between the sexes. In most raptors, the female is larger than the male bird, often as much as double the size.

In sexually monomorphic species, such as African grey parrots, many macaws and Amazons, identifying the sex of the bird has to be done by surgical sexing or DNA sexing, as there is no obvious reliable external difference between the sexes.

(2) Surgical sexing involves anaesthetising the bird and passing a fine rigid endoscope through the flank of the patient in order to examine the internal gonad(s) visually. There are risks to such a procedure, which is why the process has been largely replaced by DNA sexing.

(3) DNA sexing requires either a sample of the patient's blood or the pulp from a freshly plucked body feather. This is submitted to the laboratory to determine if the DNA is that of a male or female bird. In birds the female is the heterogametic sex, having sex chromosomes known as YZ, the male is homogametic for the sex chromosomes, being ZZ. This is the reverse of the situation in mammals where females are homogametic. In mammals, the sex chromosomes are referred to as X and Y.

Skin and feathers

Skin

Avian skin is much thinner than that of mammals, and has little or no hypodermis. This means that in general it is poorly or loosely attached to the underlying structures. However in regions such as the lower legs, the skin adheres directly to the bone.

The skin has an outer epidermal layer which is composed of three main layers, the germinatory layer, the maturation layer and the cornified layer.

The dermis is much reduced compared to mammals. It forms very little in the way of a substantial structure but it does give the skin some elasticity, although nowhere near as much as mammalian skin.

There are no sweat glands in avian skin. A bird regulates its temperature by panting, known as *gular fluttering*, and by altering feather alignment to allow heat either to escape or to be trapped against the body surface.

Claws

The tip of each toe is supplied with a claw, formed of a keratinous material similar to the beak. These may be adapted to form the basic perching claws of the Passeriformes, the multipurpose perching and grasping claws of Psittaciformes or the ripping and prey-capture implements of the raptor family.

The members of ratite family also have varying numbers of claws on their wing digits, and some falcons, such as the kestrel and peregrine falcon, have a claw on the first digit or alula of the wing.

Preen (uropygial) gland

The *uropygial gland* is situated over the synsacrum at the base of the tail. It is a highly developed structure in most waterfowl, as it is responsible for producing oil to waterproof the feathers. The oil produced from the preen gland may also act as a source of vitamin D for the bird. It has a bilobed structure with two tubular exits, one for each lobe. The preen gland is also present in many other species, but is absent in some parrots, Amazons for example, pigeons and some of the ratites.

Feathers (Fig. 1.11)

Feathers are unique to the class Aves. They are arranged in a set pattern over the surface of the body, with some tracts of skin being completely devoid of feather follicles. These areas of skin without follicles are known as *apterylae*, whilst

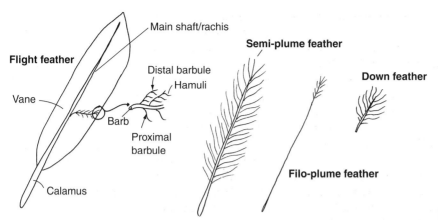

Fig. 1.11   Avian plumage.

other areas have rows of feather tracts known as *pterylae*.

There are six types of feather in most species. These are known as:

(1) The contour or flight feathers
(2) The down feathers
(3) The powder feathers
(4) The semi-plume feathers
(5) The filoplume feathers and
(6) The bristle feathers.

Contour feathers

These form the flight feathers on wings and tail, and the main feathers outlining the body. The flight feathers are subdivided into primaries and secondaries depending on whether they are derived from the 'hand' or *manus* (the carpus and digits) of the wing (the primaries), or the ulna/antebrachium of the wing (the secondaries). There are also contour feathers forming the tail, known as the *rectrices*. (The primaries and secondaries combined are referred to as the *remiges*.)

The remiges attach directly onto the periosteum of the relevant wing bone and so are deeply attached. In addition they are covered at their bases by smaller feathers on the dorsal aspect of the wing known as covert feathers (Fig. 1.12).

The structure of the contour feather is the classical quill shape. It is supported by the main shaft of the feather which is embedded in the follicle. The part of the shaft to which the vane of the feather is attached is known as the *rachis*. The vane is formed from parallel side branches set at 45 degrees to the rachis which are known as *barbs*. From the barbs arise distal and proximal *barbules*, each of which has its own smaller hooks known as *hamuli*. These form interconnections with other barbules and this allows the feather to form a solid but ultra-light structure.

The part of the shaft which is devoid of the feather vane is known as the *calamus*. This is the part which is inserted into the follicle and which, in the immature growing feather, is filled with nerves and blood vessels. This is known as the feather *pulp*. It is this area which, when emerging through the skin, is at risk of being damaged by the bird. It can then bleed profusely, giving the young feather its alternative name of 'blood feather'.

Down feathers

The down feathers provide an insulating layer below the contour feathers of the adult bird. They are also the main feather of the chick. They are much shorter in length than the contour feathers and have a 'fluffy' look, as there are no barbules to interlock the vane structure.

Powder feathers

As their name suggests, the powder feathers produce a fine white powder which is shed over the surface of the bird. This appears to act as a

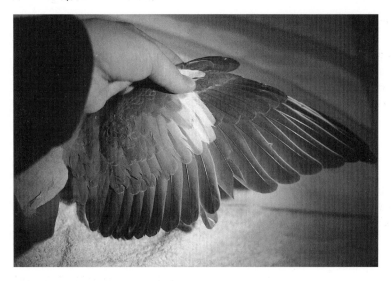

Fig. 1.12 Dorsal aspect of a pigeon's wing showing the primary, secondary and covert feathers.

semi-waterproof covering. Some species produce more powder than others, African grey parrots and cockatoos, for example. This powder may cause irritation to the airways of species which are relatively powder-free, such as Amazon parrots. This is a good reason for not mixing these species together in the same aviary/cage.

Many viral and bacterial agents may infect the powder feathers. The infection is then spread when the powder is shed. Examples of these organisms are *Chlamydophila psittaci*, the cause of psittacosis, psittacine beak and feather disease virus (a circovirus), and the gamma herpes virus which causes Mareks disease. Other feather follicles may also be affected.

Semi-plume feathers

The semi-plume feathers have long shafts, but like the down feathers, they have no barbules. This gives them a 'fluffy' appearance. They are situated below the contour feathers and are thought to provide insulation.

Filoplume feathers

The filoplume feathers are situated close to the contour feathers and possess long, fine, bare shafts which end in a clump of barbs. Their roots are surrounded with sensory nerve endings. It is thought that these feathers are responsible for sensing the positions of the adjacent contour feathers. This allows the bird to make accurate alterations of flight and body feather positions.

Bristle feathers

These are similar to the filoplumes in that they have bare shafts with a few barbs at the tip. They are however shorter and found around the beak and eyes, and again seem to have a sensory, tactile function.

Blood feathers and pin feathers

The blood feather is the young immature feather as it emerges from the follicle. It is so named because it possesses a plentiful blood supply.

At this stage, the feather is protected by an outer keratin sheath, which gives it its other name of 'pin' feather. As the feather develops inside this sheath, it is surrounded by a blood supply. As the vane forms, the blood supply retracts to the base of the feather below the skin surface. At this point the sheath should split and allow the feather to unfurl. If the sheath is damaged prior to retraction of the blood supply, then profuse bleeding will occur.

In some birds the sheath is retained long after the blood supply has regressed, and this gives the appearance of multiple, white pin-like structures over the plumage. This can be a sign of general debilitation or of a nutritional deficiency.

Moulting

Moulting occurs in most birds once a year, usually just after the breeding season in the late spring/early summer. Some species will moult more frequently, having a winter and a summer plumage which allows them to blend in with their surroundings. Many eagles and large Psittaciformes kept indoors though will moult every two years.

In general the stimulus for moulting seems to be a combination of diurnal rhythms and temperature changes. The new feather forms at the base of the old, and, like a permanent tooth pushing out a deciduous one, it dislodges the existing feather and grows in behind it.

Most species do this gradually, taking several weeks to moult all of the feathers fully. Some though, such as some ducks, become completely flightless due to the loss of all of their flight feathers at once.

Immature birds will often go through three to five rapid moults in their first year or so of life as the initial down feathers give way to more and more contour feathers and adult plumage.

Haematology: an overview

The cells in a bird's bloodstream are significantly different from those in mammals. There are five main differences:

(1) The avian erythrocyte is nucleated and oval in shape. This contrasts with the mammalian anucleate, biconcave structure.
(2) Heterophils replace the mammalian neutrophil. Their function is similar, as the first line of defence against viral and bacterial infections. Heterophils however are a rounded cell with a colourless to pale pink cytoplasm and a multiple-lobed nucleus (averaging two to three lobes). They possess brick red, cigar-shaped to oval granules, and during infection these may appear to disintegrate, with the cytoplasm becoming vacuolated or foamy. This effect is useful in assessing the presence of infection, and these cells are referred to as 'toxic' heterophils. Excessive heterophil counts ($>30 \times 10^9$/l) are associated with diseases such as psittacosis, aspergillosis, avian tuberculosis or egg yolk peritonitis.
(3) The basophil, lymphocyte and monocyte are basically similar to those in mammals and have broadly the same functions.
(4) The eosinophil has a clear blue cytoplasm with a bilobed nucleus which stains more intensely than the heterophil. It has round, bright red staining granules. It is more commonly seen in increased numbers in parasitic conditions, such as intestinal ascarid (roundworm) infestations. It may appear more basophilic in some species, such as African grey parrots.
(5) The thrombocyte (platelet) is nucleated, unlike the mammalian anucleated form.

Avian blood samples for haematological analysis may be taken into potassium EDTA tubes except in a few species. Examples of these exceptions are members of the crow, crane, flamingo and penguin families in which the erythrocytes will haemolyse. In these species heparin should be used for haematology. A fresh smear for the differential white cell count should also be made. This is because heparin samples yield inferior staining results.

Blood sampling for biochemistry testing in avian patients is best performed in heparin anticoagulant tubes.

Further reading

Braun, E.J. (1998) Comparative Renal Function in Reptiles, Birds and Mammals. *Seminars in Avian and Exotic Pet Medicine* **7** (2), 62–71. W.B. Saunders, Philadelphia.

Heard, D.J. (1997) Avian respiratory anatomy and physiology. *Seminars in Avian and Exotic Pet Medicine* **6** (4), 172–179. W.B. Saunders, Philadelphia.

King, A.S. and McLelland, J. (1975) *Outlines of Avian Anatomy*. Balliere and Tindall, London.

Klasing, K.C. (1999) Avian Gastrointestinal Anatomy and Physiology. *Seminars in Avian and Exotic Pet Medicine* **8** (2), 42–50. W.B. Saunders, Philadelphia.

Ritchie, B., Harrison, G. and Harrison, L. (1994) *Avian Medicine: Principles and Applications*. W.B. Saunders, Philadelphia.

Stormy-Hudelson, K. (1996) A Review of Mechanisms of Avian Reproduction and Their Clinical Applications. *Seminars in Avian and Exotic Pet Medicine* **5** (4), 189–190. W.B. Saunders, Philadelphia.

Chapter 2
Avian Housing and Husbandry

Cage requirements for Psittaciformes and Passeriformes

The advice given in the Wildlife and Countryside Act 1981 is that the cage should be sufficiently large enough for the bird to be able to stretch its wings in all three dimensions. This is a bare minimum requirement, and the cage sizes should be as large as is feasibly and financially possible.

Cages to avoid

It is worthwhile avoiding certain cage types:

- 'Hamster' style cages which are wider than they are high. Birds enjoy freedom of movement in a vertical plane and feel more at ease when caged accordingly.
- Tall, narrow cages which prevent lateral flight and movement.
- Cages coated in plastic which may be chewed off, as many plastics contain zinc and other compounds which may be toxic.
- Cages which have a poor metallic finish. Many cages are made of zinc alloys and if the finish of the wire surface is poor, the zinc may become available to the bird. As parrots in particular use their beaks to manoevre themselves around the cage, the tendency is to swallow the zinc dust coating the wire. The zinc builds up in the bird's body over a number of weeks and can lead to kidney and liver damage and, in severe cases, death.
- Cages with very small doors on them, which makes catching the bird difficult.

The preferred construction material for cages for Psittaciformes and Passeriformes is stainless steel. This is non toxic and easy to keep clean. Unfortunately, stainless steel cages are heavier and can be more expensive to buy.

Cage 'furniture'

Various items are necessary to provide for basic needs and to improve welfare. Consideration should be given to the type and position of perches, food and water bowls, floor coverings and toys.

Perches

Perches should be made of various different diameters, in order to provide exercise for the bird's feet and to prevent pressure sores from forming. The presence of single-diameter sized perches will lead to pressure being applied to the same parts of the bird's feet continuously. This causes reduced blood circulation and results in corns and ulcers. If not corrected, it will ultimately lead to deep foot infections, referred to as *bumblefoot*. The perches are best made of hardwood branches such as beech, mahogany, witch-hazel etc., which are relatively smooth and non-toxic. It is important to avoid using branches from trees such as ornamental cherries and laburnum which are found in many gardens, as these are poisonous. If using branches collected from hedgerows it is important to clean them to prevent contamination and disease transmission from wild birds. They should be cleaned in dilute bleach or an avian-safe disinfectant and then dried before placing them in the cage. Concrete perches should be avoided as some parrots in particular have been known to eat these, causing gastrointestinal problems or mineral over-supplementation leading to kidney problems.

Perches should never be covered with sand-paper. This does not keep their nails short, but does lead to foot abrasions which become seriously infected resulting in conditions such as bumblefoot.

Perches should be positioned so as not to allow the bird to foul the water and food bowls, and should not be stacked on top of one another as this allows any other bird in the cage to defaecate onto the one below!

Food and water bowls

Food and water bowls should not be metallic, as most are galvanised with zinc or have soldered edges, which contains lead. Both lead and zinc are highly toxic to any cage bird. Plastic or ceramic bowls are therefore preferred. Alternatively, single-pressed (i.e. no soldered seams) stainless steel food bowls can be used instead.

Floor coverings

Sawdust, shavings or bark chips should be avoided as these are difficult to keep clean and are often consumed by the cage bird. Newspaper, kitchen towel paper, or the sandpaper sold in many petshops are better options. However, certain ground-dwelling species, such as the quail, may benefit from bark chippings as a floor covering because it allows natural foraging activity. Whatever the floor covering used, it should be changed regularly, at least twice-weekly. Newspaper or other paper coverings have the advantage that they are easy to remove, so it is easier to maintain hygiene standards, and the droppings may be observed for any changes from normal.

Toys

Passeriformes, the perching birds such as canaries, finches and mynah birds, are generally less interested in toys, although providing their food in novel forms can lead to a better quality of life. Psittaciformes, on the other hand, are much more intelligent birds. On average the larger parrots have a mentality of the typical two year old human, and so benefit from toys and mental stimulation. Toys offered should of course be safe,

attractive, and of a size and number appropriate to the space allowed.

Some toys are harmful and should be avoided. These include the following:

- Open chain links: a bird's foot can easily become caught in one of these, particularly if the bird has an identification ring on its leg.
- Bells with clappers in them: birds, particularly parrots, will remove and often swallow these. The clappers are frequently made of a lead alloy, which is potentially dangerous as birds are very susceptible to lead and other heavy metal poisons.
- Human mirrors: these have various lead oxides as their backing and so present another source of lead poisoning. Polished, stainless steel mirrors are better.
- Plastic children's toys: the plastics are often too soft, and so are easily broken up and swallowed, sometimes leading to gut impaction. Some toys contain zinc, which is toxic.
- Toxic plants: many tropical houseplants, such as spider plants and cheese plants, are poisonous.

Some toys which may be safely offered include:

- Whole vegetables, such as apples, pears, broccoli, beetroot or carrots.
- Pine cones and clean hardwood branches such as beech or mahogany (cockatoos and macaws particularly love to strip bark from these). Edible fruit trees such as apple trees and grape vines may also be used. It is essential that these are well cleaned and have not been sprayed with fertilisers/pesticides/fungicides first!
- Rye grass growing in a shallow dish may be particularly well accepted by smaller Psittaciformes, and many Passeriformes, such as canaries.
- Placing favourite food items inside hollowed out pieces of wood, so the bird has to pick the food out can keep a bird occupied for hours.
- Thick ropes and closed chains may be used to suspend toys. However, no bird should be left unattended with these as they can easily become entangled.

Positioning of the cage

Correct positioning of the cage is vitally important. Wrong positioning can lead to a permanently stressed bird. Severe illness or even death may result from an incorrectly placed cage.

Birds of the Psittaciforme and Passeriforme families are prey animals rather than predators and are therefore constantly on the look-out for potential predators. If left to their own devices they will position themselves in such a way as to minimise risk. This means achieving some height (to avoid ground based predators) and getting themselves into a position where a predator can only approach from one or two sides.

Therefore, some perches should be at eye level to achieve a little height. It is important not to place the bird too far above this as the bird may then start to feel dominant to its owner and may become increasingly difficult to catch. To minimise fear of predator attack the cage should be placed in a corner of the room, rather than in its centre. For greater security, three of the four sides may be 'blocked off', for example by a wall or with a towel.

The positioning should also allow direct sunlight to fall on the cage for some part of the day, although the bird should not be in direct sunlight continuously as this will lead to heat stress. Day length should mimic that of the bird's native habitat, which often means a 12–14 hour day followed by a 10–12 hour period of darkness, and cages may be covered to provide the correct number of hours of darkness. Towels are often used to cover the cage, for this purpose, but it is important to ensure that ventilation remains adequate.

Room temperature is also important. Smaller cage birds have a large body surface area in relation to their size, and therefore lose heat rapidly. A comfortable room temperature should be maintained day and night for most species. This should be 16–20°C for most commonly kept Psittaciformes and Passeriformes. It is especially important to maintain room temperature for young birds (Plate 2.1).

The room chosen for the bird is also important. For example, the bird should not be placed in the kitchen. Many birds are potential carriers of zoonotic diseases which are more easily transmitted by close proximity to food preparation areas. In addition, many fumes produced by cooking can be life threatening to birds. Some of these toxic fumes include:

- Fumes from over-heated Teflon®-coated pans. These are lethal to birds within minutes but are completely undetectable to the human sense of smell.
- Fumes from frying fats can cause serious lung oedema and death within minutes.

With no antidote to even mild exposure to these hazards, they must simply be avoided. Supportive therapy will be discussed later on in the book.

Nor should birds be placed in bedrooms because the owner may be exposed to dander and faecal matter. This can cause allergic or anaphylactic reactions and poses a risk of zoonotic disease which many birds carry. In addition bedrooms are often the coldest rooms in the house and so not suitable for a bird. If a bird is to be housed indoors, choose the living room, or assign it a special room of its own.

Outdoor enclosures – aviary flights

One problem that occurs with indoor housing of cage birds is the lack of exposure to the ultraviolet spectrum of the sun's radiation. Ultraviolet light is required for vitamin D synthesis (Fig. 2.1). Specific ultraviolet lamps are now being sold for birds which are kept indoors. However it is becoming increasingly common to encourage owners to provide some form of outdoor enclosure for their pet birds for all or part of the year.

Exposure to the changing daylight lengths is required for setting the diurnal and seasonal body clock of the bird. Another advantage of an outdoor enclosure is that it can be made sufficiently large to allow the bird(s) room to fly and exhibit other natural display activities. These outdoor enclosures are often referred to as aviary flights by owners and breeders and may be used to house several members of the same species, or even mixed species exhibits.

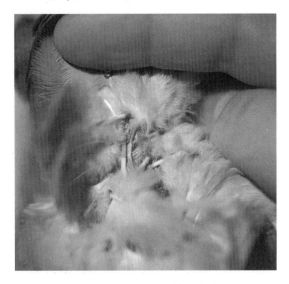

Fig. 2.1 Multiple retained feather sheaths may suggest a nutritional disease or environmental problem. The latter may include a lack of exposure to ultraviolet light and low environmental humidity.

Aviary flight construction

Construction

Aviary flights are generally constructed of wood and stainless steel. The flight flooring is made of solid concrete. This is preferable to a soil covering which can allow the build-up of pathogens and be extremely difficult to clean. The rest of the flight is usually based on four stainless steel mesh sides supported by a hardwood or stainless steel frame. The roof is also of wire mesh, or clear corrugated plastic, and some form of nest box or enclosed roosting area, for breeding and extra protection during bad weather, is provided. Many of these flights are attached to the sides of houses, providing a solid wall to one side and the additional protection that the heat and eaves of the house offer.

Any wire mesh used to form the sides of the aviary flight should ideally be made from stainless steel, rather than a galvanised alloy to avoid the risk of zinc poisoning. The size of the mesh depends on the size of the species kept.

If wood is used it should preferably be hardwood and must not have been treated with any potentially harmful wood preservatives, such as creosote.

It is sensible to provide a double door system to gain entry to the aviary flight. Usually one door gives access to a corridor, from which each aviary flight has a door branching off. This helps to minimise the risk of a bird escaping during entering or exiting.

Another potential hazard of outdoor flights is the risk of rodent and wild bird access to the system. This can cause fouling of food and water bowl contents as well as the transmission of disease. Care should be taken to ensure that the wire mesh is regularly inspected for signs of damage and that the food and water bowls are placed in a part of the cage with a solid roof over them to minimise faecal contamination by wild birds.

Positioning

Protection from the prevailing wind direction is important to prevent chilling. Equally important is to ensure that the nest or roosting box is not in direct sunlight all day. Temperatures will soar during the summer, leading to hyperthermia of adults and chicks alike. It is also useful to provide an area in the flight that protects from wind in the winter and provides shade in the summer. This allows the bird to alter its own microclimate at will, minimising environmental stresses.

Nest box

The nest or roosting box should be large enough to accommodate all birds housed in the flight and should be cleaned out regularly during the non-breeding season. During the breeding season, if breeding pairs are kept, the box should not be disturbed at all to avoid stress and mis-mothering of the eggs or young. It is also important to provide additional nest boxes if multiple pairs of breeding adults are kept together, so as to prevent intra and inter species aggression. The nest boxes should be waterproofed and positioned out of the prevailing wind and direct sunlight. They are generally constructed of marine plywood. This can lead to chewing of the boxes by the larger parrot species and so some breeders coat the inside and outside of the box with stainless steel wire. Care should be taken of the material used for this and the wire should not have sharp edges which may harm chicks inside the box.

Perches

Within the flight, perches made of hardwood should be provided. These should be of differing diameters, as discussed earlier, and be sufficient to provide all flight occupants with a perch. Food bowls may be clipped to the mesh sides of the flight or placed in an alcove recessed into one of the walls. Food and water bowls should not be placed in the roost or nest boxes, as fouling of the water and fights are much more likely to occur. Again, multiple tiering of perches, especially over food and water bowls, is to be avoided, as it may lead to widespread contamination of food and water.

Substrate

If mixed species aviary flights are used, ground-dwelling species, such as quail are often included. In these cases some form of flooring substrate is required, with bark chips, or peat being the most popular. Care should be taken in these cases to ensure that the flooring is kept very clean and that any Psittaciformes present do not start eating large quantities of substrate.

Raptors

Cage requirements

The cage requirements for raptors are different from those of Psittaciformes and Passeriformes. This is due both to the different environmental requirements of raptors and the reasons for which they are being kept. For example, many trained raptors are kept tethered for much of their lives, although there is a growing trend to keep them loose in an outside aviary system.

It is still necessary though for working raptors to be tethered for two to four weeks during their training period. The tethering device is the *jess*, a leather strap which is attached to each leg at the tarsometatarsal area just above the foot. Each jess is the same length and is attached to a metallic swivel that allows rotation. This swivel is then attached to a leash. The leash may then be used to tether the bird to a perch, which is usually positioned close to the ground. It is important to keep the leash relatively short to prevent the bird reaching sufficient flight velocity before the leash becomes taut, as this can seriously damage its legs.

Cage or shelter designs

Cages are generally all sited outdoors and vary to suit the particular raptor and the presence or absence of tethering.

As with Psittaciformes and Passeriformes, the cage design should provide protection from the weather as well as from rodents and other potential pests and predators.

Tethered raptors

Raptors should only be kept tethered during the summer months, as, by the very nature of tethering, the bird cannot move around or achieve shelter and so may die from exposure during the colder months.

During the summer months this form of housing for a tethered raptor is known as a *weathering* (Fig. 2.2). This is a three-sided, solid wooden construction, with a solid roof and open at the front. The perch is placed centrally on a floor covered with sand or gravel. Recommended dimensions for these shelters are 2.5 m × 2.0 m for Falconidae and 3.5 m × 2.5 m for hawks and eagles (Forbes & Parry-Jones, 1996).

This form of shelter is prone to two major problems. One is that during the summer, the weathering may become extremely hot and so adequate shade must be provided to prevent heat stroke. Dehydration may also be a problem as most raptors (particularly Falconidae) obtain their water from their food and will not drink free water. The second problem is the risk of predation due to the open housing and the restrained, low position of the bird.

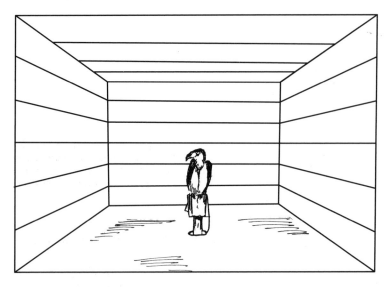

Fig. 2.2 Basic layout of a *weathering* for raptors: a three sided and roofed building, usually of wood, with a gravel floor and open at the front. The bird is tethered to a perch in the centre.

Aviary flights

These are often built along similar designs to the Psittaciformes and Passeriformes styles already mentioned. There is a major difference, though, in that raptors do not socialise well with other raptors and so aviaries tend to contain individuals or a breeding pair and no others.

One of the more successful designs is a pattern similar to the weathering, except the front is covered with a wire mesh rather than being open. Roofing materials which have been found to minimise overheating during the summer, but are waterproof, include the compound Eternit® which is a type of concrete matting (Forbes & Parry-Jones, 1996).

As with the aviary flights already mentioned, it is advisable to have a double door system so as to avoid escapees. Food is often provided on a feeding block mounted on one side of the aviary, off the ground. It is accessed either directly from inside the aviary or from outside the aviary via an access hatch. Feeding frequency is generally geared to the appetite of the individual bird, but care must be taken as overfeeding non-working raptors with fatty prey such as laboratory rats can lead to atherosclerosis and obesity.

Water should be provided fresh each day, even for those species which do not routinely drink.

Many free flight aviaries also provide some form of shallow bathing area which should be kept scrupulously clean on a daily basis.

The floor should be of solid concrete, with excellent drainage to minimise the build-up of potential pathogens.

Perches

These depend on whether the bird is tethered or free flying. In tethered situations there are two types of perch (Fig. 2.3).

The first is the block perch, which is mainly used for Falconiformes. As its name suggests, it is comprised of a block of flat wood, mounted on a short pole (usually 30–60 cm long). The block is often padded with a material such as Astroturf® to provide cushioning for the feet. This is to prevent bumblefoot or deep-seated foot infections. Raptors, particularly Falconiformes, will remain motionless on block perches for hours at a time, putting continuous pressure on the same parts of the sole of the feet. This causes reduced blood supply and necrosis of small areas of skin which may become secondarily infected leading to infection.

The second type of perch for tethered raptors is the bow perch. This is a curved rod, usually of

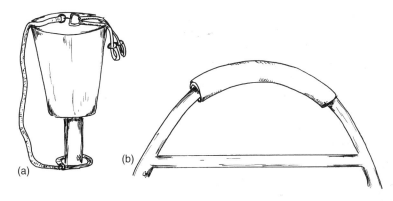

Fig. 2.3 (a) A block perch for falcons, with tether, metal swivel and jesses. (b) A bow perch for hawks with padding to prevent bumblefoot.

tubular iron or steel with padding wound around the highest point of the curve for the bird to grasp. This is the commonest perch offered to the larger raptors such as the hawks and eagles.

In both cases the length of the leash should not be so long as to allow the bird sufficient speed off the perch to be violently jerked backwards when it becomes taut but neither should it be so short that if the bird should lose its footing, it becomes suspended in mid-air by its legs.

Columbiformes

Shelter requirements

There is a huge variation in the forms of housing offered to doves and pigeons in the United Kingdom. To a large extent it depends on the reason for which the bird is being kept. Ornamental doves and pigeons are often kept in dovecotes or dove lofts, many of which are hundreds of years old. Conversely the more athletic racing pigeon is housed mostly in lofts specifically designed for the purpose and divided into breeding quarters, roosting areas and traps for racing.

Racing pigeons

A loft design will depend largely on the individual owner's preference and space available. It is recommended that the minimum space requirement in the loft area be $0.25\,m^2$ per bird with head room of around $2\,m$ for the younger stock. This requirement should be doubled for adult individuals (Harper, 1996).

The provision of wooden doweling perches is standard. It is recommended that 20–25% more perching space than there are birds be provided to avoid overcrowding stresses (Harper, 1996). The perches should be arranged side by side rather than stacked vertically. This is because, as with all birds, the dominant individuals take the highest perches leading to soiling of birds below.

Within the loft system, an owner may house his or her pigeons in several different ways.

Racing loft – natural loft system: In the natural loft system both male and female pigeons are housed together during the reproductive season. Each pair has its own nest box and perch but can mix with the other pairs in a communal area. As its name suggests, this system is the most natural, but it may be more stressful for the birds, demanding that they race and rear their young at the same time.

Racing loft – widowhood loft system: The widowhood loft houses only the males. The hen birds are housed in an adjacent loft, and this provides an additional incentive for the males to race back! To reduce fighting, it is necessary to provide more room per bird and each bird often has a double sized nest box as well as individual feeding stations. The racing season in the United Kingdom is from April to July for the older birds and July to September for the younger ones. The females are allowed into the widowhood loft just before the males to allow rearing of a single chick. After this the hens are removed and the males fed to fitness for racing.

Young loft: The young loft is used to house that year's young and so will have differing populations of pigeons throughout the year. Depending on the breeding success of the year, overcrowding can occur and the disease and stress that go with it.

Anseriformes

Shelter requirements

The Anseriformes order is a large one but there is a common requirement for all the species and that is the need for open water. The form in which it is presented, however, depends on the species. The swan family will benefit from deeper water in which they can swim and dabble than the duck family.

The type of species kept also determines the nature of the enclosure. For example, geese enjoy areas of open grassland to graze. However, they are inclined to turn grass around a pond into a mud-bath. This can lead to the rapid spread of pathogens, such as avian tuberculosis (*Mycobacterium avium*). Because of this, many waterfowl keepers will concrete the edges of ponds or place obstacles around them to prevent such damage occurring.

Other factors must be taken into account when providing ponds. One is the high incidence of bumblefoot or pedal dermatitis and abscessation, which is made worse if the standing surfaces surrounding the pond are rough and muddy (Fig. 2.4). A smooth concrete finish is therefore preferred.

Any pond should also contain an island at its centre. This is useful to encourage nesting, as waterfowl feel more secure from predation on such islands (Roberts, 2001).

Maintenance of water quality

Maintaining good water quality can be one of the most difficult aspects of keeping waterfowl. With large stocking densities or with muddied margins

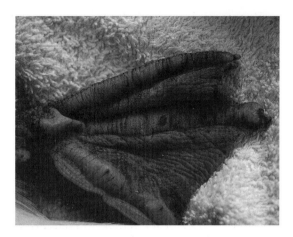

Fig. 2.4 Bumblefoot in a duck.

to the water area, the water itself can be rapidly turned into a murky breeding ground for bacteria and parasites. It is important to prevent stagnation of the water which means the standing water must move out of the pond, to be replaced by fresh water. Ideally this should be achieved by using natural resources such as local streams, but in some cases water has to be piped in and out to achieve it.

Other methods of water purification include the planting of certain marginal bog plants, which can also provide cover for waterfowl and enhance the look of a pond. A specific reed type (*Phragmites australis*) has been used for this.

Mixing species

Many waterfowl keepers will wish to keep several different species together. There are some species which cannot be kept on the same water. Examples include mixing fresh water species and salt water species. Salt-water birds can be kept on freshwater but they do need very deep water levels to enable them to dive properly.

Other combinations to avoid include:

- Mixing together more than one pair of trumpeter swans
- Mixing of Hawaiian geese with Canada geese
- Mixing of a pair of Bewick's swans with a pair of whistling swans (Forbes & Richardson, 1996).

It is generally advisable to keep any swan or shelduck as a single pair on smaller ponds as multiple pairs will always fight in the nesting season.

Other considerations

One of the main concerns of any waterfowl keeper is the loss of birds to wild predators such as foxes, cats, weasels, stoats and mink. The provision of an island in the centre of an expanse of water is one of the most useful preventive measures. Other measures include the erection of fox-proof fencing or the setting of live traps for mink, weasels and stoats. It is worthwhile noting that if non-native species of bird are allowed to escape, the owner could be in contravention of the Wildlife and Countryside Act 1981, which expressly forbids the release of non-native species into the wild in the United Kingdom.

References

Forbes, N.A. and Parry-Jones, J. (1996) Management and husbandry (Raptors). In *Manual of Raptors, Pigeons and Waterfowl* (Benyon, P.H., Forbes, N.A. and Harcourt-Brown, N.H., eds), pp. 116–128. BSAVA, Cheltenham.

Forbes, N.A. and Richardson, T. (1996) Husbandry and nutrition (Waterfowl). In *Manual of Raptors, Pigeons and Waterfowl*. (Benyon, P.H., Forbes, N.A. and Harcourt-Brown, N.H., eds), pp. 289–298. BSAVA, Cheltenham.

Harper, F.D.W. (1996) Husbandry and nutrition (Pigeons). In *Manual of Raptors, Pigeons and Waterfowl* (Benyon, P.H., Forbes, N.A. and Harcourt-Brown, N.H., eds), pp. 233–236. BSAVA, Cheltenham.

Roberts, V. (2000) *Diseases of Free Range Poultry*. Whittet Books, Stowmarket.

Further reading

Batty, J. (1985) *Domesticated Ducks and Geese*. Fanciers Suppliers Ltd., Liss, Hants.

Chapter 3

Avian Handling and Chemical Restraint

Handling the avian patient

Is there a need to restrain the avian patient?

This may seem a basic point, but it is sometimes necessary to be sure that restraint is required. A decision on whether the bird in question is safe to restrain has to be made. This is not only because of the danger to the handler's health and safety (in the case of an aggressive or potentially dangerous bird of prey), but also because of the medical aspects of the patient's own health.

Points which need to be considered include:

- Is the bird in respiratory distress, and is the stress of handling going to exacerbate this?
- Is the bird easily accessible, allowing quick, stress-free and safe capture?
- Does the bird require medication via the oral or injectable route, or can it be medicated via nebulisation, food or drinking water?
- Does the bird require an in-depth physical examination at close quarters, or is cage observation enough?

If the decision is reached that restraint is necessary, it should be remembered that many avian patients are highly stressed individuals, so any restraint should involve minimal periods of handling and captivity (Fig. 3.1).

Techniques useful in handling avian patients

The majority of avian patients seen in practice (with the exception of the owl family, Strigiformes) are diurnal, so reduced or dimmed lighting usually has a calming effect. This can be used to the handler's advantage when catching a flighty or stressed bird.

In the case of Passeriformes and Psittaciformes turning down the room lights or drawing the curtains or blinds in order to dim the room is enough. For birds of prey, there may well be access to the practice's or the bird's own hoods. These are leather caps which slot over the head and draw tight around the neck, leaving the beak free but completely covering the eyes. They are used to calm birds of prey when on the wrist or during handling or transporting.

It is also advisable to keep noise levels down when handling avian patients, as their sense of hearing is their next best sense after sight. With these two factors borne in mind, stress and time for capture can be greatly reduced.

Prior to approaching the capture of the avian patient, all items of cage furniture or other obstacles, such as toys, water bowls, food bowls, perches etc., should be removed from the cage or box. This helps to avoid self-trauma and reduces the time needed to capture the patient.

Once you have made these initial arrangements you can then confidently approach the avian patient.

Equipment used in avian handling

Birds of prey

There are two main categories of birds of prey – Falconiformes and Strigiformes.

Falconiformes: is the order of birds of prey which contains the following families – falcons, hawks, vultures and eagles. These birds are mainly

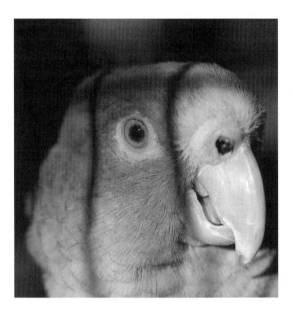

Fig. 3.1 Respiratory tract infections, such as this sinusitis in a yellow crowned Amazon (*Amazona ochrocephela*) may make restraint and anaesthesia hazardous.

diurnal and they make up the group of birds of prey most commonly seen in practice.

Strigiformes: is the order containing the owl species. They differ from falcons in two main areas:

• They rely more heavily on silent flight and excellent hearing to capture their prey.
• They are generally nocturnal, therefore the use of hoods and darkening the room will not quieten these birds.

Their saving grace is that they tend to be relatively docile and so rarely need excessive pacification. If momentary calming is required, then bright lights have a pacifying effect upon many Strigiformes.

Leather gauntlets are a must for restraint of all birds of prey, as their talons, and the power of the grasp of each foot, can be extremely strong. The feet of birds of prey and not the beak represent the major danger to the handler. It is important to note that when the bird of prey is positioned on the gauntleted hand the wrist of this hand (traditionally the left hand in European falconers) is kept above the height of the elbow. If not, the bird

has a tendency to walk up the arm of the handler with potentially serious and painful results! The type of gauntlet should be either a specific falconer's gauntlet or one of the heavier duty leather pruning gauntlets available from garden centres. To handle a bird of prey, the following steps should be taken:

• First place the gauntleted hand into the cage or box or beside the bird's perch.
• Grasp the jesses (these are the leather straps which are attached around the tarsometatarsal area of the raptor) with the thumb and forefinger of the gauntleted hand and encourage the bird to step up onto the glove.
• Once the bird is on the hand, retain hold of the jesses and slip the hood over the bird's head.

The bird of prey may then be safely examined 'on the hand' and frequently is docile enough to allow manipulation of wings and beak, small injections to be administered or for oral dosing.

If the bird of prey does not have jesses on but is trained to perch on the hand it may well step up onto the gauntlet of its own accord. If not, then it is advisable to have the room darkened for Falconiformes. Alternatively a blue or red light source could be used. This allows the handler to see the bird but prevents the bird of prey seeing normally, as their sight is limited in these light spectra.

You must then 'cast' the bird by grasping it from behind, ensuring that you are aware of where its head is. This may be done with or without a towel. Grasp the raptor across the shoulder area with the thumbs and forefingers pushing forward underneath the beak to extend the head away from the hands, then place the hood over the bird's head and place the bird onto a gauntleted hand. The majority of birds are happier and struggle less when their feet are actually grasping something, rather than when they are held in a towel with their feet hanging freely.

Alternatively the hooded bird may be held from behind, with the middle and fourth finger of each hand grasping the leg on the same side, directing the feet away from the handler and each other. This method of holding the legs prevents the raptor from grasping one foot with the other.

This can cause deep puncturing of the skin which can lead to secondary infections and bumblefoot.

If the raptor is loose in its aviary then it is advisable in the majority of cases to consider catching them at night when it is dark. Owls on the other hand should be caught during the day. The use of nets and towels is often required.

Finally, it is important to remember that the majority of birds of prey are regularly flown, so it is vital to preserve the integrity of their flight and tail feathers. A falconer may not thank you for saving his or her bird's life if they then cannot fly that bird until after the feathers have been replaced at the next moult – usually the following autumn.

Parrots and other cage birds

All of these birds will benefit from the use of subdued or blue or red light to calm the bird and to allow it to be restrained with minimal fuss.

A Psittaciforme's main weapon is its beak and powerful bite. (The hyacinth macaw, the largest in the family, can produce 330 pounds per square inch of pressure with its beak. This means that it can easily crack the largest Brazil nuts, and badly damage or even sever a finger.)

A Passeriforme's main weapon may be its beak, although this is less damaging as a biting weapon. It may still be a sharp stabbing weapon in the case of starlings and mynahs.

Heavy gauntlets are not recommended for restraint of either family group, as they do not allow for accurate judgement of grip on the patient. Instead, dish or bath towels for the larger species and paper towels for the smaller ones are advised. These provide some protection from being bitten without masking the true strength of the handler's grasp. This is very important because birds do not have a diaphragm and so rely solely on the outward movement of their ribcage for inspiration. Restriction of this with too tight a grip can be fatal.

Before attempting to restrain the patient, its cage should be cleared of all obstacles which may hinder capture or result in injury of the patient. The towel and hand are then introduced into the cage and the bird is firmly but gently grasped from behind. First grasp the head. Position the thumb and forefingers beneath the lower beak, pushing it upwards and preventing the bird from biting.

Then use the rest of the towel to wrap around the bird, gently restraining its wing movements. This will avoid excessive struggling and wing trauma (Fig. 3.2). The patient may then be cocooned in the towel with the head still held extended from behind through the towel and the rest loosely wrapped around the bird's body. Individual limbs may then be drawn from the towelling one at a time for examination, or the body accessed for medicating.

The towel technique is also better than gloves alone because the towel presents a larger surface area for the bird to try to evade. The bird is then less likely to try to bolt for freedom, whereas a bare hand is a much smaller target and encourages escape attempts.

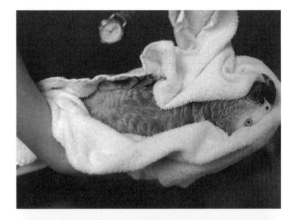

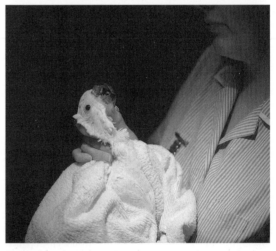

Fig. 3.2 Restraint of larger parrots may be easily performed with a towel.

For smaller cage birds, a piece of paper towel may be used and the bird transferred to a latex gloved hand. The neck of the bird should be held between the index and middle fingers. You can then use your thumb and forefinger to manipulate the legs or wings. The rest of the hand should gently cup the bird's body to discourage struggling (Fig. 3.3). It is still necessary to be cautious with this approach to prevent over-constraining the patient, as this could cause physical harm.

In the case of particularly aggressive parrots that are very difficult to handle, leather gauntlets may be used. If they are, extreme care should be exercised as too strong a grasp around the bird's body could prove fatal.

Other avian species

Toucans and hornbills

Another group of birds which is increasingly being kept in private collections is the group that includes the toucans, toucanettes and hornbills. These have an extremely impressive beak (Plate 3.1), with a serrated edge to the upper bill. Providing the head is initially controlled using the towel technique previously described for parrots, an elastic band or tape may be fastened around the bill to prevent biting. The handler still needs to be careful of stabbing manoeuvres, and it is a good idea to work with a second handler who is solely responsible for containing the beak. Otherwise, restraint is the same as for the Passeriformes (Fig. 3.4).

Columbiformes

These are restrained in a manner similar to the Psittaciformes (Fig. 3.5). The following approach may be used, with the bird's wings and feet cupped in one hand, while resting the sternum in the other.

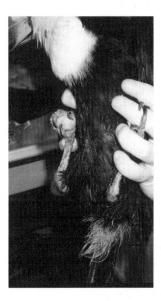

Fig. 3.4 Restraint of a red billed toucan.

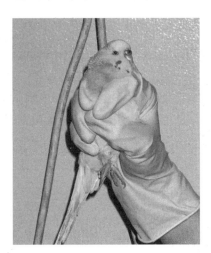

Fig. 3.3 Smaller Psittaciformes such as this budgerigar (*Melopsittacus undulatus*) may be restrained with one hand.

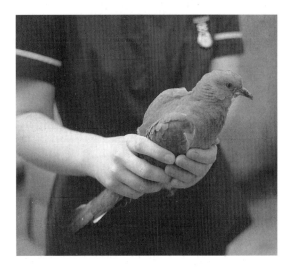

Fig. 3.5 Restraint of a pigeon

Waterfowl

Ducks, geese and swans are often found in farm situations, but are also kept by smallholders and so may well be brought to practices specialising in avian medicine.

Restraint of these species is relatively straight-forward but may become hazardous with the larger swan and goose family. The first priority is capturing the head. This can be done by grasping the waterfowl around the upper neck from behind. It is important to ensure that the handler's fingers curl around the neck and under the bill, whilst the thumb supports the back of the neck and the potentially weak area of the atlanto-occipital joint. Failing this, a swan or shepherd's crook, or other smooth metal, or wooden pole with a hook attached, can be used to catch the neck – again high up under the bill. Care should be exercised with these 'swan hooks' as overzealous handling can lead to neck trauma.

Having restrained the head and beak it is essential that you control the powerful wings before the bird has a chance to damage itself or the handler. This can be most easily achieved by using a towel, thrown or draped over the patient's back and loosely wrapped under the sternum. Many institutions have access to more specialised goose or swan cradle bags which wrap around the body, containing the wings but allowing the feet, head and neck to remain free.

The waterfowl may now be safely carried or restrained by tucking its body (contained within the towel or restraint bag) under one arm and holding this close to the torso. With the other hand, the handler may hold the neck loosely from behind, just below the beak.

Capturing escaped avian patients

Where a bird is loose in a room or in an aviary flight cage a number of methods can be used to capture it. Again, darkening the room and reducing its area, if possible, are both helpful to calm and confine the bird.

In the case of larger parrots, the use of a heavy bath towel thrown over the bird can confine it long enough to allow the handler to restrain the head from behind and then wrap the patient in the towel.

For very small birds, a fine aviary or butterfly net – preferably made of dark very fine mesh – is extremely useful to catch the bird safely either in mid-flight or against the side of the cage or room. The mesh should be fine enough to ensure that no limbs or feathers will become entangled within it, yet there should be sufficient gaps in the material to allow air to pass through to prevent suffocation. The mesh is best made of a dark or black material to restrict light and calm the bird.

It is important to ensure that the patient is rapidly transferred from the net into the handler's hands or a container, as this is the most stressful period of the capture and the inability to see whether the patient is in respiratory distress can lead to fatalities.

To recapture escaped raptors, a lure, baited with prey, can be used. Most raptors will remain within the area of their release for several days, and many captive-reared birds will not be able to kill prey for themselves. They will then become hungry and will often look for their handler to offer prey, either on the glove, if they are trained birds, or within the vicinity of their cage, if they are non-trained exhibit or breeding birds. Patience and persistence are two essential virtues when trying to recapture escaped raptors!

Aspects of chemical restraint

Assessment of the patient's status

Most avian patients are highly stressed. This means that chemical restraint, whether full anaesthesia or, less commonly, sedation, is used more and more in avian practice. All methods of chemical restraint require that the patient is first restrained manually, even though it may be for a short period, while the medication is administered. The aim is to keep the period of manual restraint to a minimum, in order to reduce stress.

Before any form of chemical immobilisation can be used, however, an assessment of the patient's status must be made. The following points need to be considered:

- Is the procedure to be performed necessary for life-saving medication or treatment, or can it be postponed if the patient's health is sub-optimal?
- Is the patient's condition likely to be worsened by the anaesthetic drugs used?

Implications of avian respiratory anatomy and physiology

Another area which must be considered and appreciated is the avian patient's normal respiratory physiology. This differs from its more well known mammalian counterpart.

There are three main differences between avian and mammalian anatomy and physiology, which are important when considering restraint:

(1) *Absence of a complete larynx.* The bird does have a glottis, but there are no vocal cords or epiglottis to worry about on intubation. The majority of the vocal sounds a bird makes come from the syrinx, which lies at the bifurcation of the trachea into the bronchi.

(2) *Presence of complete cartilagenous rings supporting the trachea.* This is important for two reasons.
   — It is relatively difficult (although not impossible) to suffocate the bird by constricting the neck.
   — There is no 'give' to the trachea and so inflatable cuffs on endotracheal tubes should not, if at all possible, be inflated, as this will cause pressure necrosis in the lining of the trachea. In some cases, such as when flushing out the crop or proventriculus of the bird to remove foreign bodies, it may be necessary to inflate the cuff in order to prevent inhalation pneumonia. This must be performed with great care.

(3) *Avian lungs are rigid structures*, attached to the underside of the thoracic vertebrae. It is the air sac system that is responsible for the movement of air through the lungs, in combination with the lateral movement of the chest wall. Therefore, if there is any form of restriction to the outward movement of chest and keel, ventilation will be reduced, leading to hypoxia.

Pre-anaesthetic preparation

Blood testing

It may be advisable to run biochemistry and haematology tests on avian patients prior to administering anaesthetics, particularly in older and obviously unwell individuals. Blood may be taken from the following vessels:

- The right jugular vein in all species (it is significantly larger than the left).
- In the larger species the brachial vein, which runs cranially on the ventral aspect of the humerus.
- In many waterfowl and raptors the medial metatarsal vein, which runs, as its name suggests, along the medial aspect of the metatarsal area.

Fasting

Because of the high metabolic rate of avian patients, extended fasting may be detrimental to their health and and their ability to recover from anaesthesia. This is because hepatic glycogen stores, which provide the most rapid form of stored energy, can be quickly depleted. Birds larger than 300 g bodyweight, which have larger glycogen stress, are slightly less likely to become hypoglycaemic with fasting.

The purpose of fasting is to ensure emptying of the crop. This is the sac-like structure which acts as a storage chamber for food and sits at the entrance to the bird's thorax. Fasting prevents passive reflux of fluid or food material from the crop during the anaesthetic. Material refluxed in this way may then be inhaled, obstructing the airway, or causing inhalation pneumonia.

Ideally, most birds are fasted between one and three hours prior to their anaesthetic, depending on their body size. The smallest (e.g. canaries, budgerigars) have the shortest period of fasting, often amounting to just one to two hours at most. Birds weighing over 300 g may be able to tolerate an overnight fast of eight to ten hours, assuming good health and body condition, and this may be necessary particularly if surgery on the gastrointestinal system or crop is intended. Whatever the period of fasting, water should only be withheld for one hour prior to anaesthesia. This is long enough to prevent regurgitation, but short enough to prevent dehydration.

Pre-anaesthetic medications

Pre-anaesthetic medications are used in cats and dogs to provide cardiovascular, respiratory and central nervous system stabilisation, a smooth anaesthetic induction, muscle relaxation, analgesia and a degree of sedation, however they are infrequently used in birds. Of those used, fluid therapy is the most important. Whether it is crystalloid or colloid, pre-, intra- and post-operative fluids can make the difference between successful surgery or failure. Fluid therapy is covered in more detail in Chapter 6.

Antimuscarinic premedicants

Atropine and glycopyrrolate have been used as pre-anaesthetic medicants to reduce vagally induced bradycardia, and to reduce oral secretions which may block endotracheal tubes. They both however may have unwanted side-effects. The two main side-effects are:

- Causing unacceptably high heart rates, increasing myocardial oxygen demand and so increasing the risk of cardiac hypoxia and arrest.
- Making oral or respiratory secretions so thick and tenacious that they make endotracheal tube blockage even more likely.

Benzodiazepine premedicants

Diazepam or midazolam may be used as premedicants in waterfowl, as these species may exhibit periods of apnoea during mask induction of anaesthesia. This is a stress response (often referred to slightly inaccurately as a 'diving response') mediated by the trigeminal receptors in the beak and nares. When this response is triggered, the breath is held and blood flow is preferentially diverted to the kidneys, heart and brain.

Induction of anaesthesia

Anaesthesia may be induced with two main categories of drugs, the injectable anaesthetics and the inhalational anaesthetics.

Injectable agents

The advantages of injectable anaesthetics include:

- Ease of administration (most birds have a good pectoral muscle mass for intramuscular injections)
- Rapid induction
- Low cost
- Good availability.

Disadvantages include the following:

- Recovery is often dependent on organ metabolism
- Reversal of medications in emergency situations is potentially difficult
- Prolonged and sometimes traumatic recovery periods may ensue
- Muscle necrosis at injection sites and lack of adequate muscle relaxation may occur with some medications.

The following are some of the injectable anaesthetics more commonly used in avian practice.

Ketamine and ketamine combination anaesthesia

When used alone, ketamine produces inadequate anaesthesia and recoveries are often traumatic, with the patient flapping wildly. Doses of 20–50 mg/kg are quoted (Forbes & Lawton, 1996). However, combining it with the benzodiazepines, diazepam (0.5–2 mg/kg) or midazolam (0.2 mg/kg) (Curro, 1998), helps with muscle relaxation and sedation, reduces flapping on recovery and allows the dose of ketamine to be reduced to around 10–20 mg/kg.

Ketamine may also be combined with xylazine (1–2.2 mg/kg) (Forbes & Lawton, 1996) or medetomidine (60–85 µg/kg) (Forbes & Lawton 1996). This improves recovery, sedation and analgesia and again allows reduction of the ketamine dosage to 10–20 mg/kg depending on the species and procedure. The medetomidine may be reversed with atipamezole (the same volume as medetomidine is given). However, the α-2 drugs have severe cardiopulmonary depressive effects and may compromise blood flow to the kidneys, risking renal damage. Sun-conures have been noted to be particularly intolerant of ketamine–α-2 combinations (Rosskopf *et al.*, 1989).

The combined medications are usually given intramuscularly. Induction will take on average five to ten minutes, but complete recovery may take two to four hours or more and is dose dependent.

Propofol

Propofol is given intravenously, preferably via a jugular, medial metatarsal or brachial vein catheter. It produces profound apnoea and is rarely used as an induction or anaesthetic agent in birds.

Inhalation agents

Nitrous oxide

This is rarely used in avian anaesthesia. It has good analgesic properties, but accumulates in large, hollow organs. There is some thought that it may therefore accumulate in the air sacs and may considerably prolong anaesthetic recovery times. Recent evidence disputes this, but it cannot be used on its own for anaesthesia. It must be used in combination with halothane or isoflurane to allow a surgical plane of anaesthesia to be reached.

Halothane

Halothane has been much used and can still be used safely in avian patients. Induction with 3–4% halothane via a face mask is recommended. When surgical anaesthesia is achieved, halothane concentration may be reduced to 2–3% for maintenance and delivered either via a face mask or, preferably, via endotracheal tubing after tracheal or air sac intubation.

Halothane, however, has several serious disadvantages. One is that it requires metabolism by the liver for recovery to occur. As many sick avian patients have some degree of impaired hepatic function, this can place the patient at some risk, and recovery is often extended. A further disadvantage is that cardiac arrest often occurs at the same time as respiratory arrest giving little response time in an emergency. Halothane is also more likely to induce cardiac arrhythmia than many injectable anaesthetics or isoflurane (see below)

Halothane also depresses the responsiveness of the bird's intrapulmonary chemoreceptors (IPC) to carbon dioxide. In the normal, unanaesthetised bird, carbon dioxide levels are monitored by the IPCs. When carbon dioxide rises above an acceptable level the IPCs trigger breathing. If the IPC sensitivity is depressed, therefore, the patient's ability to adjust ventilation in response to changes in carbon dioxide levels will be compromised.

Isoflurane

Isoflurane is the anaesthetic of choice for the avian patient. It is also licensed for use in avian species in the United Kingdom. Induction may be achieved by face mask at 4–5% concentration, reducing to 1.25–2% for maintenance, preferably via endotracheal tubing inserted into the trachea or an air sac. If using a mask for maintenance, an increase in gas concentration of 25–30% is required.

The advantages of isoflurane include:

- Low blood solubility and minimal metabolism of the drug by the bird (<0.2%). This means that the drug does not accumulate in the bloodstream, and is rapidly excreted by the patient, allowing rapid changes in anaesthetic depth.
- Minimal cardiopulmonary effects at sedative or light anaesthesia levels.
- Little or no tendency to cause cardiac arrhythmia.
- Unlike halothane, isoflurane does not require metabolism in the liver, making it suitable for sick avian cases.
- Cardiovascular arrest does not occur at the same time as respiratory arrest, allowing time for resuscitation.

Sevoflurane

This is a more recent human anaesthetic gas. Like isoflurane, it requires little or no organ metabolism and is very safe. Slightly higher percentages are required to induce and maintain the patient, but low blood solubility does allow rapid changes in anaesthesia levels (Greenacre, 1997). The high cost of this anaesthetic, and its non-licensed status, currently make it less widely used in practice in the United Kingdom.

Maintenance of anaesthesia

For prolonged anaesthetic procedures, gaseous maintenance is required. Isoflurane is currently the agent of choice.

For avian patients larger than 100 g it is advisable to intubate the bird for maintenance, as more effective control of rate and depth of anaesthesia can be achieved. Also, although isoflurane is one of the safest anaesthetics available, its respiratory depressive effects are dose dependent. This means that with prolonged procedures, the patient may become apnoeic and require either manual or positive pressure ventilation. This can be more of a risk with some species, such as the African grey parrot, than with others.

Endotracheal intubation

It is easy to intubate a bird once anaesthesia is induced using a mask. The beak must be held open, either using an avian gag, such as those sold for crop tubing, or by attaching short lengths of bandage to the upper and lower beaks. One handler can then use them to hold the beak open, while a second intubates the bird. The glottis will be easily visible at the base of the tongue, in the midline. Intubation may be made easier if the tongue is grasped with atraumatic forceps enabling it, and the glottis, to be pulled forward.

It is better not to inflate the cuff on endotracheal tubes because of the risk of causing severe damage to the lining of the rigid avian trachea. It is therefore essential to use a well fitting tube. If positive pressure is required, the very smallest inflation of the cuff may be used – enough to prevent air escaping when ventilated but not enough to traumatise the tracheal rings.

Anaesthetic circuits

Anaesthetic circuits used must be non-rebreathing and minimise dead space, as many avian patients are much smaller than the more routinely seen cats and dogs. Modified Bain circuits, or the more exotic Mapleson C circuits are useful for these reasons. Even the Ayres T-piece may be used for larger parrots and waterfowl as small as 0.5–1 kg. In any instance a 0.25–0.5 litre rebreathing bag is frequently necessary.

Air sac catheterisation

In the event of an airway obstruction, or if head or oral cavity surgery is required, it may be necessary to deliver the inhalant gases via a tube placed directly into one of the air sacs, away from the oral cavity. This is possible because many of the avian air sacs are very close to the skin's surface. These structures take no part in gaseous exchange, simply shunting the air back and forth through the rigid lung structure, but, as birds extract oxygen from the air on *expiration* as well as *inspiration*, it does not matter which direction the oxygen and gases are introduced into the respiratory system.

Air sacs which may be catheterised include the clavicular air sacs and the abdominal or caudal thoracic air sacs. A small stab incision is made in the skin over the air sac. The underlying muscle is bluntly dissected with a pair of haemostats and the endotracheal tube may then be inserted to a depth of 4–5 mm and sutured in place with a Chinese finger snare suture, or by applying zinc oxide tape around the tube and suturing it to the skin. The clavicular air sacs lie at the thoracic inlet, just dorsal to the clavicles. The caudal thoracic air sacs may be entered between the sixth and seventh ribs in Psittaciformes. The abdominal air sacs may be entered by raising the leg cranially so that the femur crosses the last ribs, and incising just caudal to the stifle.

Monitoring of anaesthesia

Monitoring of anaesthesia is crucial. The depth of anaesthesia should be adequate enough for the procedure required, while cardiovascular and respiratory parameters should remain constant. The following points should be considered:

- During the initial stages of anaesthesia (stages 1 and 2), the respiratory rate, as with cats and dogs, will be shallow and erratic. The patient will be lethargic and have drooping eyelids, a lowered head and ruffled feathers.
- As the depth increases, palpebral, corneal, pedal and cere reflexes will remain, but all voluntary movement ceases.
- As the next stage of anaesthesia (stage 3) is reached, the respiration rate becomes regular, and depth of breathing is increased. The corneal and pedal reflexes are slow and the palpebral reflex disappears. This is the light plane of anaesthesia required for minor procedures. The depth at which the pedal reflex is lost, but the corneal reflex is retained will allow most surgical procedures to be performed.
- As anaesthesia is allowed to deepen, respiratory rate and tidal volume will continue to decrease, until, if allowed, respiratory arrest will occur. Therefore monitoring of the rebreathing bag, for rate and depth of respiration, can provide valuable information to the monitoring nurse.

Equipment used for monitoring anaesthesia

A stethoscope may be used to monitor the heart rate externally, or, during anaesthesia, an oesophageal stethoscope may be inserted.

It is also possible to attach ECG leads to allow monitoring of cardiac electrical output. The attachment of the ECG leads is frequently modified in avian cases by using adhesive pads, or fine needles to attach to the avian skin rather than the more cumbersome and traumatic alligator clips. These leads may be attached to the wing web (propatagium) and the folds of skin connecting the legs to the body wall cranially. The avian ECG differs somewhat from its mammalian counterpart in that the normal QRS complex appears inverted in most species. This is actually due to a much larger RS wave than Q which creates a strong negative trace. Readers are advised to consult standard texts for further information on the ECG trace for avian patients (Lumeij & Richie, 1994; Oglesbee *et al.*, 2001).

Respiratory flow monitors can be used if endotracheal tubes are involved, although the very low flow rates of some smaller avian species may not register on machines designed with cats and dogs in mind.

Pulse oximeters may also be used to measure the relative saturation of the haemoglobin with oxygen. Reflector probe attachments are the best and may be used cloacally or orally. Again, it is important, if wishing to measure heart rates using these machines, to find an oximeter which can read the higher heart rates of even anaesthetised birds, as these will be significantly higher than those of cats or dogs. Indeed, no pulse oximeters currently available commercially will read heart rates of birds less than 150 g accurately.

Additional supportive therapy

Recumbency

Due to the unique anatomy of the avian patient's respiratory system, it is vitally important that the ribcage is unrestricted, otherwise hypoxia will develop. Common positions for surgery include lateral or dorsal recumbency.

Dorsal recumbency may be a problem in larger animals of any species when the larger digestive tract and heavier abdominal contents may press on the lungs, so increasing respiratory effort. This is exacerbated in birds because of the lack of a diaphragm and the presence of thin-walled air sacs. However, the smaller species generally do not suffer as severely from this problem and may be positioned according to need.

Intermittent positive pressure ventilation (IPPV) and resuscitation techniques

If a bird's respiratory rate becomes depressed below 15–20 seconds between each breath, then it should be given respiratory assistance. The usual anaesthetic checklist should be run through – checking flow rates, patency of endotracheal tubing, anaesthetic gas levels etc. and the emergency ABC (Airway, Breathing, Cardiovascular) protocol initiated if breathing ceases. In general, the percentage of anaesthetic gas delivered should be reduced or the anaesthetic ceased during periods of apnoea, and respiratory support started.

If the avian patient is still breathing, even sporadically, then positive pressure ventilation with 100% oxygen should be used at a rate of two to three times per minute. This is best done with a mechanical ventilator unit, as very low levels of pressure, just 100–150 mm mercury (10–15 cm of water), should be used. If using manual 'bagging' techniques, then the gentlest of touches on the rebreathing bag – enough just to allow the bird's rib cage to rise – should be used. If the bird is totally apnoeic, then a rate of 10–15 breaths per minute should be started.

Doxapram may be used orally or by injection to stimulate the central nervous system respiration centres. Doses of 10 mg/kg by injection or 0.5 mg orally are useful.

If the bird is being maintained on a mask rather than being intubated, it is possible to carry out mechanical ventilation by grasping the uppermost wing at the carpus, and gently but firmly moving it in and out at 90 degrees to the chest wall. This will simulate muscular movement of the ribcage and so allow air to move back and forth through the air sacs and lungs. Alternatively the sternum may be pushed toward the spine. This can also be useful for cardiac massage in cases of cardiac arrest.

Cardiac arrest frequently and rapidly follows apnoea and it is then extremely difficult to revive an avian patient. Adrenaline may be given at 1000 units/kg body weight – preferably via endotracheal tubing, or, directly through the glottis into the trachea. Alternatively, it may be administered intravenously via the right jugular vein or the brachial wing vein, but generally there is a poor success rate.

The likelihood of apnoea occurring depends upon the type of anaesthetic used. Xylazine is notorious as a deep respiratory depressant (Curro, 1998). Isoflurane will also produce respiratory depression in African grey parrots, even at the lowest surgical levels (Forbes & Lawton, 1996).

Maintenance of body temperature

Maintaining the body temperature is extremely important for the successful outcome of any anaesthetic procedure. It is a problem in most avian patients as they are generally small in size and therefore have a large body surface area to volume ratio. This results in loss of body heat at a much faster rate than in a larger species. Combine this with the fact that most avian species have a core body temperature between 40–44°C, as well as the fact that anaesthetic gases exert a cooling effect, and the potential for hypothermia is high.

Minimising the risk of hypothermia

To minimise hypothermia a series of procedures can be used:

- The surgical field should receive minimal plucking of feathers, and minimal soaking with surgical antiseptic solutions. (Avian skin is relatively poorly populated with contaminant bacteria and fungi in comparison to cats and dogs in any case.)
- The patient should be covered with surgical drapes, with clear drapes being preferred for ease of observation.
- The patient may be placed onto a circulating warm water blanket, the room temperature should be raised and an anglepoise lamp may also be used to increase the environmental temperature.
- Warm water filled latex gloves or other heated water containers may be placed close to the patient. However, these should not be allowed to come into direct contact with the bird, as when too hot they may scald, and as they cool they may actually draw heat away from the patient.

Although it is important to prevent *hypothermia*, care should also be taken not to induce *hyperthermia*. During the operation, cloacal temperature can be measured directly. It may be necessary to use an electronic probe, as most mercury based thermometers do not register as high as the core body temperature of many birds.

Fluid therapy and blood transfusions

Fluid therapy for disease will be covered in more detail in the chapter on avian therapeutics. However, it is worthwhile mentioning here that, as with small mammals, post-operative fluid therapy may enhance the recovery rate and improve the patient's return to normal function.

Healthy, anaesthetised birds should receive replacement fluids at 10ml/kg/hour for the first two hours, and then 5–8ml/kg/hour thereafter to prevent overhydration (Curro, 1998).

If blood loss occurs during surgery then the replacement volume of crystalloid fluid should be three times the blood loss volume. However if the volume of blood lost is greater than 30% of the normal total blood volume, then a blood transfusion should be considered. Other indicators for blood transfusions are a total plasma protein level below 25g/l, and/or a packed cell volume (PCV) below 15%.

Blood donors should at least be of the same avian family – for instance parrot to parrot, and preferably the same species, that is for example, one budgerigar to another budgerigar. It is useful to remember that on average one drop of blood is roughly equivalent to 0.05ml, and that the estimated blood volume of an avian patient is 10% of its body weight in grams. This means, for instance, that a healthy 500g African grey parrot would have roughly 50ml of blood circulating in its body. However it is equally worrying to note that a 40g budgerigar will only have 4ml of blood and thus the loss of 25% of its blood volume will occur with just 20 drops of blood (1ml). Compared to a cat or dog – in surgical terms – this is a minuscule amount.

Routes of administration of fluids will depend on the surgical procedure and the health status of the patient. Subcutaneous routes are frequently used for healthy birds undergoing minor or routine surgery. Areas that can be used for this purpose include the interscapular area, the axillae, the propatagium (wing web between the shoulder and carpus) and the fold of inguinal skin which lies cranial to each leg.

For more serious cases, the intraosseous and intravenous routes should be used. Intraosseous sites include the proximal tibia and distal and proximal ulna. Intravenous sites include the right jugular vein, and the brachial veins.

The most commonly used fluid is lactated Ringer's solution, but dextrose solutions may be used to treat hypoglycaemia in malnourished cases. Indeed, many veterinary surgeons will use a half and half mixture of dextrose solution and lactated Ringer's as a routine for surgery. All fluids should be warmed to 39–40°C, before being administered to ensure they do not further cool and cause shock.

Post-operative recovery

Recovery should always involve ventilation with 100% oxygen. The endotracheal tube should be removed once the bird starts to object to its presence, often signified by coughing and swallowing. It is important to note, however, that regardless of the anaesthetic used, practically all patients will appear disorientated and will attempt to flap their wings during recovery. Every attempt should be made to constrain them gently (without restricting respiration) to ensure that they do not damage their wings or feathers. This can best be achieved by lightly wrapping them in a towel.

Usually, with isoflurane anaesthesia, recovery is complete in five to ten minutes, and the patient is often then able to perch. However, if ketamine is used, recovery may take much longer – anything up to three to four hours. During any recovery period the environmental temperature should be kept in the 25–30°C range to prevent hypothermia developing. It also helps to keep the recovery area quiet and dimly lit to ensure minimal adverse stimulation.

The patient should be encouraged to take food as soon as it is able. This is to minimise the deleterious effects of hypoglycaemia seen in these high metabolic rate species.

Analgesia

Analgesia is a very important aspect of post-operative recovery, although it is generally under-used. Analgesia has been shown to reduce the time taken for an avian patient to return to normal eating and preening behaviour. It reduces levels of anaesthetic required, if administered pre-operatively, and results in less wound breakdown due to self-trauma.

Opioid drugs used include butorphanol, at a dose of 3–4 mg/kg (Bauck, 1990). It has been shown to be an effective analgesic in cockatoos and African grey parrots. Butorphanol does however cause some respiratory depression. It also requires metabolism by the liver for excretion. However, these disadvantages are much reduced in comparison with many other opioid analgesics.

Other analgesics which have been used and shown to have beneficial effects include the non-steroidal anti-inflammatory drug group (NSAIDs). These include: carprofen, at doses of 4–5 mg/kg subcutaneously once daily; meloxicam at 0.1–0.2 mg/kg (1–2 drops/kg body weight) orally once daily; flunixin meglumine at 1–10 mg/kg subcutaneously once daily (Curro, 1998).

It is important to point out however that NSAIDs can cause unwanted gastrointestinal and renal side-effects, just as is the case in mammalian patients. Because of their kidney structure, avian patients are more sensitive to some of these renal side-effects. Concurrent fluid therapy is therefore advised when using NSAIDs, as is the use of gastrointestinal protectants, such as sucralfate and cimetidine.

References

Bauck, L. (1990) Analgesics in avian medicine. In *Proceedings of the Association of Avian Veterinarians*, pp. 239–244.

Curro, T.G. (1998) Anaesthesia of pet birds. *Seminars in Avian and Exotic Pet Medicine* **7** (1), 10–21.

Forbes, N.A. and Lawton, M.P.C. (1996) Formulary. In *Manual of Psittacine Birds* (Beynon, P.H., ed), BSAVA, Cheltenham, Glos.

Greenacre, C.B. (1997) Comparison of sevoflurane to isoflurane in Psittaciformes. *Proceedings of the Association of Avian Veterinarians*, pp. 123–124.

Lumeij, J.T. and Richie, B. (1994) Cardiology. In *Avian Medicine: Principles and Applications* (Richie, B., Harrison, G. and Harrison, L., eds), pp. 697–711. Wingers Publishing, Lake Worth, Florida.

Oglesbee, B.L., Hamlin, R.L. and Hartman, S.P. (2001) Electrocardiographic reference values for macaws (*Ara* species) and cockatoos (*Cacatua* species). *Journal of Avian Medicine and Surgery* **15** (1), 17–22.

Rosskopf, W.J., Woerpel, R.W. and Reed, S. (1989) Avian anaesthesia administration. *Proceedings of the American Animal Hospital Association*, pp. 449–457.

Further reading

Taylor, M. (1988) General cautions with isoflurane. *Association of Avian Veterinarians Today* **2**, 96–97.

Chapter 4

Avian Nutrition

Classification of birds according to diet

Dietary preferences may be used to help classify avian species into groups, which often possess similar physical characteristics dictated by these preferences.

There are two main categories of cage and aviary birds:

- Hardbills are predominantly members of the parrot and finch families. They will eat a variety of foods, both fruit and vegetable, and also seeds and nuts. To cope with these, the parrot family has developed a powerful crushing beak, the upper part of which has a synovial joint at its connection with the skull that allows even greater pressures to be generated.
- Softbills comes from a variety of species, from the insectivorous birds, such as wild blackbirds and starlings, to the nectivorous hummingbirds and the omnivorous toucans.

In addition, there is the raptor family, which contains the main species of birds of prey, including owls, falcons, eagles and buzzards, all of which possess a sharp hooked beak used as a ripping tool for tearing prey.

In all of these cases, the individual species have become highly evolved to handle certain types of food. We also know that many of these creatures in the wild have a changing food supply throughout the year, so what may form a staple diet in the summer does not necessarily apply in the winter.

General nutritional requirements

Water

Water is a necessity. However, just as important as *providing* it, is maintaining its *quality*. Many birds will dunk their food in water, and indeed, if the water feeders are poorly situated, at low levels, may defaecate in the water bowls. This can lead to massive bacterial population explosions and gastroenteritis, sour crop and other health problems.

The quality of water that comes from the tap is also important. Many older buildings may have appreciable levels of lead in their water source. This can produce problems for humans at higher levels, but even low levels of lead can build up in a bird's body over a period of weeks causing lead poisoning. This is an insidious disease and results in the gradual weight loss, with chronic bone marrow and immune system suppression as well as liver and kidney damage. Safe levels reported for humans of $<50\,\mu g/ml$ of water are acceptable for birds.

Problems can also arise when mineral and vitamin supplements are administered in the drinking water. The enriched water will allow rapid bacterial growth over a 24-hour period, requiring owners to be rigorous about bowl hygiene if they are giving their bird any of these 'tonics'.

The amount of water consumed by individual birds will depend on the diet being offered. On dry biscuit or seed-based diets, water consumption will be higher than for birds which consume large amounts of fruit and vegetables – even so, a budgerigar, for example, may only consume 5–10 ml of water in a 24-hour period.

Maintenance energy requirements (MER)

It is extremely difficult to determine the *basal metabolic rate* (BMR) of avian patients, as this term covers the *energy expenditure when at complete rest in a thermoneutral environment after a period of sleep*. Therefore, the more useful concept of *maintenance energy requirement* (MER) is used in birds. This is the *energy usage in a moderately active adult bird in a thermoneutral environment*. This can still be difficult to calculate with accuracy, however studies of the budgerigar, for example, have revealed that current MER levels are 30 kJ per day for an adult bird.

There are times in a bird's life when this will vary. For instance, this requirement will be more than doubled in active egg-laying females, during heavy moults or during disease or growth. A formula has been devised to calculate MER. MER is dependent on the basal metabolic rate (BMR) and may be calculated from it by the following formula:

$$MER = 1.5 \times BMR$$

where $BMR = constant\ (k) \times (body\ weight)^{0.75}$

The constant, k, varies with family groups, and has been estimated at 78 for non-passerine (that is non-perching birds such as parrots etc.) and 129 for passerines (perching birds such as finches, canaries etc).

The MER of a bird gives a guide to what a bird must consume per day in order to continue to maintain good health and body weight. If the foods offered are so low in kilojoules or calories that the bird has to eat more of it than will fit into its digestive system in 24 hours, the bird will rapidly lose condition. However, many pet birds will continue eating until their digestive tracts are full, so if all they are offered is the high oilseed types then they will rapidly achieve their MER and then exceed it. This will lead to obesity.

Oilseeds, such as rapeseed or sunflower seeds, which have an energy content of 25 MJ/kg weight, have a high energy density, whereas carbohydrate-based seeds, such as millet, have a lower energy density of 17 MJ/kg weight (Harper & Skinner, 1998). This means that the bird has to consume more of the carbohydrate based seeds to gain the same energy dose. In general, though, carbohydrates are the most important source of energy for the body as they are the only source of energy the brain can use (Brue, 1994).

Protein and amino acids

Proteins are assembled from groups of up to 22 amino acids. In general terms, for humans and, it seems, for birds, ten amino acids are essential and therefore must be provided in the diet. The others may be manufactured from these ten. The essential amino acids are shown below:

- leucine
- lysine
- methionine
- phenylalanine
- threonine
- tryptophan
- isoleucine
- valine
- arginine
- histidine

In addition, it is known that if a diet is low in the amino acids methionine or arginine, an extra supplement of the amino acid glycine is required.

Proteins are assessed on their ability to provide these essential amino acids, with poor proteins supplying only non-essential ones. This is quantified by the term *biological value*. A high biological value foodstuff contains more of the essential amino acids. For companion birds, levels of 10–13% protein content in the diet have been shown to be adequate (Harper & Skinner, 1998). Most of this protein in cage birds seems to come from seeds. Some seeds are very high providers of certain amino acids. Sunflower seeds, white millet and rapeseed for example provide high levels of the sulphur-containing amino acids methionine and cystine. These amino acids are useful during moulting when new feathers are being produced rapidly.

Deficiencies in certain amino acids have been shown to cause certain diseases (Fig. 4.1). For example a deficiency in lysine has been shown to cause depigmentation of wing feathers and a lack of arginine is associated with feather picking. In some species of birds, for example the carnivorous raptors, a deficiency in essential amino acids is extremely rare.

Fats and essential fatty acids (EFAs)

Fats provide high concentrations of energy as well as supplying the bird with essential fatty acids (EFAs). The latter are required for cellular integrity and are used as the building blocks for internal chemicals. These internal chemicals, such as prostaglandins, play an important part in reproduction and inflammation. Fats also provide a carrier mechanism for the absorption of fat soluble vitamins, such as vitamins A, D, E and K.

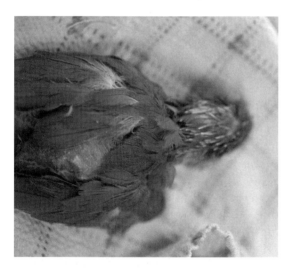

Fig. 4.1 Amino acid deficiencies may lead to feather growth abnormalities.

The primary EFA for birds is linoleic acid, as it is for mammals (Brue, 1994). The absolute dietary requirement of this fatty acid is 1% of the diet. If the diet becomes deficient in this EFA there will be a rapid decline in cell structure. This is shown clinically by the skin becoming flaky and dry and prone to recurrent infection. Linoleic acid deficiency also leads to fluid loss through the skin which in turn leads to polydipsia. It is, however, unlikely that any seed-eating bird will be deficient in linoleic acid, as it is widely found in sunflower seeds and safflower seeds amongst others.

Another EFA which is thought to be important for birds is alpha-linolenic acid which is necessary for some prostaglandin and eicosanoid production.

The problem of overconsumption of fats in cage birds which are not exercising regularly is well known, and high-fat oil seeds are prime culprits for this (Fig. 4.2). The same applies to under-worked raptors fed overweight laboratory rats. Female raptors are particularly prone to this after the breeding season when large amounts of cholesterol are mobilised for yolk production. Hyper-cholesterolaemia is hereditary as well as dietary in raptors, but it can be reduced by regular exercising and feeding of lean, low-fat prey. Saturated animal fats provide a supply of cholesterol in excessive amounts for seed and fruit eaters, causing atherosclerosis in older parrots fed on meat and fatty foods.

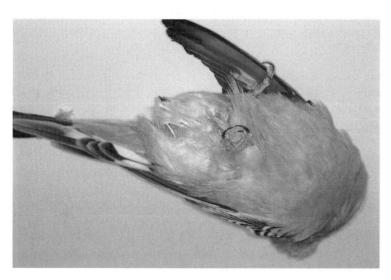

Fig. 4.2 Obesity may cause many problems, such as lipoma formation in this budgerigar.

Carbohydrates

Carbohydrates are mainly used for rapid energy production. This is particularly important in birds because they are constantly demanding rapid supplies of energy for their often hyperactive and high metabolism lives. Birds that are debilitated in some way will particularly benefit from the supply of high carbohydrate foods.

Fibre

Dietary fibre does not seem to be important for cage and aviary birds, as the presence of excessive volumes of digestive contents does not make good survival sense when trying to evade predators. As raptors are carnivorous, they do not have a dietary fibre requirement either. Only a few wild birds, such as the ratites (ostriches, emus, rheas and cassowaries) and grouse, have large fermenting caeca. The red grouse, for example, lives predominantly on heather shoots for certain times of the year.

Apart from these general dietary requirements, birds, like all animals, require a variety of vitamins and minerals for a healthy diet.

Vitamins

Vitamins are obviously an essential part of the bird's nutritional requirement.

These compounds are grouped together, although they are widely differing in nature, and all animals have a requirement for various numbers of these. They are categorised into:

- Fat soluble vitamins A, D, E and K
- Water soluble vitamins such as the B vitamin complex and vitamin C.

Fat-soluble vitamins

Vitamin A: in cage birds and waterfowl the diet frequently contains only the vitamin A precursors, which are present as carotenoid plant pigments. In birds, the most important version of these, in terms of how much vitamin A can be produced from it, is beta-carotene (Harper & Skinner, 1998). Vitamin A is needed for a number of functions, the best known of which is maintenance of

the light sensitive pigment in the retina of the eye. It is also important in the process of epithelial cell turnover and keratinisation, which is why a deficiency in vitamin A has been linked with mite infestations, such as 'scaly face'.

Hypovitaminosis A is a commonly seen problem in companion birds, particularly parrots. This is mainly due to the very low levels of beta-carotenes present in seeds, especially in the much loved sunflower seeds, millet and peanuts. An example of the requirement for vitamin A is quoted as 40 IU per budgerigar, up to a safe maximum of 2500 IU (Harper & Skinner, 1998). The lower levels may be met by as little as 0.4 g of carrot per day, but would require 200 g of millet seed to provide the same amount – that is five times a budgerigar's average weight!

If a relative deficiency in vitamin A occurs then mucus membranes become thickened. Oral and respiratory secretions dry up because of blockage of salivary and mucus glands with cellular debris. This, leads to poor functioning of the ciliary mechanisms in the airways that have a role in removing foreign particles. This, combined with vitamin A's role in immune system function, leads to respiratory and digestive tract infections (Fig. 4.3). One of the most frequently seen infections, particularly in parrots fed an all-seed diet, is the

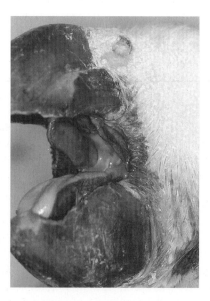

Fig. 4.3 Hypovitaminosis A may lead to increased thickening of airway mucus secretions and increased risk of respiratory disease, as in this African grey parrot.

fungal respiratory disease *aspergillosis*. Sterile pustules and cornified plaques inside the mouth are also commonly seen, with enlargement of the sublingual salivary glands.

Vitamin A is required for bone growth, for the normal function of secretary glands such as the adrenals and for normal reproductive function. On another level, coloured plumage, particularly the reds and yellows, is derived from beta-carotene pigments. Therefore, birds such as the red-factor canaries will become paler in colour if they are fed a diet deficient in this vitamin precursor.

Because it is fat soluble, vitamin A can be stored in the body, primarily in the liver. The recommended minimum dietary levels are 8000–11 000 IU/kg of food offered for both Passeriformes and Psittaciformes (Scott, 1996; Kollias & Kollias, 2000).

Vitamin D: this vitamin is primarily concerned with calcium metabolism and Vitamin D_3 compound is the most active in calcium homeostasis. Plants are not effective as suppliers of this compound.

Cholecalciferol is manufactured in the bird's skin in a process enhanced by ultraviolet light. Indoor-kept birds produce much less of this compound and this can lead to deficiencies. Exposure to just 11–45 minutes of unfiltered sunshine (glass filters out the important ultraviolet light) has been shown to prevent rickets in growing chickens (Heuser & Norris, 1929). Cholecalciferol must then be activated, first in the liver and then by the kidneys, before it becomes functional. It works with parathyroid hormone to increase reabsorption of calcium at the expense of phosphorus from the kidneys. It also increases absorption of calcium from the intestines and mobilises calcium from the bone, increasing the blood's calcium levels.

Hypovitaminosis D_3 affects with calcium metabolism and causes rickets. This is exacerbated by diets low in calcium. Typical sufferers are Psittaciformes, indoor-kept birds fed all seed diets and raptors fed all meat diets with no calcium supplementation. This produces well-muscled heavy birds, which have poorly mineralised bones. Radiographical evidence shows flaring of the epiphyseal plates at the ends of the long bones. The end result is bowing of the limbs, especially the tibiotarsal bones. The recommended minimum levels are 500 IU/kg of food offered for Psittaciformes and 1000 IU/kg for Passeriformes (Kollias & Kollias, 2000).

Hypervitaminosis D_3 is caused by over supplementation with D_3 and calcium, and leads to calcification of soft tissues, such as the medial walls of the arteries, and the kidneys. This leads to hypertension and organ failure. The recommended maximum levels are 2000 IU/kg of food offered for Psittaciformes and 2500 IU/kg for Passeriformes (Kollias & Kollias, 2000).

Vitamin E: vitamin compound is found in several active forms in plants. The most active is alpha-tocopherol. It has an important role in immune system function, particularly lymphocyte cell activity. Vitamin E is combined with selenium into the metallo-enzyme glutathione peroxidase. This mops up the free radicals that are produced in the metabolism of dietary polyunsaturated fats and which would otherwise cause cellular damage.

Hypovitaminosis E produces a condition known as 'white muscle disease' in which damage occurs to the muscle bundles and their myoglobin content, leading to pale-coloured muscles and muscle weakness. In addition, birds deficient in vitamin E, such as cockatiels may be more susceptible to the protozoal gut parasite *Giardia* spp and may pass undigested whole seeds in their droppings.

Hypovitaminosis E may occur due to a reduction in fat metabolism or absorption, as can occur with small intestinal, pancreatic or biliary diseases. It may also occur because of a lack of green plant material in the diet, as this is the main source of vitamin E. Vitamin E deficiency may also occur in birds fed on diets high in polyunsaturated fatty acids, such as fish-eating raptors fed oily fish like tuna. These diets rapidly deplete vitamin E reserves in metabolising the polyunsaturated fats.

Hypervitaminosis E is extremely rare. The recommended minimum level is 50 ppm for both Passeriformes and Psittaciformes (Kollias & Kollias, 2000).

Vitamin K: because vitamin K is produced by bacteria normally present in the gut, it is very difficult to get a true deficiency, although absorption will be reduced when fat digestion/absorption is reduced as in, for example, biliary or pancreatic disease.

The consumption of warfarin and coumarin derived compounds (such as those found in plants such as sweet clovers) can increase the demand for clotting factors. It can also be a problem for raptors that have eaten prey that has been killed by these rodenticides. The deficiency produced causes internal and external haemorrhage, but vitamin K also functions in calcium/phosphorous metabolism in the bones and this may also be affected. The recommended minimum level for raptors, Passeriformes and Psittaciformes is 1 ppm (Wallach & Cooper, 1982).

Water-soluble vitamins

Vitamin B₁ (thiamine): thiamine is found widely in plant and animal tissues alike. It is concerned with a number of cellular functions, one of which involves the integrity of the central nervous system.

Hypovitaminosis B₁ is uncommon. The most likely cause is the presence of enzymes called *thiaminases* in the diet, which destroy thiamine. A source of thiaminases is raw salt-water fish which may be fed to some raptors, such as sea-eagles and ospreys. However, there are thiamine antagonists present in foods such as blackberries, beetroot, coffee, chocolate and tea. When a deficiency occurs, neurological signs such as opisthotonus, weakness and head tremors appear. In addition, the fungal infection aspergillosis is a common sequel to B₁ deficiency. The recommended minimum levels for raptors, Psittaciformes and Passeriformes are 4 ppm (Kollias & Kollias, 2000) or 5 g of usable vitamin B₁ per day for raptors (Wallach & Cooper, 1982).

Vitamin B₂ (riboflavin): vitamin B₂ is present in particularly small amounts in seeds, and so deficiency is primarily seen in seed-eating birds. Hypovitaminosis B₂ causes growth retardation and curled toe paralysis in chicks. This is due to its function in cartilage, collagenous and nerve cell tissue growth. Birds can be supplemented using commercial powder supplements or simple brewers yeast. The recommended minimum levels for Psittaciformes and Passeriformes are 6 ppm (Kollias & Kollias, 2000), for gamebirds 3.6 mg/kg and waterfowl (Austic & Cole, 1971) 4 mg/kg of feed offered (Scott & Norris, 1965).

Niacin: niacin is found widely in many foods, but the form that occurs in plants has a low availability to the bird. It is used in many cellular metabolic processes.

Birds fed a high proportion of one type of seed, such as waterfowl overfed on sweetcorn, can become deficient. This results in retarded growth, poor feather quality and scaly dermatitis on the legs and feet. Intertarsal joint deformities can occur in the larger waterfowl. The recommended minimum requirements are 50 ppm for Passeriformes and Psittaciformes (Kollias & Kollias, 2000) or 55–70 mg/kg of feed in general (Wallach & Cooper, 1982).

Vitamin B₆ (pyridoxine): any deficiency of pyridoxine will result in retarded growth, hyperexcitability, convulsions, twisted neck and polyneuritis, although a deficiency is rarely seen. Recommended minimum levels are 6 ppm in Passeriformes and Psittaciformes (Kollias & Kollias, 2000) or 2.6–3 mg/kg of feed for game birds (Scott & Norris, 1965).

Pantothenic acid: pantothenic acid is found widely in plants and animals and so deficiency rarely occurs. When it does occur in birds, signs include crusting of the feet, eyelids and commisures of the beak, poor feather growth and general epidermal desquamation. The recommended minimum levels are 20 ppm for Passeriformes and Psittaciformes (Kollias & Kollias, 2000) or 35.2 mg/kg of feed in ducks (Scott & Norris, 1965).

Biotin: true deficiencies are rare due to gut bacterial production. Deficiencies produce a range of signs, including exfoliative dermatitis and gangrenous toes. The recommended minimum requirements are 0.25 ppm for Passeriformes and Psittaciformes (Kollias & Kollias, 2000) or

0.09–0.15 mg/kg of feed in waterfowl (Wallach & Cooper, 1982).

Folic acid: folic acid deficiency leads to severely impaired cell division. This can lead to a number of problems, such as failure of hen birds' reproductive tract development, a macrocytic anaemia due to failure of red blood cell maturation and immune system cellular dysfunction.

Folic acid is needed to form uric acid, the waste product of protein metabolism in birds. Therefore, a relative deficiency of folic acid may occur in some individuals fed a very high protein diet. In addition, some foods, such as cabbage and other brassicas, as well as oranges beans and peas, contain folic acid inhibitors. The use of trimethoprim sulphonamide drugs may also reduce gut bacterial folic acid production. The recommended minimum requirements are 1.5 ppm for Passeriformes and Psittaciformes (Kollias & Kollias, 2000) or 1.25 mg/kg of feed (Scott & Norris, 1965).

Vitamin B_{12}: vatamin B_{12} is produced by intestinal bacteria so deficiency is uncommon, although it may occur after prolonged antibiotic medication. Vitamin B_{12} is required for many metabolic pathways and neurological function and a deficiency may cause a knock-on deficiency in folic acid. It will cause slow growth, muscular dystrophy in the legs, poor hatching rates and high mortality rates in young birds, as well as hatching deformities. The recommended minimum requirements are for 0.01 ppm in Passeriformes and Psittaciformes (Kollias & Kollias, 2000) or 0.009–0.25 mg/kg of feed offered (Wallach & Cooper, 1982).

Choline: choline may be synthesised in the body, but not in enough quantities for the growing bird. Because of their interactions, the need for choline is dependent on levels of folic acid and vitamin B_{12}. Excess dietary protein increases choline requirements, as does a diet high in fats. Deficiencies cause retarded growth, disrupted fat metabolism, fatty liver damage and perosis (slipping of the Achilles tendon off the intertarsal joint groove). The recommended minimum requirements are 1500 ppm for Passeriformes and Psittaciformes (Kollias & Kollias, 2000) or

1300–1900 mg/kg of feed offered (Wallach & Cooper, 1982).

Vitamin C: there are only a few wild birds that have a direct need for vitamin C. These include the red-vented bulbul and the willow ptarmigan as well as the crimson sun-conure, a form of parrot. Birds in general do not need vitamin C in their diets as it can be produced from glucose in the liver. If a bird is suffering from liver disease, therefore, it may require a dietary source of vitamin C.

Vitamin C is needed for the formation of elastic fibres and connective tissues and is an excellent anti-oxidant similar to vitamin E. Deficiency leads to *scurvy* in which there is poor wound healing, increased bleeding due to capillary wall fragility and bone weakness.

Vitamin C also increases gut absorption of some minerals, such as iron. This may be important for chronically anaemic patients, but can be a danger for softbills, such as the mynah and toucan families, as these birds are prone to liver damage from excessive dietary uptake of iron.

Minerals

There are two main groups of minerals:

- Macro-minerals
- Micro-minerals

Macro-minerals – such as calcium and phosphorus – are present in large amounts in the body. Micro-minerals, or trace elements (such as manganese, iron and cobalt), are all necessary for normal bodily function, but are needed in far lower quantities.

Macro-minerals

Calcium: the active form of calcium in the body is the ionic, double-charged molecule Ca^{2+}. Lowered levels of this form lead to hyperexcitability, fitting and death. This can occur even though the overall body reserves of calcium are normal.

Calcium levels in the body are controlled by vitamin D_3, parathyroid hormone and calcitonin working in opposition to each other. The ratio of calcium to phosphorus is particularly important – as one increases, the other decreases and vice versa. A ratio of 2:1 calcium to phosphorus is desirable in food for growing birds and 1.5:1 for adults. In high egg laying periods though, to keep pace with the output of calcium into the shells, a ratio of 10:1 may be needed (Brue, 1994). Excessive calcium in the diet (>1%) however reduces the use of proteins, fats, phosphorus, manganese, zinc, iron and iodine and combined with a high level of vitamin D_3 may lead to calcification of soft tissue structures.

Phosphorus: phosphorus, like calcium, is used in bones. It is also used in the storage of energy as adenosine triphosphate (ATP), and as a part of the structure of cell membranes. Levels of phosphorus are controlled in the body as for calcium, the two being in equal and opposite equilibrium with each other. Nutritional secondary hyperparathyroidism may occur when dietary phosphorus exceeds calcium, and this can lead to progressive bone demineralisation and renal damage due to high circulating levels of parathyroid hormone.

High dietary phosphorus, particularly as phytates, will reduce the amount of calcium which can be absorbed from the gut, as it forms complexes with the calcium present there. This can be a big problem in cage birds which are predominantly seed eaters, as cereals are high in phosphorus and low in calcium. It may also be a problem for raptors fed pure meat with no calcium/bone supplement.

Magnesium: most of the magnesium in the body is found in the bone matrix. However, it is also essential for phosphorus transfer in the formation of ATP, and cell membranes in soft tissues such as the liver. Most magnesium is absorbed in the small intestine, and is affected by large amounts of calcium in the diet, which will reduce magnesium absorption. The recommended minimum levels are 600 ppm (Kollias & Kollias, 2000) or 475–550 mg/kg of feed (Wallach & Cooper, 1982).

Sodium: sodium is the main *extracellular*, positively charged ion and regulates the body's

acid–base balance and osmotic potential. Along with potassium, it is responsible for nerve signals and impulses.

A true dietary deficiency (*hyponatraemia*) is rare, but may occur due to chronic diarrhoea or renal disease. These disrupt the osmotic potential gradient in the kidneys leading to further water losts and dehydration. Excessive levels of sodium in the diet (greater than ten times recommended levels) lead to poor feathering, polyuria, hypertension, oedema and death. Minimum levels are quoted as 5–10 mg/kg of feed offered (Wallach & Cooper, 1982) or around 0.12% of the diet offered (Kollias & Kollias, 2000).

Potassium: as with mammals, potassium is the major *intracellular* positive ion. It is essential in maintaining membrane potentials and it is the principal intracellular cation affecting acid–base reactions and osmotic pressure. Rarely is there a dietary deficiency, however, severe stress may cause potassium deficiency, *hypokalaemia*. This is caused by an increased kidney excretion of potassium due to an elevatation in plasma proteins which is often seen at times of stress. This can lead to cardiac dysrhythmias, muscle spasticity and neurological dysfunction.

Potassium is present in high amounts in certain fruits such as bananas. It is controlled in the body in equilibrium with sodium under the influence of the adrenal hormone *aldosterone*, which promotes sodium retention and potassium excretion. The recommended minimal level is 0.4–1.1 mg/kg (Scott & Norris, 1965).

Chlorine: this mineral is the major extracellular negative ion. It is responsible for maintaining acid–base balances in conjunction with sodium and potassium. Deficiencies are rare due to its combination with sodium in the diet as salt.

Micro-minerals (trace elements)

Iron: iron is required for the formation of the oxygen-binding centre of the haemoglobin molecule. Absorption from the gut is normally relatively poor as the body is very good at recycling its iron levels from old red blood cells.

Certain species have a greater ability to absorb iron from the small intestine. The mynah and toucan/toucanette families are examples. This ability may become a problem when diets rich in iron are presented to these species. For example, rodents and day-old chicks may be fed to toucans, and so occasionally are various brands of dog or monkey biscuits. In addition, vitamin C increases iron absorption by converting the iron into the more easily absorbed ferrous (Fe^{2+}) state. This can lead to a condition known as haemochromatosis, where the liver becomes fatally overloaded with absorbed iron. The recommended minimum requirement for Passeriformes and Psittaciformes is 80 ppm, but for toucans and mynahs a maximum of 60 ppm, or less than 160 mg/kg of feed, is recommended (Worrell, 1991). Dietary deficiencies rarely occur. However, ground foraging species reared on impervious surfaces such as wire or concrete have suffered iron deficiency. This is because soil consumption, which occurs during ground feeding, is another source of iron.

Copper: copper is used for haemaglobin synthesis, collagen synthesis and the maintenance of the nervous system.

Deficiencies occur, as with iron, in some ground feeding species like pheasants and other game birds, reared on surfaces such as concrete where soil consumption during the foraging process does not occur. Signs include chronic anaemia with general weakness, limb deformities and hyperexcitability. The recommended minimum requirements are 8 ppm for Passeriformes and Psittaciformes, and 4 ppm for Galliformes (Wallach & Cooper, 1982).

Zinc: this is a vital trace element for wound healing and tissue formation, forming part of a number of enzymes.

Deficiencies can occur in young, rapidly growing birds fed on plant material high in phytates such as cabbage, wheat bran and beans. This is because, as with calcium, the phytates bind zinc and prevent its absorption from the gut. In addition, high dietary calcium itself decreases zinc uptake. Deficiencies cause retarded growth, poor feathering, enlarged intertarsal joints and slipped Achilles tendon (perosis). The

minimum recommended requirement is 50 ppm for Passeriformes and Psittaciformes (Kollias & Kollias, 2000).

Manganese: manganese is primarily found in plant materials but is often present in unavailable forms. Efficient bile salt production is required for its absorption, so birds with hepatic and biliary dysfunction are most at risk of a deficiency.

Manganese is necessary for normal bone structure, hence deficiencies are most commonly manifested by a swelling and flattening of the lateral condyles of the intertarsal joint, allowing the Achilles tendon to slip out of the groove created for it (a condition known as *perosis*). In addition, the tibiotarsus and tarsometarsus may exhibit lateral rotation. Young may be born with retracted beaks and shortened long bones. The recommended minimum requirement is 55–60 mg/kg of feed (Wallach & Cooper, 1982).

Iodine: the sole function of iodine is in thyroid hormone synthesis. Deficiencies cause the condition *goitre*, and produce effects such as reduced growth, stunting and neurological problems. It is a relatively common finding in budgerigars fed on an all seed diet without additional supplementation. They adopt a classic, hunched posture on the perch because the enlarged thyroid gland constricts the tracheal lumen. They may also be seen to regurgitate seed from the crop. Goitre is one of the differential diagnoses in a vomiting budgerigar. Levels of 4 μg per budgerigar per week prevent goitre from developing (Blackmore, 1963).

Selenium: its functions are similar to vitamin E as it is found in the enzyme glutathione peroxidase. If there is a general deficiency in both selenium and vitamin E, a condition known as *exudative diathesis* will occur. This is when the smaller, subcutaneous blood vessels become damaged and more leaky. Fluid then moves rapidly out into the subcutaneous spaces and oedema forms over the neck, wings and breast. This is often followed by stunted growth, limb weakness and death.

The selenium content of plants is dependent on where they were grown and the levels of selenium in the soil. The recommended minimum requirement is 0.1 ppm for Passeriformes and Psittaciformes (Kollias & Kollias, 2000).

Examples of food types for Psittaciformes and Passeriformes

As a rough example of food types suitable for commonly kept cage and aviary birds, please examine the list given below.

Seeds

Rape seed, millet, canary seed, hemp and linseed are useful for smaller species such as finches, canaries, budgerigars and cockatiels.

Safflower, sunflower and pumpkin seeds are useful for larger parrots but beware of addiction to sunflower seeds!

Nuts

Almonds, walnuts, brazil nuts and hazel nuts are useful for larger parrots but be careful of addiction to peanuts and *Aspergillus* spp toxin poisoning. Peanuts and pine nuts may also be fed. Nuts are high in calories.

Fruit

A wide variety of fruits are useful foods. Examples include: apple, pear, melon, mango, papaya, pomegranate, guava, apricot, peach, nectarine, oranges, bananas. Grapes and kiwi fruit should be fed sparingly due to their high sugar content, which can cause diarrhoea. Oranges should also only be fed in small amounts, since excess can cause gastric upset, and they should not be fed to toucans and mynah birds due to their high vitamin C content and iron absorption facilitation.

Vegetables

Broccoli, watercress and wild rocket are good sources of vitamin A and calcium. Other good vegetables include swiss chard, kale, sweet pepper, carrot, beetroot, boiled potato, peas, mung beans (particularly sprouted ones), cauliflower, tomato and sweetcorn.

Do not feed avocados as these cause severe fatty liver damage in birds. Lories, lorikeets and hummingbirds are all nectar feeders and so require a specialised artificial syrup food. Many are commercially produced. They may also take very ripe fruits, and enjoy eating the pollen from flowers.

Specific nutritional requirements

Nutritional requirements for growth

Embryonic growth

The egg is a perfect capsule of nutrients providing all that is needed for the developing embryo. The hen must be fed a balanced diet to ensure that she has the nutrients available to instil into the egg. If she is fed a poor or deficient diet then the egg may not be fertile. It could also undergo:

- Early embryonic death (EED). This is often signalled by a blood ring left in the yolk, which suggests a vitamin A deficiency.
- Retarded embryonic development (RED). This is often associated with vitamin B deficiencies.
- Embryonic deformities, which may be seen with manganese, zinc or other trace element deficiencies.

Post-hatch growth

Hatching occurs after the developing chick has absorbed the external yolk sac, and the chick must then be supplied within three to four days with high levels of energy and protein for the growth phase. The remaining internal yolk sac supply will last that long.

When feathers are produced, a huge demand for protein occurs, as feathers are made of keratin, a protein, and will eventually make up one tenth of the bird's weight. In addition there will be several feather changes during the first two years of life, as juvenile down plumage is replaced by adult plumage. Young birds also have a much larger requirement for calcium and vitamin D_3 for developing bones. On average, sexual maturity for the larger parrots, such as African grey parrots, macaws and cockatoos, is not reached until two to four years of age, so this growth phase may be prolonged.

If, during this growth phase, disease or low environmental temperatures are introduced, energy is diverted to immune system function and heat supply. This results in less energy for growth and in slowing of the growth rate. This may be reversed in later periods of growth, assuming no permanent damage has been caused. The obvious side-effect of this, though, is that adult weights are achieved at an older age. If a retarded bird is supplied with excess nutritional levels *after* this period of leanness, a compensatory growth spurt may occur and the chick appears to grow more rapidly than other birds of that age group.

For all of this growth to occur it has been estimated that minimum energy requirements for small Psittaciformes and Passeriformes are five times that of adults. Young chicks nearly double their weights over 48 hours, and require a protein level of 15–20%, as opposed to an adult protein need of 10–14% (Harper & Skinner, 1998). Commercial and home-prepared diets for chicks are usually preformulated mashes with this level of protein, eggs and dairy products which have a good broad spectrum of amino acids supplementation and 20% protein levels.

Excessive protein supplementation may be equally damaging. Levels greater than 25% of diet have been shown to lead to behavioural problems and claw, beak and skeletal deformities, particularly if combined with a lack of calcium. Levels of 0.6–1.2% of the diet as calcium have been quoted for chick growth (Brue, 1994) with a calcium : phosphorus ratio of 2:1 maintained.

Nutritional requirements for breeding

These requirements include those needed for egg production as well as for courtship behaviour. The requirements for egg production are high, with large volumes of fats needed for the yolk, calcium for the shell and proteins for the albumen (egg white). As egg production commences, the hen bird will increase the volume of food consumed so removing the need to increase the energy concentration of the diet being offered. It is, however, essential that the diet offered is a balanced one

with an increased protein content, particularly from methionine and cystine (the sulphur containing amino acids) and lysine.

In addition, a moderate increase in the amount of calcium and vitamin D_3 offered (an increase of 0.35% of the adult maintenance requirement for calcium) is needed, so that levels approach 1% of diet (Harper & Skinner, 1998). This not only helps to ensure proper calcification of eggshells and the developing embryo, but also to prevent egg-binding in the hen. This is when poor calcium reserves lead to low calcium blood levels, weakness, uterine muscular paresis, egg retention, shock and death.

Other compounds which, if supplied above the minimum daily requirements mentioned earlier, help with egg production, include vitamins A, B_{12}, riboflavin and the mineral zinc. In addition, it is useful for improved hatching rate, to increase the levels of the B vitamins biotin, folic acid, pantothenic acid, riboflavin (B_2) and pyridoxine (B_6), as well as vitamin E, iron, copper, zinc and manganese to above the minimum daily requirements.

Nutritional requirements for the older bird

As with cats and dogs, the aim is to provide a diet of high digestibility whilst reducing slightly the protein, sodium and phosphorus levels. This preserves renal function and prevents hypertension.

In addition, lowering cholesterol and unsaturated fat levels is important, as atherosclerosis is common in older birds. The levels of vitamins A, E, thiamine (B_1), B_{12}, and pyridoxine (B_6), the mineral zinc, amino acid lysine and fatty acid linoleic acid should also be slightly increased to ensure that any decrease in digestive function and age-related cellular damage is contained.

Special nutritional requirements for debilitated birds

Extra nutritional support for debilitated and diseased birds is vital and plays an essential role in ensuring recovery of the avian patient after disease or debility. Enteral nutrition is currently the most usual method of supporting the debilitated patient, with parenteral (intravenous) nutrition still being in its infancy in avian therapeutics.

First, fluid requirements should be assessed, as any animal will succumb to dehydration long before starvation. The reader is referred to page 90 for a more detailed discussion of this topic.

Second, energy requirements should be estimated. These can be calculated roughly from the maintenance energy requirements (MER) by multiplication as follows:

$$
\begin{aligned}
\text{Starvation} &= 0.5 \times \text{MER} \\
\text{Trauma} &= 1.5 \times \text{MER} \\
\text{Sepsis} &= 2.5 \times \text{MER} \\
\text{Burns} &= 3 - 4 \times \text{MER}
\end{aligned}
$$

From these crude estimations a rough idea of the levels of nutrition demanded and the energy concentration of the diet can be decided.

Third, protein requirements should be evaluated, as debilitation will increase amino acid and protein turnover. This may be through the increased use of proteins in the immune system response, or for repair of damaged tissue or simply after using tissue proteins as an energy source.

Birds with liver disease

Birds affected by hepatic dysfunction should be fed a diet which reduces liver use by decreasing its need to convert body tissues into blood glucose, and decreasing its need to break down the waste products of excess protein metabolism. Therefore birds should be fed a diet high in digestible carbohydrates, such as boiled rice, pasta or potatoes, for energy and sugars. Protein sources should be of a high biological value (high in essential amino acids) such as those found in whole eggs. This is in an attempt to keep to a minimum the overall amount of protein fed, particularly purine-producing proteins such as are found in fish, meat etc. These protein sources lead to the greater build up of waste products of protein digestion, which the liver then has to detoxify and eliminate via the kidneys. The feeding of frequent, small meals is also to be advocated for liver

disease patients, as is the addition of vitamin B supplements to the diet.

Birds with renal disease (Fig. 4.4)

Like the liver, the kidney is responsible for eliminating the waste products of protein metabolism. It is therefore important in renal disease to reduce protein levels, and ensure that the protein sources provided have a high biological value.

In addition, restricting phosphorus in the diet is helpful, as excess may lead to demineralisation of the bone, increased levels of parathyroid hormone and further renal damage.

Finally, restricting sodium is important to reduce fluid retention and decrease hypertension. Vitamin B supplementation can help as an appetite stimulant. It is advisable to supplement it in any case as, being a water-soluble vitamin, it can be flushed out of the body where polyuria occurs, leading to deficiency.

Birds with heart disease

Heart disease is commonly seen in older parrots and some raptors, particularly females. It is

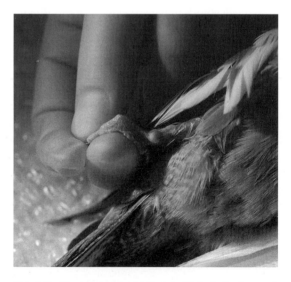

Fig. 4.4 Gout crystals may form in joints (articular gout) as in this cockatiel (*Nymphicus hollandicus*) with renal disease.

also seen as a sequel to iron storage disease (*haemochromatosis*) in toucans and mynahs. Reduction of sodium in the diet to reduce hypertension due to fluid retention is helpful. So too is lowering of cholesterol levels by removing saturated fats, such as dairy products and over-fat prey for raptors. Avoiding meat in general for birds such as parrots is advised. For toucans, mynah birds and related species, the avoidance of high-iron-containing diets is essential to prevent haemochromatosis and the cardiac damage which can ensue.

Birds suffering from maldigestion and malabsorption syndromes

Birds suffering from maldigestion and malabsorption syndromes such as pancreatic disease should be fed highly digestible carbohydrate foods such as rice, potatoes and pasta, whilst reducing all fats in the diet such as seeds, meat etc. The addition of pancreatic enzyme supplementation is to be considered, along with B-vitamin supplementation.

Birds suffering from anaemia

Anaemic patients should have their cause of anaemia investigated, as common causes include heavy-metal poisoning and chronic disease processes. Other aids to increasing red blood cell production (*erythropoiesis*) are supplementation with iron and with smaller increases in copper and cobalt levels. Vitamin B_{12}, niacin, and folic acid levels should be six times the normal minimal values to ensure that the extra demands caused by increased red cell production are met.

Other dietary factors and conditions

Other factors which are known to aid the recovery of debilitated birds are given in Table 4.1.

Hypocalcaemic tetany

A specific disease of African grey parrots commonly between the ages of two and four years is *hypocalcaemic tetany*. This is due to a failure to mobilise calcium into the blood stream. The afflicted parrot will become weak, collapse and start fitting which may progress to a coma and death. It appears to be a hereditary condition and birds often grow out of it if carefully managed. Afflicted birds appear to have plenty of calcium in their bones, but seem unable to mobilise it. Management, therefore, consists of providing sufficient dietary calcium so that blood levels remain normal.

Table 4.1 Examples of dietary deficiencies in avian species.

Vitamin A	Seems to improve the activity of the mononuclear immune system.
Vitamin B complex	Thiamine especially helps stimulate appetite, and many B vitamins are useful in protein and energy metabolism, making them important during recovery periods.
Vitamin C	Also seems to aid immune system function, and may be in short supply if the avian patient is suffering from hepatic disease, since it is the liver which manufactures vitamin C.
Vitamin D	Production of this vitamin may also be impaired due to renal or hepatic dysfunction. However, it is worthwhile noting that excess vitamin D_3 can cause soft tissue mineralisation, including in the kidney itself.
Vitamin E	Aids immune system function and helps reduce free radical oxidation of tissues.
Vitamin K	This may become deficient due to prolonged antibiotic therapy, where intestinal bacteria are depleted or where a raptor has consumed a warfarin poisoned rodent.
Zinc	This mineral helps the healing process, particularly in skin diseases, but can also help immunity, particularly with respect to phagocytosis.

Obesity

In overweight or obese birds, particularly where a fatty liver syndrome is suspected, a strict diet management is indicated.

Correcting dietary deficiencies

Attempting to encourage new food consumption

Birds are highly intelligent, particularly members of the Psittaciformes order. This means that the introduction of new foods, in an attempt to correct dietary deficiencies can be a significant problem. The following techniques may be employed to tempt a cage bird to accept new food items.

Overcoming unfamiliarity

Just because the bird was not interested in the food item today is no reason that it may not try the food tomorrow. Just like children, birds may view a new or unfamiliar food with suspicion and reject it purely for that. The key is to keep representing the food, preferably on the top of its food bowl, so that the bird has to remove it to get to the usual food underneath. The bird may eventually become used to its sight, smell and taste, and may therefore start to eat it.

Tempting the bird with food

Many birds want to eat what their owners are eating, as obviously it must be better than the rubbish in their own food bowl! This can be used to our advantage, as the owner can sample the food in front of the bird and then offer it to the bird. This can trigger acceptance.

Fooling the bird with food

Covering the food item that you wish the bird to eat in the flavour or colour of a food item it already likes can work well. An example would be honey- or peanut-butter-coated broccoli or carrot.

Pelleted commercial diets

Many excellent pelleted avian diets are now available. For all species ranging from flamingos to toucans, parrots and ducks. Their main advantage is homogeneity – that is the bird cannot pick and choose what it wishes to eat, but is rather forced to eat a balanced pre-prepared diet.

The disadvantages include the problem of selection. Some of these diets are multi-coloured and birds have good colour vision and may pick out one coloured biscuit to eat only. This is fine if all of the biscuits are of the same composition no matter what the colour, but does lead to wastage. In addition, palatability can be a problem, so getting a bird to eat some of these diets can be difficult.

Fresh water must be available at all times, as these diets are dry pellets and chronic dehydration can occur.

Avian mineral and vitamin supplements

These are very important, particularly for species fed a home-prepared diet. They are produced by many companies and cover all aspects of supplementation. Some are put in the food itself, some in water. The latter may be problematic as the taste may prevent water consumption or the vitamins may encourage bacterial growth in the water bowl. Multivitamin and mineral preparations may be used as a general supplement to a diet where the individual bird will not take a wide variety of food types, an example is the seed-obsessed parrot. They should not be used though, as an excuse to give up on offering other food types, but more to ensure nutritional balance whilst trying to encourage the bird onto a more stable diet. They may also be used, even when a balanced diet is being fed and eaten, to supplement a bird at certain times of its life when requirements for minerals and vitamins increase, such as during egg-laying, growth, moulting and old age.

Dietary requirements peculiar to specific families

Larger members of the Psittaciformes order

Larger members of the parrot family, such as cockatoos, macaws, Amazons and African grey parrots, have slightly different requirements from the smaller members of the family, such as the conures and parakeets. Many of their larger parrots require slightly more fats in their diets, to increase their calorific density, than their smaller cousins. This is not so surprising considering that the normal wild diets of these parrots involve a moderate amount of oil-based nuts and seeds. It is advisable therefore, that larger nuts, such as hazel nuts, Brazil nuts, cashews etc, should be included in the diet of these species.

An example of the maintenance energy requirements of some of the larger species of parrot include 452 kJ per day for a scarlet macaw (*Ara macau*) as opposed to 200 kJ per day (Nott & Taylor, 1993) required by the lesser sulfur crested cockatoo (*Cacatua sulphurea*). Therefore, to maintain calorific intake, a scarlet macaw will have to eat far more of a seed such as the sunflower seed, which has an energy content of approximately 24 kJ per gram of dry matter (18 g dry matter or nearly 22.5 g fresh), as opposed to the cashew nut which has an energy content of 32 kJ per gram of dry matter (14 g dry matter or nearly 17 g fresh).

However, many of the larger parrots, especially the Amazons and African grey parrots, are also prone to atherosclerosis, or hardening of the major arteries, due to cholesterol deposition in their walls. This happens if their diets are persistently high in saturated fats, such as meat and dairy products, but may also occur with chronic over-consumption of high fat nuts and seeds. Hepatic lipidosis, or the obliteration of the liver cells with fat, is also a common sequel to over-supplementation of the diet with high fat nuts and seeds in parrots. So it is important to get the balance right.

In formulating these diets it is also important that attention is paid to calcium and mineral levels, as seeds and nuts are extremely poor suppliers of these. Nuts may also be a potential source of fungal growths of *Aspergillus* spp. These can not only produce spores which may cause respiratory disease, but can also produce highly poisonous toxins, known as *aflatoxins* and *gliatoxins*, which may cause sudden death, neurological damage or chronic hepatic damage, depending on the dose consumed.

The most commonly seen deficiencies in the larger psittacines occur with vitamin A, vitamin D_3 and the mineral calcium. This is particularly the case with African grey parrots because of hypocalcaemic tetany – an inherited condition of two-to-four-year-old birds, where blood calcium levels cannot be maintained. This can lead to hypocalcaemic fits. In addition, African grey parrots fed an all-seed diet are very prone to respiratory infections, especially aspergillosis (the air sac and lung infestation with the fungus *Aspergillus fumigatus*). This is often associated with hypovitaminosis A.

However, as with so many nutrients, too much is as bad as too little. Excessive levels of vitamin D_3 commonly cause toxicosis in African grey parrots and macaws, leading to soft tissue calcification and renal damage. Excessive vitamin A can also cause problems in the large parrots and in hand-reared chicks, causing liver damage, kidney damage and haemorrhage.

Raptors

Raptors are carnivorous. They therefore require regular fresh rodent or avian prey. If fed whole, these usually provide a balanced diet. To determine the amounts of prey to be fed, a rough rule of thumb is that the larger the raptor, the smaller the food consumption is as a percentage of that bird's weight. A golden eagle, for example, may consume 5–7% of its body weight per day, whereas a sparrowhawk would perhaps consume 25% body weight per day.

For raptors in training the main aim is to keep the birds lean and slightly hungry to make it easier to hand-train them. If underfed, however, the consequence is starvation, while if overfed the bird will become obese – and atherosclerosis is a major problem in overfed raptors. To try and prevent under- or overfeeding a useful technique is to weigh the raptor on a daily basis to ensure constant weight levels. This is not always possible, however, for example when breeding the raptors when they mustn't be handled, and so at certain times of the year it may be difficult to assess their condition. During this period however it is useful, as with any animal, to increase the levels of nutrition to ensure healthy egg production. Care should be taken with egg-laying female raptors though, to ensure they are not fed obese prey items, as the presence of cholesterol and lipids for yolk production in their blood stream makes them very prone to atherosclerosis at this time.

Water consumption

Water consumption is of course vital. Dehydration may occur due to the feeding of previously frozen and then thawed prey only because the freezing process causes dehydration of the carcass. Therefore, when defrosting the rodent or avian prey item, it is advisable to soak it in water.

Food composition

Protein levels are as expected for a carnivorous family, relatively high, at 15–20% (Cooper, 1991) and this is desirable for full fitness. However excessive levels of protein (greater than 30%) should be avoided as this can lead to an excess of protein degradation products in the bloodstream, such as purines. These are converted into uric acid for renal excretion, but if the levels are excessive, the uric acid concentration will exceed that which can be dissolved in the blood. This will lead to the precipitation of uric acid causing gout.

Optimum fat levels in prey offered for raptors have been estimated at 20–25% (Cooper, 1991). Prey such as some laboratory rats and mice, as mentioned, can cause hypercholesterolaemia and atherosclerosis in underworked raptors.

Mineral supplementation may be necessary. This is especially so in chicks which are often fed small pieces of meat, rather than whole prey. This can result in calcium deficiencies, as muscle tissue is low in calcium and high in phosphorus. A ratio of calcium to phosphorus of 2:1 or at least 1.5:1 should be maintained.

Prey

The feeding of certain types of prey should be done with care. For example, pigeons fed to larger birds of prey can be a source of *Trichomonas gallinae* infestation. This is a protozoal parasite which invades the crop and digestive system, causing regurgitation, vomiting and weight loss in the affected raptor. Therefore, it is recommended that if pigeon is to be fed it be deep frozen and then thoroughly defrosted to kill any *Trichomonas* spp organisms present in the carcass.

Other parasites such as the worm *Capillaria* spp can also be transmitted from prey bird to raptor. In other avian and mammalian prey, the presence of lead shot is again a potential hazard and a cause of lead poisoning in raptors.

Other problems due to poisoning from prey offered are pesticides and herbicides, particularly the organochlorines and organophosphates. These concentrate in animal fats and so pass up through the food chain, producing highest concentrations in top predators such as raptors.

In addition, there are compounds such as the polychorinated biphenyls (PCBs). These are used for a number of purposes, including insulation and electrical circuitry, and may enter the food chain through small rodents. These also concentrate in animal fats, so concentrating their levels in the tissues of animals as one moves up the food chain. They cause problems similar to those caused by the pesticides: reproductive problems, chick mortalities and neurological tremors which can lead to death.

Food management for racing pigeons

The day-to-day feeding of racing pigeons includes the provision once or twice a day of a grain-and-pulse-based diet. For racing pigeons, one trend is the feeding of carbohydrate-based foods, such as grains, early on in the course of a week, and then increasing the protein levels with supplements and pulses as the racing day, often a Saturday, approaches. Many companies now produce homogenous pelleted feeds for racing pigeons, containing differing levels of protein depending on whether they are actively training or rearing young. Grit can be given freely. It is insoluble and aids in the grinding of grain in the gizzard. This is important in species such as pigeons which do not de-husk seed prior to swallowing it. Water is offered, as with game birds, from communal feeders, and pigeon owners will often add multivitamins, minerals and medicants to these fountain feeders.

Waterfowl

Nutrition of waterfowl receives less attention, as many geese and ducks are kept in outdoor small-holding settings and so live predominantly on grass and other herbage. Geese in particular need ample grass for grazing. It is essential to ensure that access to poisonous plants or trees, such as laburnum and foxgloves, is restricted, as these birds will eat almost anything. In poor weather, or with limited grass production, commercial pelleted food should be given. There are now commercial duck and geese pellets available. Alternatively the use of poultry 'layer' pellets can be tried.

Commercial pellets come in four main categories:

- Pellets designed for the brooding, egg-laying female, which are higher in calcium and protein
- Pellets for the very young waterfowl chick up to two to three weeks of age (known as 'starter pellets' or 'crumbs')
- Pellets for the juvenile growing waterfowl (up to four to six months)
- Adult non-breeding maintenance pellets.

The differences lie in the provision of proteins and calcium, with the highest being in the starter pellets (at around 20% protein) through to the lower end as adult pellets (14% protein). There are now companies which also produce special diets for other ornamental waterfowl such as sea duck and flamingos. (Flamingos require more protein and a selection of salts to encourage plumage colouration.)

Duck and geese enclosures need to be routinely examined for evidence of foreign objects, such as lead shot, barbed wire fragments and so on. This is because of these birds' desire to consume any and every loose potential food item they can find when foraging.

References

Austic, R.E. and Cole, R.K. (1971) Impaired uric acid excretion in chickens selected for uricemia and articular gout. *Proceedings of the 1971 Cornell Nutritional Conference November 2–3*, Buffalo, Colarado.

Blackmore, D.K. (1963) The incidence and aetiology of thyroid dysplasia in budgerigars (*Melopsittacus undulatus*). *Veterinary Record* **75**, 1068–1072.

Brue, R.N. (1994) Nutrition. In *Avian Medicine: Principles and Application* (Ritchie, B., Harrison, G. and Harrison, L., eds), pp. 63–95. W.B. Saunders, Philadelphia.

Cooper, J.E. (1991) Nutritional diseases including poisons. In *Veterinary Aspects of Captive Birds of Prey*, pp. 124–142. Standfast Press, Glos.

Harper, E.J. and Skinner, N.D. (1998) Clinical nutrition of small psittacines and passerines. *Seminars in Avian and Exotic Pet Medicine* **7** (3), 116–127.

Kollias, G.V. and Kollias, H.W. (2000) Feeding passerine and psittacine birds. In *Small Animal Clinical Nutrition 4th Edition* (Hand, M.S., Thatcher, C.D., Remillard, R.L. and Roudebush, P., eds), pp. 979–991. Mark Mervis Institute, Marceline, Missouri.

Nott, H.M.R. and Taylor, F.J. (1993) The energy requirements of pet birds. *Proceedings of the Association of Avian Veterinarians*, pp. 233–239.

Scott, M.L. and Norris, L.C. (1965) Vitamins and vitamin deficiencies. In *Diseases of Poultry, 5th Edition* (Biester, H.E. and Schwarte, L.H., eds). Iowa State University Press, Ames, Iowa.

Scott, P.W. (1996) Nutrition. In *Manual of Psittacine Birds* (Beynon, P.H., Forbes, N.A., and Lawton, M.P.C., eds), pp. 17–26. BSAVA, Cheltenham, Gloucester.

Wallach, J.D. & Cooper, J.E. (1982) Nutritional diseases of wild birds. In *Non-infectious Diseases of Wildlife* (Hoff, G.L. and Davis, J.W., eds), pp. 113–126. Iowa State University Press, Ames, Iowa.

Further reading

Heuser, G.F. and Norris, L.C. (1929) Rickets in chicks III: The effectiveness of mid-summer sunshine and irradiation from a quartz mercury vapour arc in preventing rickets in chickens. *Poultry Science* **8**, 89–98.

Stahl, S. and Kronfeld, D. (1998) Veterinary nutrition of large Psittacines. *Seminars in Avian and Exotic Pet Medicine* **7** (3), 128–134.

Worrell, A. (1991) Serum iron levels in rhamphastids. In *Proceedings of the Association of Avian Veterinarians*, pp. 120–130.

Chapter 5
Common Avian Diseases

Skin and feather disease

Feather plucking

Feather plucking can be one of the most complicated conditions in avian medicine to accurately
diagnose and treat. The causes of feather plucking
can vary tremendously as is seen in the list below
of some of the more commonly occurring causes
(Fig. 5.1):

- Ectoparasites
- Endoparasites
- Skin infections (bacterial, viral, fungal)
- Iatrogenic (for example a poor wing clip)
- Behavioural (this can be extremely difficult to
  diagnose!)
- Organopathy (damage/infection of an internal
  organ, e.g. liver)
- Heavy metal poisoning (lead, zinc)
- Psittacosis (infection with *Chlamydophila
  psittaci*)
- Salmonellosis
- Hormonal (nesting behaviour)
- Environmental contaminant (e.g. nicotine
  tainted feathers if the bird is kept in the same
  room as a smoker).

Diagnosis requires a full, detailed history to be
taken as well as a full health examination. This
often comprises feather analysis, skin scrapings
and biopsy, blood tests and radiographs. A diagnosis of a behavioural condition can only be made
accurately by extensive history taking and elimination of medical conditions from the picture.

Two different forms of feather plucker have
been identified. The first is the true feather
plucker, which actually removes the whole
feather. The second is the feather chewer, which
just mutilates the feather but leaves it embedded

in the skin. The condition is mainly seen in
members of the Psittaciformes group, although
some of the hawk family, such as Harris hawks, are
also susceptible.

Ectoparasitic

Ectoparasites are not as commonly seen in cage
birds as might be expected. There are, however,
many important skin and feather parasites of
raptors, game birds and waterfowl kept in captivity.

Mites

Cnemidocoptes: the mite most commonly seen in
avian medicine is seen mainly in the budgerigar
and canary and is a member of the genus *Cnemidocoptes*. These eat cell debris, and cause the
conditions known as 'scaly beak' and 'tassle foot'
(Fig. 5.2). The presenting signs are crusting and
enlargement of the cere at the base of the beak,
often causing beak deformities, and thickening
and proliferation of the skin of the legs. Another
mite of this genus, which is peculiar to pigeons, is
the depluming mite, *Cnemidocoptes laevis laevis*.
This mite causes disintegration of the feather
quill, causing it to break off close to the skin.
This produces bald areas over the body of the
pigeon.

Sarcoptes: scabies mites (*Sarcoptes* spp) are
uncommonly seen, but have been reported in
macaws. The symptoms are feather loss and widespread self-trauma due to rubbing, scratching and
feather plucking because of intense pruritus.

Dermanyssus: the red feather mite (*Dermanyssus
gallinae*) has been reported in raptor flights,
pigeon lofts and in some cases cage and aviary

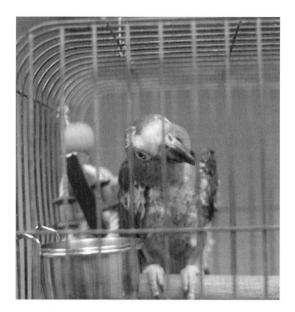

Fig. 5.1 Feather plucking may have many causes.

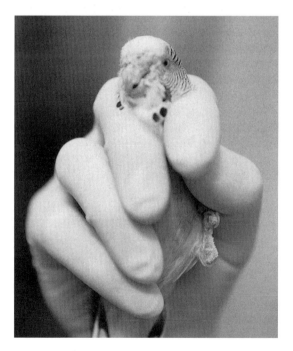

Fig. 5.2 Scaly beak in a budgerigar due to *Cnemidocoptes* spp.

birds such as parrots, particularly those in outside flights. This mite does not live on the bird permanently. It hides in the cracks and crevices of the cage or shelter during the day and crawls out to

attack the bird when it is roosting at night. This can make diagnosis difficult. It is a blood sucking mite and can cause anaemia and weakness in heavily parasitised birds.

Ornithonyssus: another blood sucking mite is the northern fowl mite (*Ornithonyssus sylvarium*). This mite does inhabit the host continuously, so it is easier to detect and to treat.

Lice

All avian lice belong to the order Mallophaga, and so cause their damage by chewing the feathers. They are generally elongated, squeezing in between the barbs of the feathers. They are more commonly seen in out-door housed birds and the main route for infestation is from wild birds.

The genus of shaft louse infesting waterfowl is *Holomenopon*. It has been associated with damage of feathers, leading to a lack of normal structure and loss of waterproofing. This causes the feathers to look bedraggled and soggy which is why the condition is often referred to as 'wet feather' disease.

In pigeons, two main types of louse are seen. These are the body louse (*Menapon latum*) and the slender louse (*Columbicula columbae*), mainly seen on the wings. They cause damage to the structure of the feather, preventing the interlocking of the barbs which keep the feather's shape intact, and so give the pigeon a somewhat ragged, and 'moth-eaten' appearance.

Raptors are particularly prone to lice and a wide variety of species-specific lice are found. The mites destroy feather integrity and this leads to poor flight. Some lice are contracted from prey species if the raptor is used for hunting, although these may not be significant.

Lice in cage birds are less common. However, some individual birds, particularly those which are unwell for some other reason and so are not preening themselves adequately, may have large enough populations to cause feather damage.

Flies

There are many different families of flies which can cause harm to avian species. The blow fly family, such as the blue, black and green bottles, may be drawn to birds with diarrhoea or with wounds. The maggots of these species then eat their way into the bird with devastating results, and allow the colonisation of the wounds by smaller species of fly maggot.

The Hippoposcidae genus contains such species as the sheep and horse keds, which are however capable of infesting aviary birds, particularly raptors. The juvenile form of the fly is flightless and so spends large amounts of time living on its host. These species can cause an unpleasant bite and will suck tissue fluids, and blood, often creating a serious infection and anaemia. They may also be able to transmit several unpleasant blood-borne parasites, such as avian malaria, and the blood parasites *Haemoproteus* spp and *Leucocytozoan* spp which may cause anaemia and immunosuppression.

Mosquitoes

Mosquitoes can also be a problem. They have been shown to cause irritation and to act as a possible vector for the transmission of avian malaria in penguins in the south of England, as well as causing the spread of other blood parasites and viruses, such as West Nile fever in the United States and Africa, and eastern and western encephalitis viruses.

Gnats

Gnats, such as the blackfly family, apart from causing intense irritation, can also transmit blood-borne parasites such as *Leucocytozoan* spp.

Ticks

These can rapidly be fatal to birds, possibly due to the presence of a toxin in the saliva of the tick. They are seen relatively uncommonly, but can occur in raptors being used for hunting, as ticks are ground dwellers. They are also common in aviary-kept birds which are overhung by surrounding trees. The ticks may be carried on wild birds and so drop off roosts and nests into an aviary beneath. Again, they may transmit many bacteria, such as members of the rickettsia family, as well as blood-borne parasites and viruses.

Endoparasitic

There are situations where internal parasites will cause a bird to exhibit feather plucking. One of these is the parasite *Giardia* which can infest cockatiels. This leads to internal irritation which causes the affected bird to pluck the feathers over its flanks and ventrum.

Viral

Psittacine beak and feather disease (PBFD)

Psittacine beak and feather disease is caused by a member of the family of viruses known as 'circoviruses'. It is transmitted by particles of feather dander. There is evidence of the presence of different strains of the virus, or differing species susceptibility. As its name suggests, it is mainly seen in Psittaciformes, although many other orders of birds have been found to be affected. In some birds, such as the lovebirds, it may cause feather loss. Ultimately the individual may fully recover and regrow all its feathers.

In many other psittacines though, the virus damages the feather follicles causing the production of deformed feathers and eventually feather loss. It also damages the structure of the beak and claws, leading to sloughing of the beak in severe cases. More importantly it can also produce immunosuppression, particularly in young birds, resulting in a low white blood cell count and anaemia, leading to multiple secondary infections such as aspergillosis. This is a common finding in young African grey parrots (Fig. 5.3, Plate 5.1).

In many parrots, the virus proves fatal. There is no cure and no preventative treatment. Diagnosis is based on the clinical signs and on either demonstrating the virus particles in a feather follicle biopsy, or by detecting the DNA of the virus in a feather or fresh blood sample by polymerase chain reaction (PCR) technology.

Polyoma virus

This has been recorded as the cause of the condition known as 'French moult' in budgerigars. This is where damage occurs, mainly to the primary, secondary and rectrice feathers, leading to deformity of their shape and fractures in their

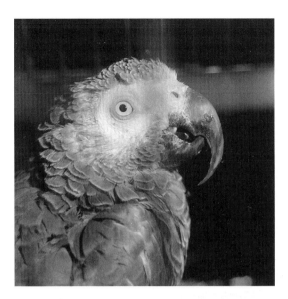

Fig. 5.3 Psittacine beak and feather disease in an African grey parrot – note the overlong beak, which is splitting, and some poor feather quality.

shafts. Some doubt has recently been cast over whether the condition of French moult may have other causes as well. Polyoma viruses, though, do infest many Psittaciformes, and its symptoms will vary depending on the age at which the bird was infected. If infected at a very young age (often less than two weeks of age), then the individual bird will often die due to heart and liver damage. Ascites and digestive disease may thus form part of this viral disease. If infected after this then the bird will develop feather abnormalities as described. The virus can be transmitted in faeces, urine and feather dander, and a bird that survives infection may then shed the virus intermittently.

There is no treatment for this condition, although some preliminary work in the United States has now produced a possible vaccine. Diagnosis is based on the clinical signs, as well as detecting virus DNA particles from a cloacal swab or faecal sample by PCR technology.

Avipox viruses

These can occur in all avian species, although none have so far been recorded in Strigiformes. Signs include pox-like lesions, occurring predominantly on the face, eyelids, feet and cere. These become secondarily infected, and may lead to more extensive lesions. Respiratory tract disease is also seen and may cause sloughing of the lining of the trachea and smaller airways, causing asphyxiation. Transmission may occur directly from bird to bird, and by flying insect vectors. The pox virus affecting canaries is particularly virulent and may cause serious mortality in canary flocks.

Diagnosis is based on demonstrating the classical Bollinger bodies, seen due to virus particles inside infected cells, as well as the clinical signs described.

Bacterial

Bacterial infections are many and varied. Examples include: *Salmonella typhimurium* var. *Copenhagen* joint infection of pigeons, which may then erupt as a boil visible on wing joints such as the elbow; *Staphylococcal* spp and *E. coli* infections of the feet of many species, which cause bumblefoot.

Bumblefoot

This is a common and difficult condition to treat. In raptors it is most frequently seen in falcons, possibly because they spend more time perching in one position than the more active hawks. This causes persistent pressure on the same parts of the sole of the foot which restricts the blood flow to these areas. This will ultimately lead to hypoxia and death of tissues in these blood-compromised areas, and the development of a shiny smooth skin with corns, followed by open sores and deep pedal infections. Many categorisations for the differing stages of bumblefoot have been described, the most basic being proposed by Cooper (1985):

- Type I: this is when the injuries are restricted to smoothing of the normally papillated underside of the foot. There may or may not be the presence of a corn and sometimes a mild scab.

- Type II: this is the next stage, wherein the mild scabs become deeply infected. This condition may also be caused by the raptor puncturing its own foot with one of its claws, for instance when it fails to grasp a prey item and the foot closes on itself. The bacteria involved include *Staphylococcus aureus*, *E. coli*, *Pseudomonas* spp and occasionally yeasts.

- Type III: this is the worst lesion, with deeper structures such as bones within the toes, ligaments etc. all becoming infected. These birds are often not possible to treat. The feet are very swollen and painful and hot to the touch.

More recently bumblefoot has been further refined in classification into 5 categories from mildest at *I*, with early devitalisation of the plantar aspect of the foot, to severe osteomyelitis of the phalangeal bones at *V* (Oaks, 1993; Remple, 1993).

Miscellaneous

Split keel

Split keel is commonly seen in young, overweight, hand-reared birds, particularly those which have been carelessly wing clipped. It occurs when the bird attempts to fly off a high perch, and, either due to poor wing muscling (such as often occurs when hand reared) or lack of flight feathers (after overzealous wing clipping), the bird drops like a stone and hits the ground with force. This often splits the thin skin covering the prominent keel area and this split may become secondarily infected. This delays healing, and may necessitate the use of antimicrobials or even surgery to achieve wound healing.

Ulcerative skin disease

Ulcerative skin disease can be due to bacterial infections, for example by *Staphylococcus* spp, or may be due to fungal infections such as infection by *Aspergillus* spp. Birds most commonly affected are species such as lovebirds, cockatoos and cockatiels.

The bird traumatises the skin underneath each wing, leading to a weeping ulcerative dermatitis. The infections may be primary or secondary. Little is known about the true initial causes of this condition, although some suggestions recently have included allergic skin conditions similar to those seen in dogs.

Psittacosis/chlamydophilosis

Systemic infection with *Chlamydophila psittaci* has been implicated in some parrots with feather plucking and generally poor feather quality (Fig. 5.4).

Changes in feather coloration and structure

This may occur due to a lack of one nutrient, such as the paler colour seen in some canary breeds, for example red factors, when deprived of vitamin A. Vitamin A in particular is required for the production of the yellow and red coloration of feathers. Other colour changes which can be seen include the following:

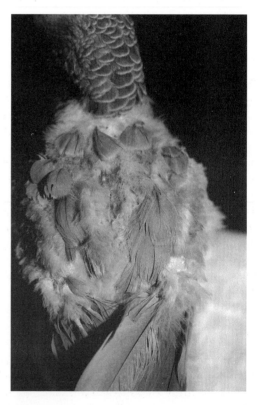

Fig. 5.4 Infection with *Chlamydophila psittaci* may cause many conditions, one of which may be feather plucking as seen here.

- Vasa parrots will develop white feathers rather than their normal grey when they are infected with PBFD virus.
- Red colouration of the grey feathers in African grey parrots may also be seen with hepatic disease and with PBFD virus (Plate 5.1).
- Black feathers appearing in green coloured birds such as Amazons can suggest liver disease.

Fret marks

Fret marks are another common feather abnormality seen in birds with a history of illness. These are breaks in the integrity of the feathers due to poor production of the interlocking barbs. This produces a noticeable band on all of those feathers which were growing at this time. The presence of fret marks suggests some systemic disease or malnutrition at the time the feathers were being produced, and can be a useful external indicator of a bird's recent past health, although they say nothing about its current health status.

Hormonal skin disease

Hypothyroidism has been recorded in birds, particularly in chickens and African grey parrots. Clinical signs include slow growth and poorly coloured feathers, which often lack the interlocking barbules and so appear ragged. Diagnosis is based on the thyroid stimulating hormone (TSH) test where 1 IU/kg of TSH is administered intramuscularly after measurement of basal T4 levels. T4 levels are then measured 24 hours later, over which time a 2.5 times increase in T4 should have occurred. Failure to do so suggests hypothyrodism. It has been suggested that an underlying cause of hypothyroidism may be a dietary deficiency of iodine.

Tumours and feather cysts

Tumours are seen regularly in avian species. The more common skin forms include subcutaneous *lipomas* in many overweight birds, and the so-called *xanthoma* seen particularly along the distal wings of birds such as budgerigars. This is more an accumulation of fat deposits within the cells, producing a thickening of the area, and a characteristic yellow colouring of the skin.

Feather cysts are seen commonly in many species, with the budgerigar and the canary topping the list (Fig. 5.5). The condition occurs when a new growing feather fails to find its way through the skin surface, and so continues to grow while trapped under the skin. The feather cyst becomes an enlarging caseous nodule, which can ulcerate and become secondarily infected. These cysts commonly occur on the wings of affected birds. It is thought that the condition is hereditary and the affected birds should be removed from breeding stock.

Oil spills

One of the commonest reasons for a major catastrophic event affecting wild birds is an oil spill. Sea birds and shore birds alike become coated with the crude oil, making them flightless and removing their water-proofing. Many also succumb to the toxic and irritant effects of the oil itself.

Treatment is based on a number of principles which include stabilisation of the often dehydrated and malnourished bird, followed by prevention of further irritation and absorption of oil across mucus membranes, and finally removal

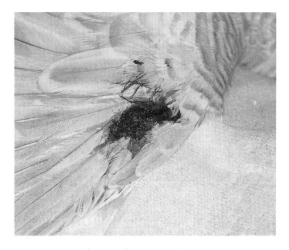

Fig. 5.5 A bleeding feather cyst on the wing of a budgerigar.

of the oil from the pelage (feathers and skin) (Chapter 6).

Digestive disease

Crop

Ingluvitis

Ingluvitis is the medical term for inflammation of the crop. It can be caused by an overgrowth of a variety of pathogens, from the yeast *Candida albicans* to bacteria such as *E. coli* and other Gram negative bacteria. It can also be due to parasites such as *Trichomonas* spp which are a common cause of regurgitation of seed in budgerigars and cockatiels.

In pigeons and raptors, *Trichomonas* spp cause a condition, known as 'canker' or 'frounce', which results in caseous yellow nodules at the corners of the oropharynx and the proximal oesophagus (Fig. 5.6). The feeding of wild-caught pigeons to raptors is a prime means of transmitting this particular pathogen from one species to the other. If a raptor owner is to feed wild-caught pigeon, then it should first be frozen for three to four weeks and then thoroughly defrosted before being fed, so as to kill off any *Trichomonas* spp present. Diagnosis of the causal agent is by crop wash. Sterile saline is flushed into the crop via a crop tube and syringe, the crop manipulated from the outside, and the saline immediately withdrawn. The volume of saline to use varies from 0.5 ml in the case of a budgerigar up to 10 ml in the case of a large macaw. The sample should then be examined using both Gram's stain and Diff-Quik® style dichrome stains. *Trichomonas* spp may be difficult to pick up using this method, as it is often in the lining of the crop. Treatment may therefore have to be given on the *assumption* that this disease exists, once all of the other possibilities have been ruled out.

Sour crop

Sour crop is associated with juvenile birds. It occurs when the contents of the crop ferment, producing a foul smelling acidic environment. This condition may be life threatening because of the possibility of an acute toxic reaction to the chemicals thus produced. Psittaciformes and raptors in particular are prone to this condition.

Crop impaction

Crop impaction occurs in juvenile birds that may overeat. Alternatively, they may eat the floor covering, and, if this is composed of shavings or sawdust, impaction may occur (this is particularly common in pheasants and other young game birds).

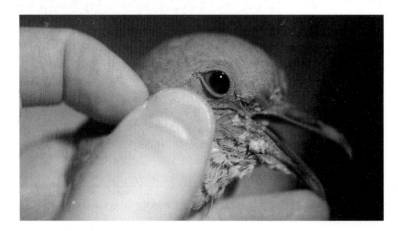

Fig. 5.6 *Trichomonas* spp infection in and around the mouth of a pigeon.

Capillariasis

Capillariasis is the name given to the infestation of the crop lining with the parasitic worm *Capillaria* spp. This tends to be mainly a problem for pigeons and raptors, but it is also seen in Passeriformes, such as finches and canaries, as well as species of Galliformes, such as pheasants and grouse. It is much rarer in Psittaciformes.

A raptor affected by capillariasis continually flicks its head from side to side when eating, and will regurgitate food. In pigeons, acute infections are associated with a high mortality rate because of intense vomiting.

The parasite *Streptocara* spp has been associated with oesophageal damage in waterfowl similar to that caused by *Capillaria* spp in other birds.

Crop burns

These are frequently seen in hand-reared Psittaciformes. They occur when the owner has fed the juvenile bird a rearing formula porridge that has been microwaved and not thoroughly stirred and allowed to stand. This results in 'hot spots' within the mixture, which, when fed, will cause local burns. These can be full thickness, causing the skin to slough after seven to ten days (Plate 5.2).

Associated crop disorders

Goitre is a condition, seen in budgerigars fed an all seed unsupplemented diet, which mimics crop disease. The lack of iodine in an all seed diet will cause thyroid gland enlargement (goitre). This enlarged gland will press on the crop and proximal oesophagus, so limiting its ability to empty and fill. The bird will then adopt the classic horizontal posture as it lies across the perch with the head slightly raised. There is frequent intermittent regurgitation of seed.

Proventriculus

Proventriculitis

Proventriculitis is inflammation of the proventriculus, the true avian acid-secreting stomach. It can be caused by a number of pathogens, including the yeast *Candida* spp and the bacteria *Megabacterium* spp. Signs can include the vomiting of food, the passing of undigested seed in the faeces, in the case of Psittaciformes, anorexia, diarrhoea and weight loss. In budgerigars the incidence of megabacteriosis (caused by *Megabacterium* spp) is relatively high. Many birds are carriers with no clinical signs (*asymptomatic*), but a percentage of a flock will show a 'going light' syndrome typical of megabacteriosis. They will eat voraciously, yet lose weight, often passing undigested seed in their faeces.

Psittacine proventricular dilatation syndrome (PPDS)

This syndrome is also known by the names 'gastric dilatation syndrome' (GDS), and 'macaw wasting syndrome' (MWS). It is now known to be caused by a virus, and is invariably fatal in those affected. The condition occurs in members of the Psittaciformes (not necessarily macaws) and presents as a bird which chronically loses weight, often passing undigested seeds in its faeces and vomiting food more and more frequently (Fig. 5.7). The

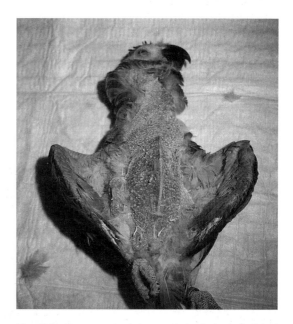

Fig. 5.7 Severe emaciation and death is the clinical outcome of proventricular dilation syndrome (breast feathers have been manually removed to show extent of weight loss).

virus attacks the nerves supplying the crop and proventriculus, leading to their progressive paralysis. Food and fluid sit in these two organs, ferment and are often vomited.

Diagnosis is made on the clinical appearance and confirmed by proventriculus or crop biopsy demonstrating the typical nerve damage (Fig. 5.8). There is no vaccination available and no treatment for this condition. The bird will eventually die of malnutrition.

Endoparasitic

Helminths

Helminths comprises the worm families, including the roundworms or *ascarids*, as well as the 'tapeworms' or *cestodes*.

Ascarids are commonly seen in cage and aviary birds, particularly those that have a deep litter or earth floor to their aviary, as this allows maturation of any worm eggs that are passed in the faeces. Infected individuals may show no external signs, but if parasitised heavily enough they may lose weight, have diarrhoea or, in severe cases, may experience intestinal blockage and death. Ascarids have a direct life cycle. This means that the eggs passed in the faeces of an infected bird, can, after a few days, be directly infectious to another bird without having to be taken up by an intermediate host. Diagnosis is made by finding the thick-walled eggs in the faeces of the affected bird.

Capillaria *spp*

In pigeons, *Capillaria obsignata* burrows into the lining of the intestine where it can cause severe diarrhoea and regurgitation, often with fatal consequences. *Capillaria* spp are less commonly found in cage and aviary birds, but symptoms are similar to those already described. Diagnosis is by demonstrating the presence of the bi-operculate eggs in the faeces or regurgitated material produced by the infected bird. Its life cycle is direct, as with the ascarid family.

Other digestive system worms seen in birds

Other species of worm found in the digestive system are largely *nematodes* and include *Ornithostrongylus quadriradiatus* which is found in the intestine of pigeons. It is a blood-sucking worm, similar to the hookworm families seen in cats and dogs, and causes weight loss, anaemia and death. Its eggs are thin walled and more spherical than the *Capillaria* spp eggs.

Waterfowl: in waterfowl there are many different species of nematode worms. Some of these include *Echinuria* spp which cause a high mortality rate in young ducks and swans. It is transmit-

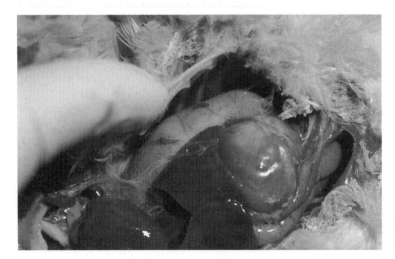

Fig. 5.8 An enlarged proventriculus (cream structure pointed to at top of picture) is seen on examination.

ted via the intermediate host *Daphnia*, the barely visible water flea. It can produce tumour-like lumps in the lining of the proventriculus and gizzard, which may lead to partial blockage of these organs.

Other waterfowl worms seen commonly in geese are the *Epomidostomum* and *Amidostomum* spp which infest the gizzard. They cause bleeding into the lumen of the gizzard, diarrhoea, enteritis and weight loss. In young birds it causes growth retardation and even death.

Gamebirds: in gamebirds, turkeys and hens, the roundworm *Heterakis* spp has been reported. *Heterakis isolonche* is a significant cause of mortality in young pheasants, causing severe damage to the caecal lining. In many Galliformes, such as turkeys and chickens, this worm carries another pathogen with it as it migrates through the body. Known as *Histomonas meleagriditis*, this is a single celled protozoan parasite that can cause significant focal liver necrosis, giving the disease its name of *black spot*.

Non-helminth digestive system parasites

The non-helminth parasites include the single celled protozoan parasites such as *Giardia* spp, *Hexamita* spp, *Trichomonas* spp, and the coccidia such as *Caryospora* spp and *Eimeria* spp.

Protozoan parasites
Giardia spp are commonly found in cockatiels and budgerigars, but may be found in other species, such as toucans, as well. Signs of the disease vary, and in the case of the cockatiel has been associated with a deficiency in vitamin E, producing feather plucking.

Diagnosis is by finding the parasites on faecal smears. The sample is suspended in saline and examined using the × 400 microscope lens. The sample must be fresh, as the parasite disintegrates rapidly once the faeces dry. When fresh, diagnosis is aided by the movement of the organism which has eight flagellae.

Hexamita spp are commonly found in pigeons. It produces weight loss and diarrhoea. It is frequently observed in young birds towards the end of the breeding season when environmental con-

tamination is high. Diagnosis is by finding large numbers of the motile, eight-flagellae-bearing, elongated protozoa using the × 400 microscope lens on on a slide of fresh faeces suspended in saline.

Trichomonas spp may affect the intestines as well as the crop.

Coccidiosis
Eimeria spp infest many species, from pigeons and cage birds to Galliformes and waterfowl. They present a major intestinal parasite problem, contributing to the 'going light' syndrome wherein the bird loses condition rapidly.

Caryospora spp are a less commonly seen blight of raptors, where they cause crop and intestinal damage. There is often high mortality in young birds, with adults exhibiting abdominal discomfort.

In canaries and other Passeriformes, the coccidial parasites *Atoxoplasma* spp or *Isospora* spp may be found. *Isospora* is confined to the gut whereas *Atoxoplasma* spreads into the mononuclear white blood cells and so is carried through the bloodstream. The parasite is filtered out of the blood by organs such as the liver, causing organ enlargement. (This condition is known as 'black spot' because it is visible through the thin skin of the canary's abdomen. It is not to be confused with the disease seen in Galliformes mentioned earlier!). Diarrhoea may be seen, or the disease may be a symptomatic. On the other hand, in severe cases, death from liver failure may ensue.

Diagnosis of coccidiosis is by finding the oval to round oocysts in the bird's faeces using sugar flotation methods, or by direct smear with the × 400 microscope lens.

Bacterial

Bacteria such as *E. coli, Campylobacter* spp, *Clostridia* spp, *Pseudomonas* spp, *Salmonella* spp and *Chlamydophila psittaci* may all cause diarrhoea and even toxaemia, septicaemia and death. *Salmonella* spp may be particularly difficult to treat as the bacteria becomes entrenched in the lining of the intestines. Culture and sensitivity testing using specific *Salmonella* spp culture medium should always be performed on avian faecal samples in cases of diarrhoea and weight loss.

In addition, the mycobacterium *Mycobacterium avium*, the cause of avian tuberculosis, is often seen in waterfowl and raptors. It inhabits the gut and associated organs and is thus spread via the faecal–oral route. It is often implicated in chronic wasting diseases, and produces classical caseous nodules throughout the gut. Diagnosis is made on Ziehl-Neilsen stains demonstrating the acid-fast bacteria, and bacterial culture of the faeces. It is not treatable and, as it is a zoonotic disease, affected birds should be euthanased.

Viral

Duck plague virus

The duck plague virus is a member of the herpes virus family. It affects both ducks and geese. It is spread in the faeces and oral secretions and may be carried latently with no clinical disease, or can cause death with no premonitory signs. Alternatively it may cause violent diarrhoea, anorexia and neurological tremors. Death usually occurs within three to twelve days of infection, and one to ten days after developing clinical signs. Diagnosis is made on the clinical signs and isolation of the virus from faeces, in the live bird, or on demonstration of intranuclear inclusion bodies in the gut wall on post mortem.

Avian papillomatosis

This condition is thought to be due to a papovavirus. It occurs in members of the Psittaciformes family commonly, causing papillomas throughout the digestive system from the crop through the proventriculus, intestine and frequently the cloaca. In the latter situation it often leads to irritation and eversion of the cloaca, or even prolapse due to repeated straining. Other clinical signs include regurgitation, recurrent bouts of enteritis, passage of blood in the faeces and infertility. Papillomatosis is also linked with a high incidence of liver and pancreatic cancer in affected birds.

Diagnosis is made in the live bird by visualising the papillomas. This is aided in the cloaca by applying 5% acetic acid to the lesion, which will cause the papillomas to turn white while normal mucosal folds will remain pink.

Liver

Haemochromatosis

Haemochromatosis is a condition in which excessive amounts of iron are deposited in the liver parenchyma. Birds affected are commonly members of the toucan, toucanette, mynah and starling families. In the wild these species often live in iron poor soil areas, and their digestive systems are therefore adapted to absorb as much iron as possible. When presented with an iron rich diet, especially with high levels of vitamin C, which encourages iron absorption from the gut, too much iron is absorbed. This iron is then deposited in the liver, leading to liver damage and failure.

Clinical signs include ascites, dullness, dyspnoea (due to the ascites pressing on the air sacs), abdominal swelling and sudden death. Diagnosis is based on breed predilection and clinical signs, but frequently requires a liver biopsy to assess iron levels. This can be a dangerous procedure, particularly if the bird has ascites. There is then a real danger of rupturing air sacs and drowning the bird.

Avian tuberculosis (Mycobacterium avium *infection*)

Avian tuberculosis may produce liver disease, causing classical caseous nodules throughout the structure, and is also associated with intestinal disease.

Hepatic lipidosis

Hepatic lipidosis is usually diet related. High fat diets (such as the all-seed diets so beloved of Psittaciformes) and lack of exercise lead to obesity and fat deposition in the liver cells or *hepatocytes*. Liver function suffers as a consequence. This condition may be seen in raptors that are not working, but are still being well fed.

Affected birds are often sleek, plump birds, which then become dull and lethargic, and may exhibit signs varying from ascites, to respiratory distress and clotting defects.

Other bacterial diseases

Any bacteria, such as *Salmonella* spp, *E. coli* and *Pseudomonas* spp, that breaches the gut wall may affect the liver directly via the enterohepatic circulation. In addition, the pansystemic infection of *Chlamydophila psittaci* will cause hepatitis manifested, as with so many hepatic disorders, by green to yellow coloured urates. Diagnosis is based on clinical signs, biochemistry and isolation of the bacteria from the gastrointestinal tract and, if possible, from hepatic swabs.

Viral liver diseases

Pacheco's disease (herpes virus infection of Psittaciformes): Pacheco's disease is spread in the faeces and oral secretions of infected birds. The condition is highly infectious, and may rapidly spread through a flock. Many birds will die within a matter of days of contracting the disease, the incubation period varying from two to twelve days. Some birds will, however, remain latently infected and will shed the virus into the environment.

Clinical signs include watery green to orange-red faeces, due to large amounts of blood being shed from the gut, and abdominal swelling. However, a bird may die suddenly without warning. Terminally there are often neurological signs including leg paresis, paralysis, opisthotonus, seizures and torticollis. Diagnosis is made by detecting the virus using PCR techniques (as for *C. psittaci*) in faeces, the clinical signs and finding intranuclear inclusion bodies in the liver cells.

Falcon herpes virus: another member of the herpes virus family affects Falconidae and occurs mainly in Europe and the Middle East. It is usually fatal and causes liver and spleen swelling and necrosis, bone marrow necrosis and gut inflammation with haemorrhage. It is transmitted directly from bird to bird and via prey items. The drug acyclovir appears not to be effective in treating this herpes virus.

Owl herpes virus: this virus causes liver, spleen and bone marrow necrosis and is specific to the owl family. It is invariably fatal within three to nine days. Yellow nodules may be found in the gut and the pharyngeal mucosa. It is spread in urine and faeces, as well as respiratory secretions. Some birds which survive will remain latently infected. There is no treatment or vaccine available.

Duck viral hepatitis: duck viral hepatitis affects chiefly young ducklings under three weeks of age and is caused by a member of the Picornoviridae. It is rapidly fatal and produces severe liver damage and haemorrhage from the liver surface.

Avian leukosis/sarcoma virus: this family group of viruses is known to induce a tissue borne leukaemia in Psittaciformes, Galliformes (such as the domestic chicken) and Passeriformes (such as the canary). It destroys the liver and kidneys, which become infiltrated by rapidly dividing lymphocytes. Hen birds seem more susceptible to this virus than cock birds, and it is shed in the faeces, oral/respiratory secretions and semen. It is also passed in genetic material from mother to young in the egg. Clinical signs include hepato- and renalomegaly, ascites (Plate 5.3), respiratory distress, weight loss, green coloured urates, polydipsia and polyuria. There is no treatment.

Toxic liver conditions

Toxins from a number of sources may cause hepatic damage in the avian patient. These include the heavy metal toxicoses such as lead and zinc poisoning. It may also include other metals such as copper, chromium and mercury.

Lead poisoning: Lead poisoning is one of the two commonest seen in birds. Lead poisoning is frequently seen in waterfowl, particularly swans, which have inadvertently eaten lead shot from hunting or fishing. However Psittaciformes are frequently affected by lead poisoning, as they will consume or destroy many household items which contain lead. These include:

- Metal strips used for creating a lead window effect on kitchen units
- Lead weights in window curtain or blind drawer cords
- Lead in the foil used for wine bottles
- Metallic cloths used for sanding/polishing metals
- Lead paints in older houses.

Clinical signs include:

- Weakness (the classic S-shaped neck of the swan)
- Lethargy, vomiting, passage of blood in the faeces (very common in Psittaciformes)
- Passage of lime green faeces (very common in raptors, Plate 5.4)
- Chronic non-regenerative anaemia (due to bone marrow suppression)
- Seizures
- Kidney and liver damage
- Death.

Diagnosis is by finding blood lead levels in excess of 0.2 ppm (12.5 µmol/l). Those in excess of 0.4–0.6 ppm (25–37.5 µmol/l) are diagnostic. In addition, radiography will often show lead particles as radiodense areas in the proventriculus and ventriculus.

Zinc poisoning: Zinc poisoning is the second of the two commonest poisonings. It is mainly seen in Psittaciformes shortly after they have been moved into a new cage, and has thus attracted the synonym 'new wire cage disease'. This is because the finish on many cages is a compound of zinc. Occasionally the finish of these cages is of a poor quality and a fine powder of zinc oxide forms on the surface of the wires. The parrot manoeuvres itself around the cage with feet and beak, and takes in small volumes of this powder on a daily basis. After four to six weeks, liver and kidney damage will occur, and the bird may present as for lead poisoning, weak, lethargic, having seizures and with anaemia (Fig. 5.9). Other sources of zinc include some forms of coin, some plastics and other alloys. Diagnosis is made on clinical signs, history and finding zinc blood levels above 2 ppm (2000 µg/l).

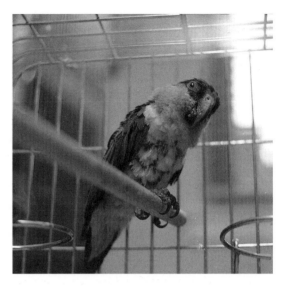

Fig. 5.9 Zinc poisoning may cause a number of signs, from weakness and fitting to feather plucking. The bird exhibited feather plucking and neurological signs.

Other poisons

Organic poisons, such as the aflatoxins released by *Aspergillus* spp, are known to be hepatotoxic and carcinogenic, as are the organic poisons found in rapeseed, ragwort and the castor bean. Treatment is rarely possible, the aim being to avoid the toxin in the first place. Supportive therapy and the use of adsorbants, such as activated charcoal, are suggested.

Pancreas

Diabetes mellitus is a common condition in budgerigars and cockatiels. It seems that the condition may be hereditary, although pancreatitis can result in the development of this disease.

Clinical signs are similar to those of mammals, with polydipsia and polyuria being the most commonly seen, often with dramatic weight loss despite a healthy appetite.

Diagnosis is made on the clinical signs in conjunction with a persistently raised blood glucose (often above 25 mmol/l up to 44 mmol/l). Some glucose may be found in the urine normally, but high levels (>1%) are strongly suggestive of disease.

Respiratory disease

Upper respiratory tract

Nostrils

Often feathers are stained just above the nares, and there may be sneezing and head flicking due to the discharge. The causes of this are many and varied, and may be purely confined to the upper airways, or may hint at more generalised respiratory disease.

Rhinoliths are a common finding in Psittaciformes. These are concretions of dried secretions that form a ball of solid material, blocking the entrance to the nasal passages. They may be caused by dietary insufficiencies such as hypovitaminosis A, and/or may involve local or deeper infections due to bacteria such as *Mycoplasma* spp particularly in pigeons, or *Chlamydophila psittaci*, the cause of psittacosis.

Fungi, such as *Aspergillus* spp, or viruses, such as the avipox virus group, are also causes. In budgerigars and other cage birds, as well as raptors, the presence of scaly face/beak (the mite *Cnemidocoptes* spp) may also contribute to the blockage of the nostrils.

Some species of parrot, such as the Amazons, are particularly susceptible to nasal irritation in dry arid environments, and in the presence of other species of bird which produce large amounts of feather dander, such as African grey parrots and cockatoos.

A not uncommon congenital defect in some birds is the absence of a patent internal choanal slit. This prevents the normal nasal secretions from draining ventrally into the oropharynx, where they are swallowed. The secretions then present as a clear nasal discharge.

Theromyzon tessulatum is the duck nasal leech and is a common parasite in Anseriformes. It may lead to secondary infections of the nasal passages.

Pigeon herpes virus (PHV) is a common disease of young (<6 months) pigeons. It causes a nasal discharge, sneezing and necrotic plaques to form inside the mouth and upper airways. It may also cause the cere to become discoloured and crusty. In severe cases death may occur. There is no specific treatment or vaccine available, although sup-portive therapy should be performed as many birds will survive.

Sinusitis may be seen in conjunction with rhinoliths and nasal discharges. It may be visible as a swelling on the face, often ventral to the eye in the area of the infraorbital sinus.

Lower respiratory tract

Trachea

The following conditions may be associated with the avian trachea.

Gape worm infection: the gape worm, *Syngamus trachea*, is found particularly in Galliformes, as well as in pigeons and raptors such as buzzards. This parasite uses the earthworm as its intermediate host before finally maturing in the windpipe of the afflicted bird. There it causes irritation and secondary infection, and may be present in sufficient numbers to suffocate the bird. Diagnosis is made by finding the characteristic Y-shaped worms (the male and female worms are permanently joined in copulation!) in the mucus of the mouth and trachea.

Avipox virus: in Amazon parrots, a severe form of avipox virus may cause the sloughing of the lining of the windpipe, resulting in dyspnoea, pneumonia and even death from secondary infection. All avipox viruses cause pox lesions on the face, particularly around the eyes and mouth, the pharynx and trachea, but may also produce lesions on the feet. Secondary infections are common. In pigeons there are vaccines available. Diagnosis is confirmed by finding the characteristic Bollinger bodies which are the reproductive centres of virus replication within the host cells. There is no treatment for avipox viruses other than supportive therapy and antibiosis for secondary infections.

Aspergillosis: aspergillosis, due to the fungus *Aspergillus* spp, can produce a growth which blocks the windpipe in a matter of days. This condition is particularly common in raptors and many Psittaciformes such as African grey parrots. Diagnosis is based on history, which is often of a cough and a change in voice in Psittaciformes. In raptors it may suddenly present with dyspnoea. Rigid endoscopic examination of the trachea is recommended, with sampling for culture of any material that is identified.

Air sac mites: Air sac mites, *Sternostoma tracheacolum* are common in Passeriformes such as canaries where they prefer the trachea and bronchi, despite their name, and cause dyspnoea. The mites may be seen easily if the feathers of the neck region are wetted and a bright, but cold light, is shone from behind the bird. The mites are silhouetted as dark pin-heads crawling up and down within the trachea. Another form of air sac mite, known as *Cytodites nudus*, is seen in waterfowl, and produces dyspnoea, often with a cough.

Avian cholera: avian cholera is a disease seen in waterfowl caused by the bacterium *Pasteurella multocida*. It causes a thick mucoid discharge from the mouth and trachea, dyspnoea and often death in young birds. A related bacteria, *R merella* (*Pasteurella*) *anatipestifer*, will cause tracheal and upper airway discharge in ducklings and a condition known as duck septicaemia. It is a common cause of mortality.

Lungs and air sacs

The absence of a diaphragm in avian species means that any disease causing fluid retention or production, such as liver damage, has the potential to affect breathing. This is particularly so when a thin walled air sac ruptures and allows fluid to access the respiratory system. The bird may then become suddenly severely dyspnoeic.

Chlamydophila psittaci infection: chlamydophilosis, ornithosis and psittacosis are all terms for the same infectious condition – that caused by the zoonotic bacterium *Chlamydophila psittaci*.

Psittacosis refers to the condition in Psittaciformes, ornithosis to the condition in other avian species and chlamydophilosis may be applied to both. The bacterium is of great significance in pet cage and aviary birds first because of its widespread presence, particularly in the smaller species such as cockatiels and budgerigars, and

second because birds may act as carriers of the bacteria for months to years without necessarily showing any signs of disease. Indeed they may shed the bacterium into their faeces and oral secretions only intermittently, which can make detection of carriers extremely difficult. This is thought to be because *Chlamydophila* can live inside the host's cells, more like a virus than a traditional bacteria.

The disease is spread via faecal, oral and respiratory secretions and feather dander, and different strains of the bacteria affect different species of bird. Not all strains are as potent, either to the bird, or to man.

Pigeons are commonly affected by chlamydophilosis. Often this is shown by relatively mild signs of persistent conjunctivitis and sneezing. Conversely, in species such as the macaw family, the first sign of psittacosis may be death!

Other symptoms include a clear nasal discharge, sneezing, conjunctivitis, greenish diarrhoea, dyspnoea and the classical 'sick bird syndrome' of a hunched and fluffed up, dull bird.

C. psittaci can infect almost every internal organ, including the spleen, the liver and the kidneys. It would be more accurate therefore, in species such as the Psittaciformes, to consider chlamydiosis as a systemic disease with respiratory symptoms.

Diagnosis of chlamidophilosis: the methods of diagnosing chlamydiosis are not all guaranteed to detect the bacteria even if present. This is because of the intermittent shedding of the bacteria into the environment that frequently occurs in carrier status individuals. Traditional methods employing radiography and white blood cell counts are useful, as infected Psittaciformes often have markedly enlarged spleens on radiography and white blood cell counts in excess of $30 \times 10^9/l$ if actively infected.

The most reliable test is the PCR test used to detect the bacteria in droppings, or, on postmortem, from internal organs. It is extremely sensitive, but due to intermittent shedding may not pick up all infected birds.

The Clearview® test (Unipath) has been designed to pick up particles of the bacteria shed in oral or faecal samples and again is relatively sensitive, but will not detect the bacteria if the bird is not actively shedding it through these routes when tested.

The Immunocomb® test (Biogal Labs) detects the antibodies (IgG_1) produced by the bird's immune system against the bacterium, and so is beneficial in testing birds which may be carriers of the disease and not shedding it into the environment. The disadvantage of the test is that the bird may not be currently infected, and yet still have antibodies against the disease if it was infected in the past.

Chlamydophilosis as a zoonosis: all humans are susceptible, but those most at risk include:

- The very young
- The very old
- Those on immunosuppressive medication such as high dose corticosteroids (e.g. asthma sufferers) and chemotherapy
- Those with immunosuppressive diseases, such as diabetes mellitus and AIDS.

If the owner falls into one of these categories then serious thought should be given to rehoming or even euthanasing the bird.

In a pet shop situation, where the public are at risk, the affected livestock must be removed from public areas into a specific quarantine area. All handlers of birds during the treatment period should wear face-masks and protective clothing when in the same air space as the birds. Faeces should be incinerated.

The owner should also be informed of the symptoms of chlamydophilosis in humans, and advised to contact his or her doctor immediately to receive testing or medication if any of these occur.

The symptoms of chlamydophilosis in humans include all or some of the following:

- A dry, non-productive cough
- 'Flu-like muscle pains and fever
- Migraines
- Kidney and liver damage
- Dyspnoea
- Heart damage
- Occasionally death.

Despite all of these problems, chlamydophilosis is not a notifiable disease. This does not, however, diminish the veterinary surgeon's responsibility under Health and Safety guidelines to ensure that all staff, as well as owners, are aware of the risks and health hazards, and that all precautions are taken to ensure adequate protection of staff dealing with infected birds is taken.

Veterinary nurses and technicians are equally obliged to follow practice protocols and health and safety procedure, when dealing with positive cases.

Aspergillosis: aspergillosis is the fungal condition caused by *Aspergillus* spp frequently *Aspergillus fumigatus*. This fungus is found as an environmental contaminant and so any bird may be affected. It is not however infectious from one bird to another. Certain environments will contain more air-borne microscopic spores of this fungus. These include areas near rotting vegetation, which includes the bottom of a parrot cage which has not been cleaned out recently!

Certain species are very susceptible, including most raptors, but particularly gyrfalcons, golden eagles, the northern goshawk and snowy owls. In addition, all species of penguin are extremely susceptible. In Psittaciformes, all species can suffer from this condition, but African grey parrots particularly are more likely to suffer from it than other species.

Younger birds are more commonly affected than adults. Aspergillosis may also be seen in birds which are immunosuppressed due to concurrent illness, or are stressed or where immunosuppressive medication such as corticosteroids are used. Indeed it is now standard therapy to start treatment for aspergillosis whenever a bird from a susceptible species is likely to be stressed. This might be when moved from one owner to another, or when undergoing treatment for other conditions or surgery. This is because once the disease has got a firm hold within the airways of the bird, it is extremely difficult to treat.

The fungal spores settle out on the surface of the respiratory tract, particularly in the region of the syrinx, the abdominal air sacs and the lung structure itself. If the number of spores is low and the bird is in good health and unstressed, its own cellular immunity will mop up these spores. If, however, the bird has any of the problems already mentioned, the spores will germinate into the spreading fungal hyphae and invade the surrounding structures. This can lead to blockage of the airway in the case of the syrinx, or it can lead to the production of large balls of fungus, known as 'fungal granulomas', within the air sacs.

The fungus progressively blocks airways leading to dyspnoea and death through asphyxiation, or it invades the bloodstream and is transported to other organs, such as the liver, kidneys and central nervous system. This can then produce a variety of signs depending on the system affected.

Aspergillus spp can also produce a toxin known as aflatoxin. This is highly toxic to birds and rapidly causes liver damage, failure and death. In addition, a gliatoxin may also be released causing central nervous system damage, with paresis, fitting and other neurological signs being observed.

There is some evidence to suggest that, due to its important role in cellular turnover of the airway linings and local immunity, hypovitaminosis A may play a part in the disease.

Diagnosis of aspergillosis: Full blood cell counts are useful as the condition will often cause a markedly elevated white blood cell count (greater than 30×10^9/l). Radiographs are useful to show thickening of the normally transparent air sacs, and the growth of any fungal granulomas within them, or in the area of the syrinx.

Rigid endoscopy is frequently essential to examine the syrinx and the internal air sacs. This method not only allows the user to examine the affected areas visually, but also to sample them to enable culture and microscopic examination for a definitive diagnosis.

Tracheal and lung washes may be performed with small volumes of sterile saline (0.5–1 ml kg of bird) flushed into the trachea of the anaesthetised bird, and then immediately aspirated. This is a useful technique to collect samples for suspected bacterial pneumonias as well. However it often requires that an air-sac tube be placed (page 98).

Recently, studies have shown that an *Aspergillus* spp antibody test has been useful, although often affected birds do not produce antibodies to the fungus until quite late on into the course of the disease (Redig *et al.*, 1997; Cray, 1997).

Paramyxovirus/Newcastle disease: this is a condition seen primarily in pigeons, and is important, as Newcastle disease and Paramyxovirus 1 (PMV-1) are notifiable in the United Kingdom. That is, the local government animal health office must be informed if they are diagnosed. This is due to their ability to cause mortality and debility in commercial poultry.

Symptoms of paramyxovirus disease are varied and may include:

- Dyspnoea
- Tachypnoea
- Oedema around the eyes
- Listlessness and neurological signs such as wing drooping
- Head tilt and circling (torticollis)
- Sudden death.

The virus is thought to be transmitted via droppings. Diagnosis is based on the symptoms and confirmation is made using viral haemagglutination inhibition tests.

Bacterial pneumonias and air sacculitis: bacterial pneumonias are common in all species of bird. Some occur due to primary pathogens such as *Chlamydophila psittaci*. Others are due to secondary bacterial infections such as those occuring in raptors after infestation by the raptor air-sac mite *Serratospiculum* spp.

Diagnosis is made on clinical signs, full blood cell counts and full body radiographs. Treatment will depend on the bacteria involved, and it would be sensible to take a sample for culture and sensitivity testing. Nebulisation therapy may be used to administer antibiotics as well as antifungal agents to the air sacs.

Teflon® and smoke-inhalation toxicity: birds are extremely sensitive to the odourless fumes given off by overheated Teflon® coated pans. The consequence can be a reaction causing pulmonary oedema with severe dyspnoea and often death before treatment can be initiated. A similar situation is seen with poisoning due to the toxic fumes from smoke, or cooking fat inhalation.

Cardiovascular disease

Congenital heart defects

With the success of breeding programmes to produce colour variants, the incidence of congenital heart defects has increased.

Atherosclerosis

In recent years the incidence of atherosclerosis has increased both in cage birds, such as Psittaciformes, and in raptors. It is often because of lack of exercise and inappropriate, high fat diets. The major arteries become thickened with cholesterol deposits, their lumen diameter decreases and they become less elastic, so blood pressure increases (Fig. 5.10).

Arterial calcification

Some birds, oversupplemented with calcium and vitamin D$_3$, may suffer from calcification of the walls of the major blood vessels. This leads to loss of elasticity and increased blood pressure, heart failure and organ damage.

Vegetative endocarditis

Chlamydophilosis can lead to myocardial damage, as can a number of septicaemic and bacteraemic conditions. It can also lead to vegetative endocarditis. This is when one or more heart valves become infected with bacteria and cease to function efficiently. More bacteria may seed off into the bloodstream as septic emboli which can spread the condition to other organs.

Haematological disease

Anaemia is a frequent finding in any debilitated bird. It may also be due to heavy metal, such as lead or zinc, poisoning, or due to bloodparasites. *Leucocytozoan* spp inhabit red and white blood cells and is thought to cause disease not only in the bloodstream where it causes intravascular haemolysis leading to anaemia, but also in the spleen and liver where the parasite multiplies. It is transmitted by blackflies and is known to cause serious problems in young Galliformes, raptors and Anseriformes.

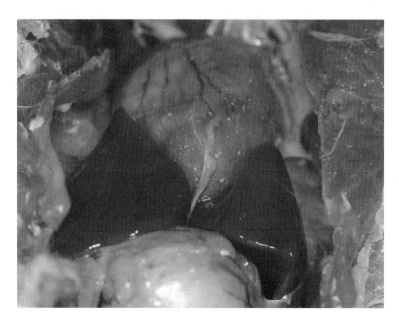

Fig. 5.10 An enlarged heart in an African grey parrot due to atherosclerosis. Note also the white granular gout crystals covering the pericardium due to secondary renal failure

Other significant blood parasites include the malarial parasites, *Plasmodium* spp, which can cause severe anaemia, lethargy, vomiting, seizures and death, particularly in penguin species. Plasmodium is transmitted by mosquitos of the *Anopheles* spp or by direct blood to blood transfer during fighting. Treatment is difficult, but human antimalarial agents have been used.

A common haemoparasite, *Haemoproteus* spp, which inhabit the avian red blood cell, generally does not cause disease.

Urinary tract

Acute renal disease

Acute renal disease is often due to bacterial conditions, such as chlamydophilosis, or *E. coli* septicaemia. It may also be caused by poisons such as zinc, antifreeze and chocolate (theobromine). Diagnosis is often difficult. It is based on clinical signs such as anuria or oliguria, and extreme depression, with a history of exposure to the relevant poison. Another cause of acute renal disease in geese is the coccidial parasite *Eimeria truncata*, which causes lethargy, rapid weight loss and diarrhoea with high mortality rates.

Chronic renal disease

As with acute renal disease, chronic renal disease has a number of causes, including poisons, chronic low-grade infection, excessive calcium and vitamin D_3 supplementation, and excessive levels of dietary protein in Psittaciformes.

Gout

Anything that causes renal failure will lead to a build-up of the main kidney excretory product, uric acid, which rapidly reaches its saturation point. After this, crystals of uric acid form in the bloodstream and become deposited in and around vital organs.

The organs in which uric acid deposits form preferentially include the kidneys themselves, the heart and pericardial sac and the liver. Ultimately all aspects of the avian body can be affected by gout. The joints, particularly the distal leg joints, may develop deposits of white uric acid crystals which cause joint swelling and pain, known as articular gout. The bird is often lame, and the white crystals may be seen through the skin surface.

Renal urolithiasis

Renal urolithiasis is a common condition in laying hens. It can lead to renal failure due to blockage of the renal tubules. It happens because of the high levels of calcium that circulate during egg laying, some of which spills over into the urine. The situation may be exacerbated if the bird becomes egg-bound, pressing on the kidneys, restricting renal blood flow and creating renal ischaemia.

Renal tumours

Renal tumours are common in species such as budgerigars. Clinical signs usually involve unilateral paralysis of the leg on the affected side. This is because the sciatic and ischiadic nerves that supply the leg run through the kidney, where the tumour impinges on them.

Diagnosis of chronic renal disease

Blood tests: the biochemical parameter uric acid may be measured in a heparinised blood sample. If levels exceed $500\,\mu mol/l$ then there is a high possibility that renal disease is present. The sample should be taken from a fasting bird, as (particularly in the meat-eating raptors) a recent meal can falsely raise the levels. Excessively high levels of calcium ($>3\,mmol/l$) may suggest dietary oversupplementation. An exception is an in-lay hen, whose blood levels may rise this high normally due to calcium mobilisation for shell production.

Radiography: radiography may show kidney enlargement in the case of nephritis and tumours. It will also show increased radiodensity in cases of calcinosis.

Urinalysis: sampling of the urine portion of the faeces is possible, but must be performed carefully to avoid contamination with the faecal portion.

The urate, or solid urinary waste product (the white portion of the dropping) is less useful, but the liquid section can be used for analysis.

Presence of haematuria is an important sign, often associated with heavy metal poisoning, severe renal disease or the haemorrhagic syndrome of Amazons and conures. Faecal contamination of the urine though, often confuses the issue.

Low levels of glucose are seen in the urine of healthy birds, so this is an unsafe test for diabetes mellitus. The presence of ketones suggests a severe catabolic disease, such as liver failure. The specific gravity should be around 1.005–1.020, with polyuric birds often dropping below 1.005.

Traces of protein (probably from faecal contamination) are common. The urine should also be clear in colour. In diseases that affect the liver, such as chlamydophilosis, the excretion of large amounts of biliverdin through the kidneys results in a green yellow tinge to the urine.

Histology: renal biopsy techniques can be used to ascertain definitive diagnoses of the condition afflicting the bird.

Reproductive tract disease

Egg-binding

This is the commonest complaint of the avian reproductive system in caged birds. The hen bird often presents with a history of compulsive egg laying and is often a budgerigar or cockatiel, although any species is susceptible. There is also frequently a history of poor diet, high in seeds and low in calcium. The hen bird becomes lethargic, dull and sits on the floor of its cage. The causes of egg-binding in these cases can vary from low blood calcium levels due to persistent egg laying and a low calcium containing diet, to primary muscle hypomotility, deformed eggs and uterine rupture. These can be exacerbated by failure to provide suitable nesting facilities. Or by keeping

the hen in poor environmental conditions, such as too cold a position within the house.

Diagnosis of egg-binding

In addition to the above clinical signs, it is often possible to palpate the egg if it is situated in the lower reproductive tract, just caudal to the sternum. Radiography is useful for more cranially situated eggs, although it may be necessary to perform a barium study to highlight the digestive system to differentiate it from the reproductive system.

Salpingitis

Salpingitis is also known by the name of vent gleet because of the discharge from the cloaca which accompanies it. It is due to infection of the uterus, or, more correctly, the portion of the uterus corresponding to the salpinx. Signs may vary from non-specific malaise, with a bird becoming intermittently dull and lethargic, to an obvious purulent discharge.

Musculoskeletal disease

Hypocalcaemic syndrome of African grey parrots

This is seen in African grey parrots between the ages of two and four years. It occurs where, although bone calcium quality is adequate, the parrot is unable to mobilise calcium reserves to maintain blood calcium levels. This is often compounded by a low calcium, that is all seed, diet. This leads to hypocalcaemia, muscular weakness, tremors, collapse, fits and death.

Carpometacarpal luxation

This condition is often known by its colloquial name of angel wing and is seen commonly in budgerigars, macaws and geese and other waterfowl. It is when the carpometacarpal joints in either wing rotate and subluxate so that the distal primary feathers point dorsally giving a fanlike appearance. It is thought that the condition may have a connection with vitamin D_3 deficiency (rickets) and excess dietary protein levels, as it is a growth deformity.

Nutritional osteodystrophy/metabolic bone disease

Nutritional osteodystrophy is due to a deficiency in vitamin D_3 and calcium. Several syndromes are seen. The commonest is bowing of the tibio-tarsal and tarsometatarsal bones. This is because the weight of the growing bird cannot be properly supported by poorly mineralised bones. Often the diets of the birds have high levels of protein as well as low calcium and vitamin D_3, promoting rapid growth and further exacerbating the situation.

Pinwheel

Pinwheel is a developmental deformity of the stifle joint of young pigeons. It occurs around two to four weeks of age. The squab cannot flex its stifle, and since only one leg is usually affected it leads to the circling or pinwheeling which gives the condition its name. It seems to occur in well fed chicks reared in flat bottomed nests with little nesting material. Prevention is the key to success. Treatment is usually ineffective.

Articular gout

Articular gout is seen commonly in older cage and aviary birds and has been discussed under chronic renal disease.

Neurological disease

Fitting

This condition has many aetiologies, including:

- Trauma (flying into glass windows etc.)
- Nutrition (hypoglycaemia, hypocalcaemia, hypovitaminosis B_1)
- Heavy metal poisoning (lead and zinc primarily)
- Plant and pesticide poisons
- Meningoencephalitis (bacterial, viral or protozoal)

- Organopathy (particularly hepatic disease)
- Idiopathic epilepsy (reported in red-lored Amazons)
- Vestibular disease
- Cardiovascular disease (fat emboli during egg production, atherosclerosis)
- Cancer
- Congenital CNS disease (cerebellar hypoplasia seen in lutino colour birds).

The breed of bird may suggest a condition, for example a fitting African grey parrot between the ages of two and four years may well have hypocalcaemia syndrome, and waterfowl are prone to lead poisoning from lead shot and fishing tackle weights.

Other causes of neurological disease

Kidney tumours

Unilateral leg paralysis is a common peripheral neuropathy in budgerigars. It is often due to tumours of the kidneys, through which the major nerves innervating the legs have to pass. Radiographs are useful in diagnosing this condition.

Kidney disease

Any form of kidney disease which results in swelling of the renal parenchyma can theoretically place pressure on the leg nerves and so produce varying signs of paresis and paralysis.

Egg-binding

Egg-binding is a common cause of bilateral hindlimb paresis and paralysis in hen birds. The egg becomes stuck in the pelvic inlet, placing pressure on the nerves in the roof of the pelvis that innerve the legs. Radiography will aid in diagnosing this condition.

Wing paralysis

Wing paralysis is common after flying injuries or fracture of the humerus. This fracture results in rotation laterally of the distal fragment, often lacerating the radial nerve.

Spinal abscesses and fungal infection

Spinal abscesses and fungal infection can occur in birds. Spinal abscesses may occur from bacteria which have spread there via the bloodstream, particularly after spinal trauma, such as bruising after a flying injury. Fungal granulomas are common in cases of aspergillosis, and may invade the spinal cord as many vertebrae are pneumonised and so connected to the air sac system.

Paramyxoviruses/Newcastle disease

These are important to note because of their significance with respect to the poultry industry. Paramyxovirus is frequently isolated from pigeons. The condition is preventable by vaccination, which is compulsory in pigeons presented at races and shows under the Disease of Poultry Order 1994 (SI 1994/3141) (page 101). In addition to respiratory problems, the virus can also cause neurological disease. Signs of this include wing drooping, circling, torticollis and opisthotonus.

An overview of avian biochemistry

Biochemical parameters may be measured using heparinised blood or clotted blood samples. Bile acid and protein electrophoresis results are best performed on serum gel collected blood samples. As mentioned in the section on anatomy and physiology, haematological parameters are best measured in potassium edetate collected blood samples.

Liver biochemical parameters

The most reliable test for liver function in avian species is that for bile acids. Normal ranges vary from species to species, but commonly range from 20–80 μmol/l.

Other useful tests include aspartamine transaminase (AST) rather than the mammalian AST. Alkaline phosphatase (ALKP) is too non-specific for birds to be of great use. AST activity is also found in muscle tissue, so often the two other biochemical tests of lactate dehydrogenase (LDH) and creatinine phosphokinase (CPK) are performed. This allows some differentiation between liver and muscle damage, as CPK is only found in muscles. LDH is released in the early stages of liver disease, but also has some skeletal and cardiac muscle distribution. The enzyme glutamate dehydrogenase (GLDH) is released when liver and kidney cells die or are disrupted. As the renal source of this enzyme goes into the urine directly, and not the bloodstream, blood levels of GLDH reflect any hepatocyte damage. Levels greater than 2 IU/l are considered elevated in psittacines (Hochleithner, 1994).

Kidney biochemical parameters

The only reliable test for renal function is uric acid. Neither urea nor creatinine are useful in avian species. Uric acid is not, however, a sensitive test, and is only elevated once the majority (>75%) of the renal mass ceases to function. Levels may be falsely elevated in raptors immediately after feeding, so samples should be taken in the fasted bird. Levels greater than 420 μmol/l in psittacines, 550 μmol/l in fasted raptors and 750 μmol/l in racing pigeons are suggestive of renal problems.

Calcium and phosphorus

Levels of calcium and phosphorus depend on nutritional levels and renal function as well as on the presence of vitamin D_3 and functional parathyroid glands. Normal values quoted for calcium are 2–2.8 mmol/l in most psittacines and 1.9–2.6 mmol/l in pigeons, and 0.9–5 mmol/l in psittacines and 0.57–1.33 mmol/l in pigeons for phosphorus. Elevated phosphorus and calcium may suggest renal dysfunction. Low calcium and high or normal phosphorus suggest nutritional deficiency or the hypocalcaemic syndrome seen in African grey parrots.

Total proteins

These are very useful in birds to allow an assessment of nutrition and hepatic function. To gain accurate values for albumin and globulins though, it is necessary to perform protein electrophoresis.

The practice laboratory dry chemistry systems used for mammals are not accurate enough for this. Protein electrophoresis is a useful technique to assess whether the bird is mounting an immune response, when the values of some acute phase proteins may rise, and the pattern of this can be suggestive of some types of disease.

Blood glucose

Blood glucose measurement is useful in raptors, where the values should range between 17–22 mmol/l. If levels fall below 15 mmol/l, hypoglycaemic fitting and coma may develop in small species of raptor. If levels exceed 27 mmol/l, hyperglycaemic fitting can occur. Diabetes mellitus is seen in Psittaciformes such as budgerigars. Here values greater than 30 mmol/l may be observed. It is worth noting though that small elevations in blood glucose commonly occur in stressed birds and should not necessarily be taken to suggest clinical disease.

References

Cray, C. (1997) Application of aspergillus antigen assay in the diagnosis of aspergillosis. *Proceedings of the Annual Conference of the Association of Avian Veterinarians*, pp. 219–220.

Hochleithner, M. (1994) Biochemistries. In *Avian Medicine: Principles and Applications* (Ritchie, B., Harrison, G. and Harrison, L., eds), pp. 223–245, W.B. Saunders, Philadelphia.

Oaks, J.L. (1993) Immune and inflammatory responses in falcon staphylococcal pododermatitis. In *Raptor Biomedicine* (Redig, P.T., Cooper, J.E., Remple, J.D. and Hunter, D.B., eds), pp. 72–87. University of Minnesota Press, Minneapolis, Minnesota.

Redig, P.T., Brown, P.A. and Talbot, B. (1997) The ELISA as a management guide for aspergillosis in raptors. *Proceedings of the 4th Conference of the European Committee of the Association of Avian Veterinarians*. Pp. 223–226.

Remple, J.D. (1993) Raptor bumblefoot: A new treatment technique. In *Raptor Biomedicine* (Redig, P.T., Cooper, J.E., Remple, J.D. and Hunter, D.B., eds), pp. 154–160. University of Minnesota Press, Minneapolis, Minnesota.

Further reading

Beynon, P.H., Forbes, N.A. and Lawton, M.P.C. (1996) *Manual of Psittacine Birds, 2nd Edition*. BSAVA, Cheltenham.

Beynon, P.H., Forbes, N.A. and Harcourt-Brown, N. (1996) *Manual of Raptors, Pigeons and Waterfowl*. BSAVA, Cheltenham.

Coles, B.H. (1997) *Avian Medicine and Surgery, 2nd Edition*. Blackwell Science, Osney Mead, Oxford.

Cooper, J.E. (1985) Foot conditions. In *Veterinary Aspects of Captive Birds of Prey, 2nd Edition*, pp. 97–111. Standfast Press, Gloucestershire.

Forbes, N.A. (1996) Fits and incoordination. In *Manual of Raptors, Pigeons and Waterfowl* (Beynon, P.H., Forbes, N.A. and Harcourt-Brown, N.H., eds), pp. 197–207. BSAVA, Cheltenham.

Forbes, N.A. and Parry-Jones, J. (1996) Management and husbandry (raptors). In *Manual of Raptors, Pigeons and Waterfowl* (Beynon, P.H., Forbes, N.A. and Harcourt-Brown, N.H., eds), pp. 116–128. BSAVA, Cheltenham.

Forbes, N.A. and Richardson, T. (1996) Husbandry and nutrition (waterfowl). In *Manual of Raptors, Pigeons and Waterfowl* (Beynon, P.H., Forbes, N.A. and Harcourt-Brown, N.H., eds), pp. 289–298. BSAVA, Cheltenham.

Harper, F.D.W. (1996) Husbandry and nutrition (pigeons). In *Manual of Raptors, Pigeons and Waterfowl* (Beynon, P.H., Forbes, N.A. and Harcourt-Brown, N.H., eds), pp. 233–237. BSAVA, Cheltenham.

Lightfoot, T.L. (1998) Approach to avian obstetrics. In *Proceedings of the North American Veterinary Congress*, pp. 757–778.

Malley, A.D. (1996) Feather and skin problems. In *Manual of Psittacine Birds* (Beynon, P.H., Forbes, N.A. and Lawton, M.P.C., eds), pp. 96–105. BSAVA, Cheltenham.

Meredith, A. and Redrobe, S. (2002) *Manual of Exotic Pets, 4th Edition*. BSAVA, Cheltenham.

Ritchie, B., Harrison, G. and Harrison, L. (1994) *Avian Medicine: Principles and Applications*. W.B. Saunders, Philadelphia.

Roberts, V. (2000) *Diseases of Free-Range Poultry*. Whittet Books, Stowmarket, Suffolk.

Chapter 6

An Overview of Avian Therapeutics

FLUID THERAPY

Maintenance requirements

To maintain fluid levels, a bird must take in enough fluid to replace everyday losses through urine, insensible losses such as panting (gular fluttering in birds) and tears.

In birds there is almost no water lost as sweat as they have no proper skin sweat glands. However there are greater losses compared with cats and dogs, due to their increased metabolic rates and because of their high body surface and lung area to body weight ratio. This means that proportionately large amounts of fluids are lost through respiration.

To compensate for this, birds can conserve water more efficiently than mammals. Unlike urea, their waste protein excretory product, uric acid, requires very little water to be excreted. However the losses and gains equal out, so that maintenance levels in companion birds have been estimated as 50 ml/kg/day which is the same as for cats and dogs.

The effect of disease on fluid requirements

With any disease the need for fluids increases, even if no obvious fluid loss has occurred. This may be due to a number of factors. The disease process may affect the kidneys, causing increases in the glomerular filtration rate or reduction in water reabsorption by the collecting ducts, leading to increased urine output. Or there may be a loss of absorption of water from the small or large intestine. For example, the endotoxins produced in cases of *E. coli* septicaemia or enteritis cause

a reduction in the response of the renal collecting ducts to arginine vasotocin (AVT) (the avian equivalent of antidiuretic hormone (ADH) released from the pituitary). This will lead to less concentration of the urine, more fluid loss and dehydration.

Respiratory disease is common in avian patients, especially in cases of chlamydophilosis, hypovitaminosis A and aspergillosis, all of which may lead to fluid loss.

Individuals suffering from diarrhoea will experience fluid loss and often metabolic acidosis due to prolonged loss of bicarbonate. There may also be chronic losses of potassium, due to the reduced absorption of this electrolyte by the large intestine.

Most avian patients have the potential to regurgitate, for example in cases of sour crop and trichomoniasis in psittacines. Fluid loss by this route is therefore not uncommon. The secretions of the crop are mainly neutral to alkali, and so losses are more likely to give straightforward neutral water loss. However, more severe true vomiting will occur in birds with proventricular disease, such as 'macaw wasting syndrome' or megabacteriosis, and metabolic alkalosis due to loss of hydrogen ions will ensue.

Another less obvious route of fluid and electrolyte loss is through skin disease. Lovebirds and cockatiels in particular are prone to ulcerating skin conditions, particularly under the wings. This is often due to self-trauma with secondary infection by environmental bacterial organisms such as *Pseudomonas* spp or fungi such as *Aspergillus* spp. These produce lesions which resemble chemical or thermal burns, and leave large areas of weeping, exudative skin which allow fluid and electrolyte loss.

Post-surgical fluid requirements

Surgical procedures are being more and more frequently performed on birds for both routine and emergency reasons. These bring their own requirements for fluid therapy. There is the possibility of intrasurgical haemorrhaging, necessitating vascular support with an aqueous electrolyte solution or, in more serious blood losses (>10%), colloidal fluids or even blood transfusions (Fig. 6.1).

Even if surgery is relatively bloodless, there are inevitable losses via the respiratory route because of the drying nature of the gases used to deliver the anaesthetics commonly used in avian surgery. The smaller birds have larger surface areas in relation to volume, and this applies to the lung fields as well as the skin. To exacerbate the situation, avian patients also have an air-sac system which increases the surface area for fluid loss even further.

Many patients are not able to drink immediately after surgery. The period without food or water intake may stretch to a few hours, enough time for any avian to start to dehydrate. Finally, some forms of surgery, such as prosthetic beak repair procedures, will lead to inappetence for a period.

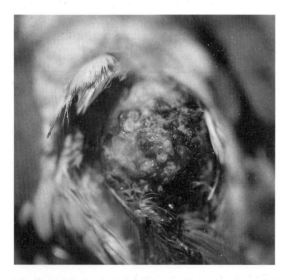

Fig. 6.1 Removal of tumours, such as this uropygial gland tumour from an African grey parrot, will result in blood loss and require fluid replacement therapy.

Electrolyte replacement

In cases of chronic fluid loss, electrolytes as well as fluids will often need replacing. Chronic diarrhoea, such as in megabacteriosis or giardia infestations where gut pathology leads to maldigestion and malabsorption, will cause loss of food, water and electrolytes to waste. The main electrolyte losses involve bicarbonates and potassium.

Because they have a crop between the mouth and the true stomach, birds may well regurgitate rather than vomit. The crop contents are alkaline to neutral, and so metabolic alkalosis is unlikely to occur with regurgitation or crop problems, indeed metabolic acidosis is more likely. However, in serious proventriculus disease, such as the viral condition 'macaw wasting syndrome', stomach megabacteriosis or ulcers, loss of hydrogen ions will occur and metabolic alkalosis can ensue.

Fluids used in avian practice

Lactated Ringer's/Hartmann's

Lactated Ringer's solution is useful for rehydration and to supply maintenance needs. It is particularly useful for avian patients suffering from metabolic acidosis, such as those with chronic gastrointestinal disease and bicarbonate loss, but it can also be used for fluid therapy after routine surgical procedures. The quantity of potassium present in lactated Ringer's solution is unlikely to cause a problem in birds with hyperkalaemia (such as those suffering from rapid weight loss or with serious skin or tissue trauma). The use of calcium gluconate (5 mg/kg) or the addition of a glucose-containing fluid will help drive the potassium ions into the cells and so reduce the hyperkalaemic threat.

In hypokalaemic birds (such as those suffering from chronic diarrhoea, vomiting, burns or on longterm glucose/saline fluids) the addition of potassium to the fluids at rates of 0.1–0.3 mEq/kg body weight may help stimulate appetite and reduce the risk of cardiac arrhythmias.

In birds which are in metabolic acidosis an assessment of bicarbonate ion loss can be made from a blood sample. However, in many cases it is not possible in practice to measure it. Therefore, if persistent vomiting or chronic weight loss or trauma occur and metabolic acidosis is suspected, a rough approximation may be made. Give a sodium bicarbonate supplement at 1 mEq/kg at 15–30 minute intervals until a maximum of 4 mEq/kg has been reached. (This supplement must not be given with the lactated Ringer's solution as it will precipitate out.)

Glucose/saline combinations

Glucose/saline solutions are useful for small avian patients. These may well have been through periods of anorexia prior to treatment and therefore may be borderline hypoglycaemic. The principles for use of these fluids is the same as for cats and dogs. The concentration to start with when dehydration is present is 5% glucose, 0.9% saline. Once dehydration has been reversed, the avian patient may be moved on to the 4% glucose, 0.18% saline concentration for maintenance purposes.

Protein amino acid/B vitamin supplements

Protein and vitamin supplements can be very useful for nutritional support. Products such as Duphalyte® (Fort Dodge) may be given at the rate of 1 ml/kg day. They are particularly useful to replace nutrients in cases where the patient is malnourished or has been suffering from a protein-losing enteropathy or nephropathy. They are also good supplements for patients with hepatic disease or severe exudative skin disease such as thermal burns.

Colloidal fluids

Colloidal fluids have been used in avian practice only by the intravenous route, although there is some evidence that they may be used via the intraosseous route. This may limit their use, as some birds are just too small to gain full vascular access. They are used in the same way as with cats and dogs:

- For when a serious loss of blood occurs
- Where severe hypoproteinaemia is seen
- In order to support central blood pressure.

This is due to their ability to stay in the blood stream for several hours after administration, whereas crystalloids remain in circulation for just 15–30 minutes on average. Colloids may be used as a temporary measure whilst a blood donor is selected, or, if a donor is not available, the only means of attempting to support such a patient. Bolus treatment with gelatin colloids such as Gelofusine® (Millpledge) and Haemaccel® (Hoechst) may be given at 10–15 mls/kg intravenously four times over a 24-hour period to aid in the treatment of hypoproteinaemia.

Blood transfusions

Blood transfusion should be considered if the PCV (packed cell volume) drops below 15%. Birds in general are far more tolerant of blood loss than their mammalian counterparts as the oxygenation of their blood through the rigid lung structure is more efficient. However transfusions are sometimes required. Donors are best selected from the same species, for example African grey parrot to African grey parrot, or budgerigar to budgerigar. Blood can be collected from the donor into a container or syringe with acid citrate dextrose anticoagulant or, in an emergency, a heparinised syringe may be used. Ideally a blood filter should be used before blood is transfused into the recipient bird, but frequently this is not possible in general practice, and so collection and administration should be done with care, to reduce haemolysis and clumping.

It is useful to remember that one drop of blood is roughly equal to 0.05 ml and that the estimated blood volume of an avian patient is 10% of its body weight in grams. Volumes which can be transfused range from 0.25 ml in a budgerigar to 5 ml in an African grey parrot.

Oral fluids and electrolytes

Oral fluids may be used in avian practice for those patients experiencing mild dehydration, and for 'home' administration. Many products are available for cats and dogs and may be used for birds. One electrolyte in particular may be useful and that is Avipro® by VetArk. This is a probiotic, but used at the correct concentration may also be used as an oral electrolyte solution. The lyophilised bacteria are useful to aid digestion, which is also often upset during periods of dehydration.

Calculation of fluid requirements

A critically ill avian patient is assumed to be at least 5–10% dehydrated. As with cats and dogs, you should assume that 1% dehydration is equal to needing to supply 10 ml/kg body weight of fluid in addition to maintenance requirements. Assumptions then have to be made on the degree of dehydration of the bird concerned. Roughly this works out as:

- 3–5% dehydrated – increased thirst, slight lethargy, tacky mucous membranes, increased heart rate
- 7–10% dehydrated – increased thirst, anorexia, dullness, tenting of the skin and slower return to normal over eyelid or foot, dry mucous membranes, dull corneas, red or wrinkled skin in chicks
- 12–18% dehydrated – dull to comatose, skin remains tented after pinching, desiccating mucous membranes, sunken eyes.

These deficits may be large and the volume required for replacement difficult to administer rapidly. Indeed, it may be dangerous to overload the patient's system with these fluid levels all in one go. To spread the deficit evenly it is advised that the following protocol be used:

- Day one: Maintenance fluid levels +50% of calculated dehydration factor
- Day two: Maintenance fluid levels +50% of calculated dehydration factor
- Day three: Maintenance fluid levels.

If the dehydration levels are so severe that volumes are still too large to be given at any one time, it may be necessary to take 72 rather than 48 hours to replace the calculated deficit.

To add to the problem, debilitated avian patients may also be anaemic, and therefore PCVs may appear misleadingly normal, so total protein levels are an additional parameter to look at when assessing dehydration. Uric acid levels may also be measured, as these will often increase in cases of moderate to severe dehydration. Other useful parameters include weight measurement and of course fluid intake and urine output. Table 6.1 gives some normal PCV and total protein values.

Equipment for fluid administration

The equipment required to administer fluids to birds is often very small in size. For example, the blood vessels available for intravenous medication are often 30–50% smaller than their cat or dog counterparts and tend to be highly mobile and much more fragile and prone to rupture.

Crop tubes

Crop tubes are often used in avian patients in order to provide nutritional support in as stress-free a manner as possible. They are also useful as a route for fluid administration. Crop tubes

Table 6.1 Normal packed cell volumes (PCV) and total blood proteins for selected avian species.

Species	PCV l/l	Total protein g/l
Budgerigar	0.45–0.57	20–30
Amazon parrot	0.41–0.53	33–53
African grey parrot	0.42–0.52	26–49
Macaw	0.43–0.54	25–44
Cockatoo	0.42–0.54	28–43
Cockatiel	0.43–0.57	31–44
Mallard duck	0.42–0.56	32–45
Canada goose	0.35–0.49	37–56
Mute swan	0.32–0.5	36–55
Chicken	0.24–0.43	33–55
Pheasant	0.28–0.42	42–72
Pigeon	0.36–0.48	21–35
Peregrine falcon	0.37–0.53	25–40
Barn owl	0.42–0.51	29–48
Tawny owl	0.36–0.47	27–46

come either as straight or curved metal tubes, both with blunt ends. To insert a crop tube, extend the bird's head. Starting from the left side of the inside of the lower beak pass the tube down the proximal oesophagus into the crop at the right side of the thoracic inlet. Maximal volumes which may be given vary from 0.5 ml in a budgerigar to 15 ml in a large macaw (Fig. 6.2).

Catheters

Because they have a length of tubing attached to the needle, butterfly catheters are extremely useful for the small and fragile avian vessels. If the syringe or drip set is connected to this piece of flexible tubing, rather than directly to the catheter, there is less chance of the catheter becoming dislodged should the bird draw back after the catheter is inserted. Also the piece of clear tubing on the catheter allows you to see when venous access has been achieved, as blood will flow back into this area without having to draw back on the syringe (which would collapse the fragile veins anyway).

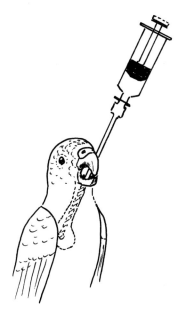

Fig. 6.2 Method of inserting a crop tube. Approach from left side of beak and aim towards the lower right neck region.

It is advised to flush any catheter with heparinised saline prior to use to prevent clots forming. 25–27 gauge sizes are recommended and will cope with venous access for budgerigars through to small conures. 23–25 gauge will suffice for larger parrots and some of the bigger waterfowl and raptors.

Ordinary over-the-needle catheters may also be used for catheterisation of jugular veins. The latex catheter is useful for long-term maintenance of venous access, as butterfly catheters tend to rupture the vessels if left in for long periods. It is better to use an over-the-needle catheter which has plastic flanges so that it can be sutured to the skin at the site of insertion to prevent removal.

Hypodermic or spinal needles

Spinal needles have a central stylet to prevent clogging of the lumen of the needle with bone fragments after insertion and are therefore useful for intraosseous catheterisation. 21–25 gauge spinal needles are usually sufficient for most cage birds. Straightforward hypodermic needles may also be used for the same purpose, although the risks of blockage are higher. Hypodermic needles may also be used, of course, for the administration of subcutaneous fluids. Generally 21–25 gauge hypodermic needles are sufficient for cage birds.

Syringe drivers

For continuous fluid administration, such as is required for intravenous and intraosseous fluid administration during anaesthesia, syringe drivers are becoming more widely used. They are less useful in the conscious bird due to poor tolerance of drip tubing, hence bolus fluid therapy is more commonly used in avian practice.

Elizabethan collars

It may be necessary to place some of the psittacine family into an Elizabethan style collar as they are the world's greatest chewers! There are also a selection of lightweight perspex neck braces which may be better tolerated. These however are not so useful when jugular vein catheters are used.

Routes of fluid administration

There are four main routes available for administration of fluids to birds. They are:

- Oral
- Subcutaneous
- Intravenous
- Intraosseous

The advantages and disadvantages of the four routes are given in Table 6.2. The intraperitoneal route used in mammals is not available for use in birds, due to the lack of a diaphragm and the presence of air sacs. This means that any injection into the body cavity (or coelom) may inadvertently enter an air sac and thence on to the bird's airways, resulting in drowning.

Oral

Lactated Ringer's solution, probiotic or electrolyte solutions such as VetArk's Avipro® and Critical Care Formula® or 5% dextrose solutions may be used. The maximum volumes which may be administered via crop tube are given below.

Budgerigar – 0.5–1 ml
Cockatiel – 2.5–5 ml
Conure – 5–7 ml
Cockatoo – 10 ml
African grey – 8–10 ml
Macaw – 10–15 ml

Subcutaneous

Table 6.2 gives the advantages and disadvantages of subcutaneous fluid therapy. The sites for subcutaneous fluid administration are located in the inguinal web of skin which attaches the leg to the body cranially, the axillary region immediately under each wing, and the dorsal interscapular area. Fluid absorption may be increased significantly by the addition of hyaluronidase to the fluids.

Intravenous

Table 6.2 gives the advantages and disadvantages of intravenous fluid therapy in avians.

Table 6.2   Advantages and disadvantages of various avian fluid therapy routes.

	Advantages	Disadvantages
Oral	• Reduced stress (if competent handler) • Physiological route • Less trauma • Home therapy possible	• Increased stress (if inexperienced handler or untamed patient) • Not useful in cases of digestive tract dysfunction or disease • Risk of inhalation pneumonia or regurgitation • Slow rate of rehydration • Inaccurate method of dosing unless crop tubing
Subcutaneous	• Faster uptake of fluids than oral route • Volumes given may be large, reducing dosing frequency	• Reduced uptake in severe dehydration or peripheral vasoconstriction • May be painful in smaller species • Only hypotonic or isotonic fluids may be used
Intravenous	• Rapid rehydration and support of central venous pressure • Use of hypertonic and colloidal fluids possible	• Venous access may be difficult in some species • Veins may be fragile • Some species will not tolerate permanent, indwelling, intravenous catheters
Intraosseous	• Rapid rehydration and central venous support • Useful in smaller species where venous access is difficult • May be better tolerated for indwelling catheters than intravenous routes • Hypertonic and colloidal fluids may be administered	• Potentially painful procedure requiring analgesia and local or general anaesthetic • Risk of bone fracture and osteomyelitis • Bolus fluids take longer to administer due to rigid confines of bone marrow cavity • Avoid use of Pneumonised bones (e.g. humerus and femur) as will cause drowning

Blood vessels used for intravenous therapy

Veins which may be used for intravenous therapy include the basilic and ulnar veins, which run on the underside of the wing in larger species. The right jugular vein may be used for bolus injections in all species down to the size of a canary. In raptors, a jugular vein catheter is very well tolerated for repeated bolus injections. In waterfowl, such as swans and ducks, raptors and some larger parrots, the medial metatarsal vein, which runs along the medial aspect of the lower leg, can be used. Avian species will tolerate catheterisation of this vessel extremely well for several days.

Volumes of fluid which may be administered intravenously

Isotonic solutions may be given at 10–15 ml/kg per bolus, although volumes up to 30 ml/kg rarely cause problems. Maximum intravenous bolus volumes are given below:

Finch – 0.5 ml
Budgerigar – 1 ml
Cockatiels – 2 ml
Conure – 6 ml
Amazon parrot – 8 ml
Owl – 10 ml
Cockatoo – 14 ml
Buzzard – 12–14 ml
Macaw – 14 ml
Swan – 25–30 ml

Placement of intravenous catheters

Right jugular vein catheterisation: the following steps will allow catheterisation of the right jugular vein.

(1) Sedate or lightly anaesthetise the avian patient, preferably with isoflurane, to ensure no trauma occurs and to minimise stress.
(2) The feathers overlying the area should be wetted and parted. An area of no feather growth (known as *apterylae*) lies over the immediate area of the right jugular vein.
(3) Raise the vein at the base of the neck with a thumb and swab the area lightly with surgical spirit.

(4) Use a 23–25 gauge over-the-needle catheter, pre-flushed with heparinised saline. Insert it in a caudal direction, as these are often better tolerated than cranially pointing ones, particularly when administering fluids.
(5) Once in place, suture the cather securely to the skin on either side with fine nylon and reflush to ensure it is properly in the vein. Then attach the intravenous drip tubing or catheter bung to the end of the catheter.
(6) Sometimes a light bandage may be necessary to protect the catheter. In severe cases an Elizabethan bird collar may be used (although the latter may catch on the catheter). Many avian patients will tolerate a catheter unprotected at this site for 24–48 hours.

Medial metatarsal catheterisation for waterfowl: this procedure may be used for larger Psittaciformes and raptors. It may also be performed with the bird conscious, particularly in waterfowl as the blood vessel is less mobile and likely to rupture. You should however sedate or give a light anaesthetic to fractious or highly-stressed birds.

(1) Wipe the inside of the lower leg with surgical spirit or povidone-iodine just above the intertarsal joint.
(2) The vessel runs from the anterior aspect distally to a more medial aspect proximally, and is obvious without digital pressure.
(3) Use a 23–25 gauge over-the-needle catheter inserted in a proximal direction (i.e. in the direction of blood flow up the leg).
(4) Tape the catheter in place using zinc oxide tape and apply a catheter bung after flushing with more heparin saline.

Intraosseous fluid therapy

Table 6.2 gives the advantages and disadvantages of intraosseous fluid therapy in avians.

Bones used for intraosseous fluid therapy

The two bones most commonly used for intraosseous fluid therapy are the ulna and the tibiotarsus. The ulna may be accessed from a distal or proximal aspect, and the tibiotarsus is accessed from a cranial proximal aspect through the crest just distal to the stifle joint.

Placement of intraosseous catheters

Proximal tibiotarsus: this is the procedure for placing a tibiotarsal intraosseous catheter.

(1) Sedation or anaesthesia is needed for conscious animals. In all cases good analgesia must be administered.
(2) Pluck the area overlying the cranial aspect of the tibial crest and surgically prepare this with dilute povidone-iodine.
(3) Insert a 21–25 gauge needle through the tibial crest (depending on the size of the patient), screwing it into the bone in the direction of the long axis of the tibiotarsus distally.
(4) Flush the needle with heparinised saline. The advantage of using a spinal needle is that it has a central stylet which helps prevent it from becoming plugged with bone fragments.
(5) Tape the needle securely in place and apply an antibiotic cream around the site. Radiographing the area to ensure correct

intramedullary placement of the needle is advised.
(6) Once correct placement has been assured, attach the needle to intravenous tubing and a syringe driver and bandage this securely in by wrapping bandage material around the limb. If the catheter has merely been placed for use later, insert a catheter bung and bandage in place.
(7) Finally, fit an Elizabethan collar or avian neck brace if the patient shows signs of trying to remove the catheter.

Distal ulna in all species (Fig. 6.3): sedation or isoflurane anaesthesia is often required.

(1) Pluck the feathers over the distal aspect of the carpal joint of the wing to be used.
(2) Surgically prepare the site with povidone-iodine or surgical spirit and flex the distal tip of the wing caudally. This flexure exposes the distal aspect of the radius and ulna bones within the carpal joint. The ulna is the larger of the two bones, unlike in mammals, but as with mammals it lies caudal to the radius.

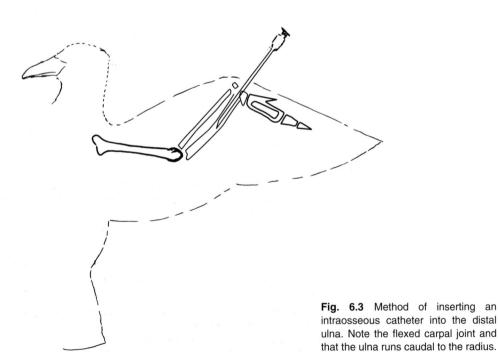

Fig. 6.3 Method of inserting an intraosseous catheter into the distal ulna. Note the flexed carpal joint and that the ulna runs caudal to the radius.

(3) Palpate the end of the ulna with the carpal joint maximally flexed, and using a 23–25 gauge hypodermic or spinal needle, screw into the medullary cavity of the bone along the long axis of the ulna from a distal to proximal direction.

(4) Flush the catheter with heparinised saline and place a catheter bung over the end. Radiographs may be taken to ensure accurate placement, and antibiotic cream can be used at the site of insertion.

(5) Bandage the wing to the side of the bird to immobilise it. Encircle the thorax and pass both cranial and caudal to the opposite wing's attachment at the chest wall, otherwise the bird may flap wildly and loosen the catheter or traumatise itself.

(6) The catheter may then be used for either intermittent slow bolus injections or for attachment to a syringe driver for continuous perfusion.

Treatment of avian diseases

As this text is aimed at the veterinary technical nurse it is not intended to give exhaustive lists of treatments or drug dosages, rather to give an idea of the treatments possible and the techniques useful to aid recovery. For drug dosages the reader is referred to one of the many excellent texts listed in the additional reading list at the end of this chapter.

Avian dermatological disease therapy

Table 6.3 highlights some of the treatments and therapies commonly used for the management of avian skin diseases. In addition, the management of the bacterial pododermatitis problem known as 'bumble-foot' is also discussed.

Treatment and prevention of bumblefoot

This condition is not restricted to raptors but is seen in almost any species, and prevention is better than cure. Some methods to prevent bumblefoot from developing include the following:

- Provide a variety of different diameter natural wood perches for cage and aviary birds. These will allow the feet of the bird to expand and contract as they grip the differing perches. This allows blood to be pumped through the foot, preventing devitalisation, and also applies pressure to different areas, preventing corns.
- For falcons and raptors perches should be covered in padding such as Astroturf®, particularly if they are tethered for days at a time.

Table 6.3 Treatment of avian skin diseases.

Diagnosis	Treatment
Ectoparasites	*Mites* (e.g. *Cnemidocoptes* spp.): ivermectin injectable at 0.2 mg/kg once, repeat after 10–14 days. *Lice*: fipronil sprayed onto a cloth and wiped over feathers or pyrethrin based powders. *Dermanyssus gallinae* will require treatment of cage/aviary environment as they only live on the host at night
Avipoxvirus	no specific treatment. Antibiosis and topical treatment with dilute povidone iodine are useful
Pigeon poxvirus	Vaccine available for prevention. Columbovac PMV/POX® (Fort Dodge) given subcutaneously over dorsal neck. Nobivac Pigeon Pox® (Intervet UK Ltd) given by removing 6–8 feathers from lower leg/breast and brushing vaccine into feather follicles
Ulcerative dermatitis	Appropriate anti-fungal (e.g. enilconazole washes) or antibiotics advised. Behavioural aspects, e.g. environmental enrichment or exposure to UV light, need to be considered. Possibility of allergic skin disease

This cushions the foot and again prevents excessive pressure which causes restrictions of blood flow.

- A good quality diet is vital. Vitamin A is particularly important for skin integrity and local immunity, as well as the vitamin B complex and minerals such as calcium. Preventing obesity is also important as this will lead to increased pressure on the feet.

Once these have been adopted and bumblefoot still develops, the following may be useful:

- For type I–II lesions (Cooper, 1985; Oaks, 1993), padding the perches is a simple solution. In the case of raptors, increasing the time spent flying helps, and the use of antibiotics has been recommended where inflammation is present.
- If a scab exists, it should be debrided under sedation with antiseptic such as povidone iodine, followed by padding of the foot. The padding is formed from a non-adherent dressing such as Coflex®/Vetband®, which is wound in small strips around the base of each digit. This lifts the plantar aspect of the foot off the perch, thus allowing increased circulation.
- For type III–IV lesions (Oaks, 1993), it is recommended that a culture of the lesion is taken whilst the bird is anaesthetised in order to choose the correct antibiotic. The wounds should be repeatedly debrided with dilute povidone iodine and the toes bandaged. In more severe cases, the application of a ball bandage (where a wad of padding is placed in the grip of the foot and the foot bandaged to this ball) may be necessary (see Fig. 6.4). Alternatively, casting materials may be used to create a large but lightweight 'corn plaster' which removes pressure from the affected area of the foot. It is usually necessary to do this to both feet to avoid putting pressure on the non-affected foot.
- For type V–VI lesions (Oaks, 1993), the process is the same as for type III–IV. If bone is involved the outlook is poor but antibiotic-impregnated polymethylmethacrylate (PMMA) beads have been shown to improve healing and recovery rates. These beads are implanted and sewn into the wounds where they release antibiotic slowly at the site of the infection over a period of weeks. Alternatively, drains may be placed in the affected foot, exiting proximally on the caudal aspect of the tarsometatarsus. This allows the wounds to be flushed with antibiotics for a number of days. The foot should be placed into a ball bandage dressing, which should be changed after each flush.

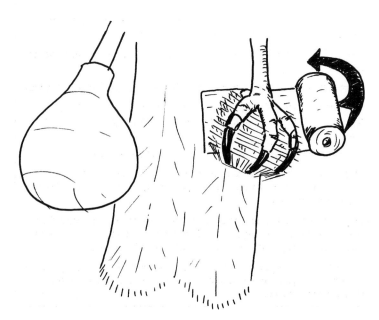

Fig. 6.4 Application of a ball bandage to the feet of a raptor with bumblefoot. Note gauze packing to support the foot before using elasticated bandage material.

Avian digestive tract disease therapy

Table 6.4 highlights some of the treatments and therapies commonly used for the management of avian digestive tract diseases.

Avian respiratory tract disease therapy

Table 6.5 highlights some of the treatments and therapies commonly used for the management of avian respiratory tract diseases. In addition, the procedure for flushing the avian nasal sinuses is described, which is useful in the treatment of upper respiratory tract disease. The procedure for placing an avian air sac tube is also covered. This may be necessary during surgery or treatment of tracheal/syringeal disease, or when a tracheal/syringeal obstruction occurs.

Performing a sinus flush

Apply the hub of a syringe (minus its hypodermic needle!) to one external nostril. To make a

Table 6.4 Treatment of diseases of the digestive system of avians.

Diagnosis	Treatment
Nematodes (e.g. *Capillaria* spp.)	Fenbendazole 15–20 mg/kg orally daily for 5 days (may need 20–50 mg/kg for *Capillaria* spp.) – care during moult as will damage growing feathers. Ivermectin 0.2 mg/kg once, repeat 14 days
Protozoa (e.g. *Trichomonas* spp., *Hexamita* spp., *Giardia* spp.)	Metronidazole 10–30 mg/kg orally twice daily 3–5 days
Coccidiosis	Carnidazole (pigeons) 25 mg/kg orally once, clazuril (*Caryospora* spp.) 5–10 mg/kg orally every other day, 3 doses
Bacterial/fungal infections	Based on culture and sensitivity results. *Megabacteria* **spp**. – amphotericin B 1 ml/kg orally twice daily 3–5 days or ketoconazole 10 mg/kg twice daily for 10 days *Candida albicans* – nystatin 300,000 units/kg orally twice daily. Associated with lack of vitamin A
Sour crop	Food should leave crop after 3–4 hours. If not crop wash and remove manually. May need antibiosis + sodium bicarbonate (antacid) + metoclopramide
Crop impaction	Crop wash under sedation with warm water and milk contents out. Advise intubation as there is a risk of inhalational pneumonia
Crop burns	Leave until skin sloughs. Then surgically debride and suture + antibiosis and supportive therapy
Duck plague	No treatment – prevention vaccine is Nobilis Duck Plague® (Intervet UK Ltd)
Haemochromatosis	Iron chelation agent deferoxamine 100 mg/kg once daily. Phlebotomy (bleeding 1–2 ml blood per kg once weekly). Diet should contain <60 ppm iron levels
Cloacal papillomas	Surgical removal, caustic silver nitrate under sedation/anaesthesia
Hepatic lipidosis	Reduce proteins, but increase biological value. Vitamin B and K supplements and lactulose syrup 0.3 ml/kg orally once daily. *Spirulina* diet supplement advised
Lead/zinc poisoning	Heavy metal chelation agent sodium edetate 20–50 mg/kg twice daily for 5 days (beware renal toxicity), or D penicillamine 50–55 mg/kg orally twice daily. Flush foreign body out of proventriculus under anaesthesia.
Diabetes mellitus	Protamine zinc insulin 0.5–1 unit/kg. Dilute in saline accurate dosing. Rarely controls blood glucose. Aim is rather to stop weight loss. Twice daily dosing often required.

Table 6.5 Treatment of respiratory system disease.

Diagnosis	Treatment
Upper respiratory tract disease	Antibiosis based culture/sensitivity, swab from choanal slit. Surgical removal of rhinoliths, sinus flushes (see below), parenteral antibiosis
Respiratory parasites	*Syngamus trachea* **(air sac mites)**: ivermectin 0.2 mg/kg once
Ornithosis/psittacosis/infection with *Chlamydophila psittaci*	Use of doxycycline advised, treatment for 42–45 days (this is the lifespan of the alveolar macrophage). This can be administered in water (relatively inaccurate), or by intramuscular injection of 100 mg/kg doxcyline (Vibravenos® Pfizer). Always a danger of *Candida* spp. over-growth of GI tract
Aspergillosis	Difficult. Surgical debridement of granulomas, possible air-sac tube placement (see blow). Nebulisation with amphotericin B/itraconazole. Intravenous amphotericin B 3–5 days, 1.5 mg/kg initially (beware of renal toxicity – always give bolus fluids as well). Oral itraconazole 5–10 mg/kg twice daily (beware toxicity in African grey parrots). Treatment for 3–12 months.
Paramyxovirus	No treatment. Prevention is by vaccination of young pigeons, using, for example, Columbovac PMV® (Fort Dodge), Nobivac Paramyxo® (Intervet UK Ltd). Essential for racing pigeons in UK by law (Disease of Poultry Order 1994 (SI 1994/3141))
Smoke inhalation toxicity	Supportive, furosemide 1–4 mg/kg intravenously/intramuscularly (beware nephrotoxicity). Oxygen enriched environment is advised, and in severe cases give prednisolone 6 mg/kg for lung oedema (beware immunosuppressive side effects)

snug fit between syringe and nostril it is often helpful to remove the rubber stopper of a 2 ml syringe, pierce a hole through its centre and attach this to the hub of the syringe containing the medication.

The bird is held inverted and the contents of the syringe (0.5 ml for a budgerigar, up to 5–7 ml for a large macaw or raptor) is expelled into the nostril. The mixture should exit through the infraorbital sinus and out through the eye, and through the internal choanal slit and out of the mouth. Holding the bird upside down minimises aspiration of this mixture.

Repeat the procedure for the other nostril.

Air sac tube placement

In many cases of syringeal aspergillosis or when performing tracheal washes in a dyspnoeic bird, the placement of an air sac tube may be vital to keep a patent airway. This may be inserted as follows:

(1) Place the bird in the right lateral recumbancy position. The bird may first be anaesthetised, or in emergencies this may be performed in the conscious bird.

(2) Elevate the uppermost wing (left). Another operator pulls the uppermost leg caudally.

(3) Make a small skin incision just caudal to the last rib, and just ventral to the pelvis at its conjunction with the spine.

(4) Pass either a specifically designed air sac tube and cannula through the body wall or a short length of 2–3.5 gauge endotracheal tubing is grasped with a pair of haemostats and pushed through the body wall. The cuff on the endotracheal tube or air sac tube may be inflated and the tube sutured to the body wall.

(5) The outlet of the anaesthetic circuit may then be attached to the free end of the tube to administer anaesthetic or oxygen. Alternatively, in the conscious bird the air sac tube is cut short and may be left in place for normal breathing for 3–4 days whilst the bird's condition is treated.

The air sac tube works so well because of the unique physiology and anatomy of the avian airway. Birds can extract oxygen on both inspiration and expiration so air entering caudally and exiting cranially can still oxygenate the bloodstream.

A nebulisation circuit may be used to administer oxygen or drugs in aerosol form to avians with respiratory disease (Fig. 6.5).

Avian reproductive tract disease therapy

Table 6.6 highlights some of the treatments and therapies commonly used for the management of avian reproductive tract diseases.

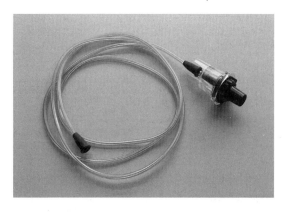

Fig. 6.5   A nebulisation circuit which may be attached to an oxygen supply or preferably a nebulisation unit to administer drugs in aerosol form to avian patients with respiratory disease.

Table 6.6   Treatment of reproductive system diseases.

Diagnosis	Treatment
Egg binding	Provision suitable nesting material. If hypocalcaemic treat with 100 mg/kg calcium gluconate intramuscularly once. Fluid therapy advised – treat with oxytocin 0.1–1 unit/kg once intramuscularly. May need to collapse egg with needle and syringe either per cloaca if visible or, if not, via midline through the abdominal wall.
Compulsive egg-laying	Reduce daylight length to a maximum of 10 hours. Leave eggs in with hen, or use plastic egg-replacers to inhibit further laying. Progesterone injections may be administered – medroxyprogesterone actetate 5–50 mg/kg once only (side effects include increased risk diabetes mellitus, liver damage, immunosuppression). Human chorionic gonadotrophin may be administered on days 1, 3 and 5 at 500–1000 IU/kg intramuscularly (Lightfoot, 1998) with fewer side effects. Surgical spaying may be required if no success.
Salpingitis	Antibiosis based on culture and sensitivity. Surgical spaying may be the only option.

Table 6.7   Musculo-skeletal system diseases.

Diagnosis	Treatment
Fracture management	Fracture repair is rapid in birds, with callus formation in 7–10 days. For small birds, canaries and budgerigars with distal pelvic limb fractures use zinc oxide tape splints ('Altman splint') (see Fig. 6.6) Surgical repair may be necessary, and use of external transcortical pins advised for narrow bones with small medullary cavity. Intramedullary pins allow rotation and stack pins (multiple small diameter pins implanted) help prevent this. For wild birds achieve a 100% successful repair, otherwise there will be welfare aspects if re-released into the wild. It may be better to euthanase if conditon is severe. Splinting is satisfactory for temporary stabilisation and wound management (see Fig. 6.7).
Carpometacarpal luxation	Bandage wings to body wall for 4–6 weeks if early on in condition. Once rotation of joint has occurred the only option is surgical.
Nutritional osteodystrophy	Once bones are deformed and mineralised the only options are surgical. Prevention geared to adequate diet, calcium supplementation, etc., and not providing excess proteins which generate too rapid growth rates.

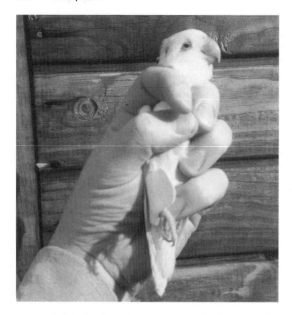

Fig. 6.6   An Altman splint applied to the tibiotarsus of this lovebird for a simple closed fracture. Two pieces of heavy zinc oxide tape are used to sandwich the proximal and distal fragments together.

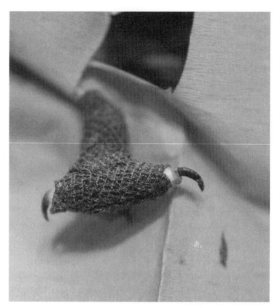

Fig. 6.7   A light padding and elasticated bandage support for a toe amputation.

Avian musculoskeletal system disease therapy

Table 6.7 highlights some of the treatments and therapies commonly used for the management of avian musculoskeletal system diseases. The process for splinting a fractured wing is also described.

Temporary wing splinting

Splinting of wing fractures may be performed with bandage material. It should be noted, though, that when a bird's joint is kept immobilised for a few days it starts to stiffen and fibrose. This can be disastrous for raptors and wild birds. Bandaging techniques are therefore more suitable for cage and aviary birds, and also for emergency support dressings, or where it is possible to maintain joint movement.

The technique for humeral/radial/ulna fractures is described below.

- Flex the wing using coflex/vetwrap.
- Starting from the point of the elbow take the bandage over the dorsal aspect of the wing to a point just distal to the point of the carpus.
- Place the bandage over the ventral aspect of the wing, heading back to the point of the elbow.
- Cover the dorsal aspect of the wing to a point just proximal to the carpus.
- Put the bandage onto the ventral aspect of the wing towards the digits.
- Roll it over the leading edge of the wing and the dorsal aspect once more and back to the elbow.

This 'figure of eight' technique bunches the primary feathers together and so uses them as a splint.

Avian neurological system disease therapy

Table 6.8 highlights some of the treatments and therapies commonly used for the management of avian neurological system diseases.

Miscellaneous conditions

Oil spills

Stabilisation: this involves the administration of fluid therapy to correct dehydration, which is commonly seen because diarrhoea results from the

Table 6.8 Treatment of nervous system diseases.

Diagnosis	Treatment
Hypocalcaemic syndrome of African grey parrots	Slow intravenous/intramuscular injection of 100 mg/kg calcium gluconate. Diazepam/midazolam to control fitting. Prevention – adequate dietary calcium, supplementation with calcium in water and small volumes of dairy products, e.g. bioyoghurts and cottage cheese. Will grow out of condition by 5–6 years of age.
Seizuring	Treatment is based on diagnosis of cause. For heavy metal toxicity see Digestive System Diseases. For hypocalcaemic syndrome see condition above. Also seen in young raptors. Symptomatic treatment – dimmed lighting, reduced noise levels, careful handling, diazepam/midazolam 0.3–1 mg/kg intravenously/intramuscularly. If the condition occurs in a small raptor, it may be hypoglycaemia. Administer 40% glucose w/v intraveneously and slowly at 0.25–1 ml per bird depending on size. Northern goshawks are prone to hyperglycaemia at the start of the training season. Diagnosis is blood glucose >30 mmol/l. To treat use protamine zinc insulin 0.1 unit and repeat until glucose levels fall below 15 mmol/l (Forbes, 1996b).
Newcastle Disease/ PMV-1	Treatment is not possible but vaccination for PMV-1 is compulsory in racing pigeons in the UK. Vaccines include Columbovac® (Fort Dodge) and Nobivac Paramyxo® (Intervet).

bird consuming oil. In addition, birds are often hypothermic because they are unable to move properly. Gentle warming in a stream of warm air, such as that from a hairdryer, can be used to bring body temperature to near normal. Heated cages with dimmed lighting to reduce further stress are also advisable. As these birds may have been unable to feed for days readily digestible liquid food should be provided. This can be easily crop tubed into the bird if necessary. Various preparations are available, such as Critical Care Formula® (VetArk).

Initial treatment: this involves the oral administration of adsorbents, such as activated charcoal, to prevent further absorption of oil. Covering antibiotics and further fluid and nutritional support may also be necessary. Due to the extreme stress of the situation many birds succumb to systemic fungal diseases such as aspergillosis and this may necessitate additional treatment.

Cleaning: The best cleaning agent for removal of oil is washing-up liquid, which should be diluted 1 part to 50 parts water. This should be lathered into the oil and sprayed off using a shower head attachment. The water supply should be kept at around the bird's own body temperature (between 40–45°C) to reduce further loss of body heat. This is important as it may take up to an hour to clean some birds. Attention must be paid to thoroughly cleaning all of the feathers, so a cleaning pattern or routine should be used. Washing can stop when the water starts to form small, bead-like droplets on the feathers.

Once the oil has all been removed, the feathers should be dried initially using a hairdryer, and then by placing the bird in a heated cage. After cleaning and ensuring that the birds are feeding properly and maintaining condition, it is often necessary to retain waterfowl in captivity for a few days to ensure that they are regularly preening to waterproof their feathers.

Lead poisoning

This is still a common problem in wild waterfowl, particularly swans. It is often caused by the bird consuming lead shot from shotgun discharges or old lead weights from coarse fishing (which are now banned but can still be found in the environment). Commercial mining may also occasionally contribute to discharges of lead and other heavy metal discharges, such as zinc and tin.

Diagnosis of lead poisoning should be made by radiographing the affected bird to demonstrate radio dense particles, often in the gizzard or ventriculus of the patient. However, many affected birds no longer have lead particles in their digestive system but are still suffering from lead poisoning. Therefore, a blood sample to demonstrate elevated levels of lead is required. Normal levels are below 0.4 ppm, while levels over 0.5 ppm, and particularly over 2 ppm, are diagnostic for lead poisoning.

Raptors often present with green diarrhoea, they are weak, and adopt a classical 'holding hands' posture wherein they rock back on their intertarsal joint, and one foot grasps the other. Waterfowl will often be weak, may have wing droop and a curved S-shaped neck, particularly swans.

References

Cooper, J.E. (1985) Foot conditions. In *Veterinary Aspects of Captive Birds of Prey*, 2nd edn, pp. 97–111. Standfast Press, Gloucestershire.

Forbes, N.A. (1996a) Respiratory problems. In *Manual of Raptors, Pigeons and Waterfowl* (Beynon, P.H., Forbes, N.A. and Harcourt-Brown, N.H., eds), pp. 147–157. BSAVA, Cheltenham.

Forbes, N.A. (1996b) Fits and incoordination. In *Manual of Raptors, Pigeons and Waterfowl* (Beynon, P.H., Forbes, N.A. and Harcourt-Brown, N.H., eds), pp. 197–207. BSAVA, Cheltenham.

Lightfoot, T.L. (1998) Approach to avian obstetrics. In *Proceedings of the North American Veterinary Congress*, pp. 757–778.

Oaks, J.L. (1993) Immune and inflammatory responses in falcon staphylococcal pododermatitis. In *Raptor Biomedicine* (Redig, P.T., Cooper, J.E., Remple, J.D. and Hunter, D.B., eds), pp. 72–87, University of Minnesota Press, Minneapolis, Minnesota.

Further reading

Benyon, P.H., Forbes, N.A. and Lawton, M.P.C. (1996) *Manual of Psittacine Birds*. BSAVA, Cheltenham.

Benyon, P.H., Forbes, N.A. and Harcourt-Brown, N.H. (1996) *Manual of Raptors, Pigeons and Waterfowl*. BSAVA, Cheltenham.

Coles, B.H. (1997) *Avian Medicine and Surgery*. Blackwell Science, Oxford.

Cooper, J.E. (1991) *Veterinary Aspects of Captive Birds of Prey*. Standfast Press, Glos.

Cooper, J.E. (2002) *Veterinary Aspects of Captive Birds of Prey*, 2nd edn. Standfast Press, Glos.

Forbes, N.A. and Parry-Jones, J. (1996) Management and husbandry (raptors). In *Manual of Raptors, Pigeons and Waterfowl* (Beynon P.H., Forbes, N.A. and Harcourt-Brown, NH., eds), pp. 116–128. BSAVA, Cheltenham.

Hochleithner, M. (1994) *Biochemistries*. In *Avian Medicine: Principles and Application* (Ritchie, B., Harrison, G. and Harrison, L., eds), pp. 223–245. Wingers Publishing, Lake Worth, Florida.

Ritchie, B., Harrison, G., and Harrison, L. (1994) *Avian Medicine: Principles and Applications*. Wingers Publishing, Lake Worth, Florida.

Roberts, V. (2000) *Diseases of Free-Range Poultry*. Whittet Books, Stowmarket.

Samour, J. (2000) *Avian Medicine*. Mosby, London.

Reptiles and Amphibians

Chapter 7

Basic Reptile and Amphibian Anatomy and Physiology

SERPENTES (SNAKES)

Like the bird, the snake has no diaphragm, so no separate thorax and abdomen. Instead it has a *coelomic*, or common, body cavity.

Musculoskeletal system

All true snakes have no limbs. This distinguishes them from species such as the slow-worm, which is actually a lizard with vestigial limbs. There are some remnants of limbs in one or two of the older evolutionary species of snake such as the boiid family (pythons and boa constrictors). These can possess vestigial pelvic remnants, having claw-like spurs either side of the vent representing the hind limbs.

The snake skull possesses a small cranial cavity containing the brain and a large nasal cavity. The maxilla has 4 rows of teeth, two on either side. The mandible has the more normal two rows of teeth (Fig. 7.1). The teeth vary somewhat between the genera. The more commonly seen non-poisonous species, such as the colubrid family (containing the kingsnakes and ratsnakes) and the boiid family, have simple, caudally-curved, peglike teeth. Some of the more poisonous species have specialist adaptions. Rattlesnakes, for example, have hinged, rostrally situated fangs which swing forward as they strike. All teeth are replaced as they are lost, including fang teeth in poisonous species. It is worth mentioning that owners (other than zoos) of poisonous species of snake, such as pit vipers and rattlesnakes, must be licensed and registered in the United Kingdom under the conditions of the Dangerous Wild Animals Act of 1976.

The anatomy of the snake's head has a number of adaptations that allow it to swallow large prey. In all snakes, the two halves of lower jaw are loosely held together rostrally and the mandibular symphysis can separate. In addition, the snake has no temperomandibular joint. Instead it possesses a quadrate bone, which articulates between a mandible and the skull and allows the mandibles to be moved rostrally and laterally, 'dislocating'. The maxilla also hinges only loosely with the rostral aspect of the cranium so allowing the nose of the snake to be raised, increasing the oral aperture.

The skull articulates with the atlas vertebra via a simple joint containing only one occipital condyle, rather than the mammalian two. The coccygeal vertebrae (those caudal to the vent) are the only vertebrae with no ribs attached. Instead they have paired, ventral, haemal processes between which the coccyeal artery and vein run. This vein can be used for venipuncture both for sampling and for intravenous injections. The site for this is one third the distance from the vent to the tail tip on the ventral aspect.

The ventral scales, known as *scutes* or *gastropeges*, overlie the muscular casing of the snake's torso. This muscle is segmental and supplied by intervertebral nerves. It is by alternately contracting and relaxing these segmental muscles that the snake can propel itself across the ground, the caudal edge of each ventral scute providing friction.

A very few species of snake, such as the glass snake, exhibit *autotomy*. That is, they will shed their tail if roughly handled or caught by a predator. They will regrow their tail later.

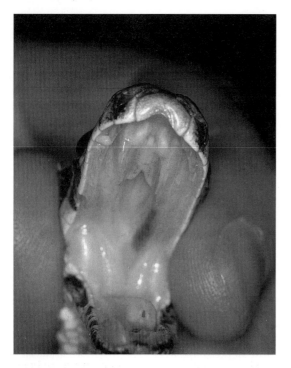

Fig. 7.1 Intraoral view of a young Burmese python showing the four upper and two lower rows of teeth, as well as the glottal tube and tracheal entrance, rostral to which is the tongue sheath.

Respiratory system (Fig. 7.2)

Upper respiratory system

The nostrils are paired and open into the roof of the mouth. Snakes, like all reptiles other than crocodilians, do not have a hard palate. When the mouth is closed, the internal nostrils are positioned directly above the entrance to the trachea. This is guarded by the glottis. An epiglottis may be present in vestigial form, but there is often fusion of the cartilages here to form a glottal tube. This tube is rigid enough to withstand the pressures placed upon it when the snake is swallowing whole prey. At rest the glottis is held closed, only opening when the snake breathes. The glottis then opens into the trachea which, in the snake family, is supported by C-shaped cartilages similar to those of the cat and dog.

Lower respiratory system

In the majority of colubrid species, such as ratsnakes and kingsnakes and some Viperidae, the right lung is the major lung, the left having regressed to a vestigial structure. The vestigial left

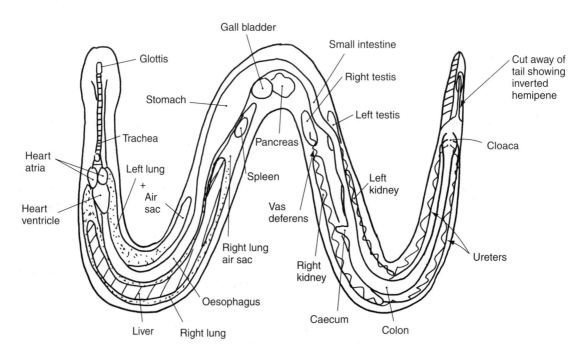

Fig. 7.2 Diagram of a male snake (ventral aspect).

lung is often replaced by a vascularised air sac and so can take part in gaseous exchange. In the evolutionarily older species such as the Boiidae there are two lungs.

The trachea bifurcates at the level of the heart. The lungs occupy the first half of the middle third of the body of the snake. As there is no diaphragm, inspiration is purely due to the outward movement of the ribs and intercostal muscles. This is aided by elastic tissue present within the lung structure, which allows the lungs to expand and recoil. Expiration is facilitated by contraction of abdominal and intercostal muscles, and the elastic recoil of the lungs themselves. A 'tracheal lung' is often present as an outpouching of the lining of the trachea from the open part of the C-shaped cartilages. This is thought to aid respiration when main lungs are being compressed during the swallowing of large prey items.

The stimulus for respiration is a lowered partial pressure of oxygen, rather than an increase in the partial pressure of carbon dioxide, as is the case in mammals.

Digestive system

Oral cavity

The tongue sits in a basal sheath at the rostral end of the oral cavity just in front of the glottis and can be pushed out through the lips even when the mouth is closed through the labial notch. The tongue is *bifid* (split into a forked end) and is used to catch odours on its moist surface. These are then pushed into the roof of the mouth into the *vomeronasal organ*. The vomero-nasal organ is connected to the olfactory region of the brain and is a primitive but effective pheromone and scent detector. The oral cavity contains salivary glands which are stimulated to release saliva during mastication. The mouth is normally free of saliva at other times.

The oropharynx passes on into the oesophagus, which is an extremely distensible muscular tube traveling ventral to the lungs and entering the stomach in the second half of the middle third of the snake's body.

Stomach, associated organs and intestine

The stomach is a tubular organ, populated with compound glands secreting both hydrochloric acid and pepsin (mammals having two separate cells) and separate mucus secreting glands. There is no well-defined cardiac sphincter. The majority of the digestive process occurs in the stomach and is continued by the small intestine. The only substance which cannot be digested is the hair of the prey, known as the 'felt', which is passed out in the stool.

The stomach empties into the duodenum, which is poorly defined from the jejunum and ileum. The spleen, pancreas and gall bladder are found at the point where the pylorus empties into the small intestine. Some snakes have a fused splenopancreas. The gall bladder is found at the most caudal point of the liver, which is an elongated structure extending from the mid-point of the lungs to the caudal stomach.

The small intestine empties into the large intestine, which is distinguished from it by its thinner wall and larger diameter. In the Boiidae there may be a caecum at this junction.

The large intestine empties into the coprodeum portion of the cloaca, which, as with birds, is the common emptying chamber for the digestive, urinary and reproductive systems.

Urinary system

There are paired elongated kidneys (Fig. 7.3), situated in the distal half of the caudal third of the snake's body, attached to the dorsal body wall. The right kidney is cranial to the left and both each has a single ureter which travels across their ventral surface to empty into the urodeum of the cloaca, caudal to the proctodeum. There is no urinary bladder in snakes. The caudal portions of the kidneys in male snakes are the 'sexual segments', enlarging during the breeding season as they provide seminal fluid.

Renal physiology

As with the majority of reptiles, snakes are *uricotelic*, that is that like birds their primary

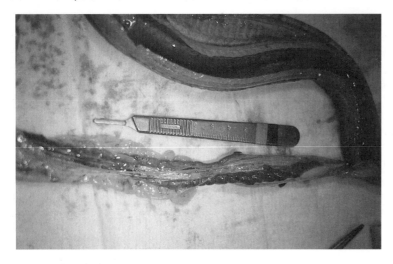

Fig. 7.3 Post mortem showing the elongated lobular right and left kidneys of a corn snake (*Elaphe guttata guttata*) adjacent to scalpel handle.

nitrogenous waste product is not urea but uric acid. This compound is relatively insoluble allowing conservation of water. This is particularly important for reptiles, as they have no loops of Henle in their kidneys therefore they cannot create hypertonic urine as mammals can. To further conserve water, urine in the urodeum portion of the cloaca can be refluxed back into the terminal portion of the gut where more water reabsorption can occur. If the reptile becomes dehydrated, or renal blockage or infection occurs, then excretion of uric acid is reduced and can lead to gout as is seen in birds.

Cardiovascular system

Heart

The heart is three chambered, with two atria and a common ventricle situated within the pericardial sac, but it despite this functions as a four chambered organ. The heart lies in the caudal half of the proximal third of the snake's body, and is mobile, to allow the passage of large food items through the oesophagus above it. There are two cranial vena cavae and one caudal vena cava entering via the sinus venosus (a narrow tube leading to the right atrium from which it is separated by the sinoatrial valve).

Blood vessels

The snake family has paired aortae. They exit one from each of the two sides of the single ventricle of the heart and then fuse into a single abdominal aorta. The pulmonary artery that leads to the lung(s) also arises here.

As with birds, snakes have a renal portal system. The blood supply from the caudal portion of the snake in the coccygeal artery splits into two and can enter the renal circulation or may bypass it via a series of valves. This is important when administering drugs which are nephrotoxic or which may be excreted by the kidneys, as it means they might be concentrated there. They should therefore be administered in the cranial part of the snake.

There is also an hepatic portal system from the intestine to the liver. A ventral abdominal vein lies in the midline, just beneath the ventral abdominal musculature, and must be avoided when performing surgery.

Two external jugular veins run just medial to the ventral cervical ribs, and may be reached to place catheters for intravenous fluid administration via a surgical cut-down procedure. The ventral tail vein has already been mentioned and is useful for venipuncture for blood collection.

Lymphatic system

There are no specific separate lymph nodes as seen in mammals, a situation similar to birds. Instead, as with birds, there are discrete accumulations of lymph tissue within most of the major organs, particularly the liver and intestines. There is also a spleen, as mentioned above, which has loosely arranged red and white pulp. Lymphatic vessels are found throughout the body. A lymphatic sinus, for example, runs the length of the snake just ventrolateral to the epaxial musculature immediately below the skin surface on either side of the body. This may be used for small volumes of fluid administration. In the walls of many of the lymphatic vessels there are muscular swellings known as 'lymph hearts' which aid in the return of the straw coloured lymphatic fluid back to the true heart.

Reproductive system

Male (Fig. 7.2)

The paired testes lie intracoloemically (within the coelom or common body cavity, as snakes like most reptiles have no diaphragm and so no separate thorax and abdomen only a common coelomic cavity). They are situated cranial to each kidney, and caudal to the pancreatic tissue, with the right testis slightly cranial to the left, and are oval in shape. The testes enlarge during the breeding season, often reaching two to three times their quiescent state. Close to the testes lie the adrenal glands. Each testis has a solitary vas deferens leading down to the urodeum portion of the cloaca, where seminal fluids from the reproductive sexual segment of the kidneys are added.

The male snake also has paired penises, known as *hemipenes* in its tail. At rest they are like two inverted sacs either side of the midline and lie ventral to two other small invaginations in the tail which form the anal glands. When a hemipene's lining becomes engorged with blood, it everts, forming a finger-like protrusion through the vent. As with the domestic cat, the hemipenes are often covered in spines and barbs, and they each have a dorsal groove into which the sperm drops from the cloaca, and so is guided into the female's cloaca. The hemipenes therefore do not play any part in urination.

Female

The female has paired ovaries, cranial to the respective kidneys, with the right ovary cranial to the left. There are two coiled oviducts starting with the fimbriae opposite each ovary, and moving through the tubular portion of the infundibulum and on into the magnum. From here the tract merges into the isthmus and then the shell gland or uterus before opening into the muscular vagina. This organ ensures that the eggs are layed only when the timing is correct. The vagina empties into the urodeum section of the cloaca. The vascular supply is from the dorsally suspended oviduct mesentery, rather than the caudocranial route employed in mammals.

Most females are stimulated to reproduce in the spring when the weather warms and the daylight length increases. The tropical boas (such as the *Boa constrictor*) and the Burmese python (*Python molurus*), however, start breeding when the temperature *drops* slightly during the cooler portion of the year.

Some species of snake are *oviparous* (that is they lay eggs), others are *viviparous* (that is they bear live young). The latter are, for example, the garter snakes (*Thamnophis sirtalis*) and the boiid family, which have a vestigial egg structure more closely resembling a placenta. Other species make nests, and some species of python will incubate eggs by contracting and relaxing skeletal muscles, so creating warmth.

Sex determination and identification

Snakes are chromosomally dependent for sex determination, as with most mammals. This is in contrast with the Chelonia, Crocodylia and some Sauria, in which sex may be temperature dependent.

Sex identification is best made by surgical probing. A fine, sterile, blunt-ended probe is inserted through the vent and advanced just to one side of the midline in a caudal direction. If the snake is a male, then the probe will pass into one of the inverted hemipenes to a depth of 8–16 subcaudal scales. In the female, there are anal glands in this region, and so the probe may be inserted only to a depth of two to six subcaudal scales. In some species, such as the boiid family, the males possess a paracloacal spur. This is the remnant of the pelvic limb and may be found on either side of body, ventrally, at the level of the cloaca. In very young snakes it may be possible carefully to evert the hemipenes manually, a technique known as 'popping'.

Skin

The outer epidermal layer in snakes is thrown into a series of folds forming scales, which cover the whole surface of the snake. There are different sizes of scale over the body, with smaller, less raised ones covering the head, to larger and more raised scales over the main portion of the body. Some species have scales with ridges on their surface to add greater grip, other species have smooth scales. In some snakes, such as the sea snakes, the skin is very loose fitting, and apparently has few elastic fibres. Other snakes have elastic skin which relatively quickly returns to its normal shape. The reptile skin has little or no skin glands. Its outer layer, or *stratum corneum*, is heavily keratinised, and composed of three layers of dead cells filled with keratin. These cells become progressively more flattened as they approach the surface. On the ventral surface of the snake there is a single row of scales which span the width of the snake, and are known as the ventral scutes or gastropeges. The caudal edge of each overlaps the cranial edge of the following scale (Fig. 7.4).

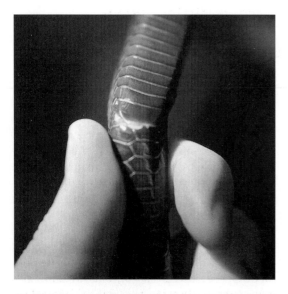

Fig. 7.4 The vent of a ratsnake showing the division of the ventral scales from single scutes cranial to the vent to paired scales caudally.

Ecdysis

Ecdysis is the regular shedding of the entire skin. Other reptiles also shed their skin, but the Chelonia and Crocodylia shed individual scutes, and the Sauria shed in patches. Only the Serpentes shed all of their skin (including the clear, fused eyelids, or spectacle) in one go. The stimulus can be dependent on time of year, health status and age of the snake and the process is partly controlled by the thyroid gland.

First the new layer of skin is formed deep to the old one. Once it is complete, the snake secretes a proteinaceous lymph fluid between the new layer of skin and the old one. At this time the snake will become dull in colour, and often exhibits blueing of the eyes. The fluid forces the outer layer of old skin to separate away from the new, and often contains enzymes to help in this process. Once separation has been achieved the fluid is reabsorbed and the snake's eyes may be seen returning to normal. A few days later the snake will shed the old skin. It starts the process by rubbing the corners of its mouth on some abrasive surface. The shedding proceeds with the head skin first and the snake then rolls the old skin back until the tail is the last to emerge.

In a healthy snake all of the skin should come away at once (Plate 7.1). If the skin does not shed the condition is known as dysecdysis. There can be many reasons for this. Disease, dehydration (which causes too little fluid to be produced), scars on the skin surface or lack of an abrasive surface upon which to remove the skin can all be factors. Regular bathing and soft but abrasive damp surfaces may be needed to aid shedding, and any underlying disease should be attended to.

Special cutaneous adaptations in snakes

There are one or two special structures associated with the skin of snakes. These include the lateral spurs of the Boiidae, which have been mentioned earlier. The male possesses larger spurs than the female.

Snakes do not have mobile eyelids. Instead, the eyelids have become fused together and transparent, forming the so-called 'spectacle'.

Many snakes also have special sense organs on the head. The older snake families such as the Boiidae have labial pits – a series of depressions running along the dorsal border of the upper jaw. These function as rudimentary heat sensors. In the more evolutionarily advanced species, such as the pit vipers, the heat sensing organs can actually focus on their prey, and are composed of bilateral, forward-facing pits midway between the nares and the eyes. They are supplied by branches of the trigeminal nerves, and, in the case of pit vipers, may be sensitive enough to detect changes of heat as small as 0.002°C!

Snakes do not possess an external eardrum or middle ear. They can however hear airborne sounds and can of course detect ground tremors.

SAURIA (LIZARDS)

Musculoskeletal system

Lizards have a musculoskeletal system more familiar to those used to dealing with mammalian forms. They possess in the majority four limbs, an axial skeleton and much of the anatomical layout of small mammals. There are some exceptions, one being the slow worm, a native of mainland Britain and northern Europe which resembles a snake, having no obvious external limbs. It is actually, however, a highly evolved lizard with rudimentary limbs.

The skull is more rigid than its snake counterpart, having less mobile jaws. There are four rows of teeth, one to each jaw. These are peg-like in shape and are continually replaced in the Sauria except for the Agamidae and Chameleonidae. There are no fang teeth in Saurians, but the beaded lizard (*Heloderma horribilis*) and the gila monster (*Heloderma suspectum*) have hollow teeth which allow the venom from sublingual venom glands to ooze through them into the prey when they bite them. These two species are therefore currently classified as dangerous wild animals under the Dangerous Wild Animals Act 1976, in the United Kingdom requiring a special licence to keep them in captivity outside of a zoological collection.

The skull articulates with the atlantal cervical vertebra via a single occipital condyle. The thoracic vertebrae and lumbar vertebrae generally have paired ribs either side. The coccygeal vertebrae possess ventral haemal arches between which it is possible to access the ventral tail vein for venipuncture.

In many saurians the tail possesses fracture planes which allow the tail to break off during escape from a predator. These fracture planes occur in the mid to caudal portions of the tail, but not proximally, where vital structures such as the male reproductive organs and fat pads are stored. Only certain species exhibit this tail autotomy. These include most of the Iguanidae, but does not include the Agamidae, monitor lizards and true chameleons. When the tail is regrown in these species, the coccygeal vertebrae are not replaced, instead a cartilagenous rod of tissue forms the rigid structure. In addition the rows of scales over the new tail surface are often haphazardly arranged and do not match the size and shape of the rest of the tail (Fig. 7.5).

Respiratory system (Fig. 7.6)

Upper respiratory system

Lizards have paired nostrils situated rostrally on the maxilla. To the side, or just inside the nares, particularly in iguanids, there is often situated a pair (one on each side) of salt-secreting glands. These are responsible for excreting excess sodium as sodium chloride so helping to conserve water. The sodium chloride may be seen as a white crystalline deposit around the nostrils which is often sneezed out by the lizard. The nostrils enter into the rostral part of the oral cavity, there being no hard palate.

The entrance to the trachea is guarded by a rudimentary larynx which often lacks an epiglottis and vocal folds. Some species, such as the Geckonidae, do possess vocal folds and are capable of producing a variety of sounds. In most species the trachea is supported by incomplete cartilaginous C-shaped rings similar to those of the cat and dog.

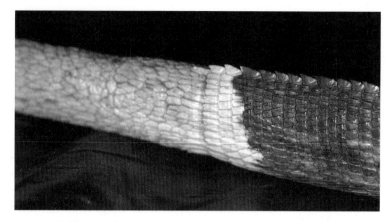

Fig. 7.5 Regrowth of the tail is possible in many species of lizard, but the scales which regrow are arranged haphazardly, and the vertebrae lost are replaced by a rod of cartilage.

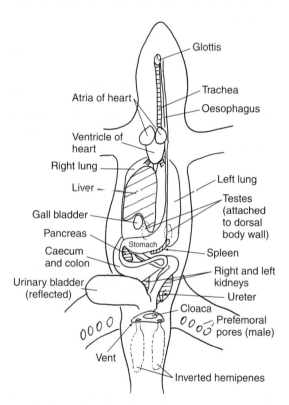

Fig. 7.6 Diagram of male green iguana (ventral aspect).

Lower respiratory system

The trachea bifurcates into two main bronchi in the cranial thorax to supply two lungs. In more primitive lizards the lungs are sac-like structures with large bulla-like divisions and alveoli. In the more advanced lizard species the lungs are more like the mammalian sponge-like system, with finer divisions and more structured alveolar systems. Lizards will often overinflate their lungs, in an attempt to make themselves look bigger, when threatened.

There is no diaphragm in any lizard species, so there is no clear distinction between the thorax and abdomen, rather there is a common body cavity, known as the coelom, as in snakes and birds.

Respiration is thought to be stimulated by falling partial pressures of oxygen in the blood stream. The act of inspiration is due to the mechanical contraction of the intercostal muscles causing an upwards and outwards movement of the rib cage. This is aided by the elastic tissues that are present within the lung structures themselves. Expiration is by contraction of the abdominal and intercostal muscles, and by the elastic recoil of the lung tissue.

Digestive system

Oral cavity

The majority of lizards have a large, fleshy tongue which is frequently mobile. In some species however, such as the chameleons, the tongue has become specialised. It lies coiled in the lower jaw and can be projected out at a flying insect or other potential prey item. The green iguana has a more traditional fleshy tongue, which has a much darker tip. This is not to be confused with pathological changes. A vomeronasal organ is present.

Stomach, associated organs and intestine

The stomach is a simple sac-like structure in most species. The glands are combined hydrochloric-acid- and pepsin-secreting glands lining the walls. There are also separate mucus-secreting glands for lubrication.

The small intestine is better developed in more carnivorous species such as the monitor lizards and the insectivorous water dragons. In herbivorous species it is relatively short. It is poorly divided into jejunum and ileal structures. In a few, mainly herbivorous, species, at the junction between the small and large intestines, lies the caecum. The liver is roughly bilobed in structure and is situated ventral to the stomach and lungs. There is usually a gall bladder, with the primary bile pigment being biliverdin, as with birds, rather than the bilirubin of mammals.

The large intestine is more highly developed in herbivorous species than in carnivorous or omnivorous species. Examples include the green iguana and the chuckwalla. These have a large intestine which is often sacculated and divided into many chambers by leaf-like membranes. These increase the intestinal surface area so that microbes, upon which these species depend for vegetation digestion, may colonise it.

The large intestine then empties into the coprodeum portion of the cloaca. The cloaca itself is then continued, as with birds and snakes by the other two segments, the urodeum which receives the urogenital openings, and the proctodeum which is the last chamber before waste exits the cloaca through the vent.

Urinary system

The kidneys are paired and often bean-shaped organs. Their position is variable depending on the species. In some, such as the green iguana, they are both situated in the pelvis, attached to the dorsal body wall (see Fig. 7.6). Other species, such as chameleons, have longer kidney structures which extend cranially into the coelomic cavity. As with snakes, the males of some species have a specially developed caudal portion of the kidneys, known as the 'sexual segment' which enlarges during the breeding season and contributes to the production of seminal fluid. The kidneys empty into the ureters which empty into the urodeum portion of the cloaca.

Many lizards have a bladder. This is not however like the sterile bladder of mammals, as it is not connected directly to the ureters. Instead, it is joined to the cloaca, and so urine has to enter the cloaca, before entering the bladder. There is some evidence that the bladder is able to absorb some fluid from its contents, or it may function as a fluid storage chamber, flushing its contents back into the caudal large intestine for further fluid absorption.

Renal physiology

The renal physiology is similar to that already described for snakes. The main differences lie in the variable presence of the urinary bladder which may have some water reabsorption capabilities.

Cardiovascular system

Heart

The saurian heart is very similar to the snake model, with paired atria and a single common ventricle which nevertheless functions as two. The majority of the deoxygenated blood is channelled to the pulmonary arteries and the oxygenated blood enters the paired aortae. (Plate 7.2).

Blood vessels

The two aortae fuse dorsally, after giving off paired carotid trunks, to form the abdominal aorta. Lizards also possess a hepatoportal venous supply and a renal portal system, hence, as with birds and snakes, intravenous injection into the caudal half of the lizard of medications which are excreted through the renal tubules, could result in their failure to reach the rest of the lizard's body. It could also increase the toxicity of substances known to be renally toxic if given by this route.

Lizards, like snakes, also possess a large ventral abdominal vein which returns blood from the tail area and passes just beneath the body wall, ventrally and in the midline. This must be avoided when performing abdominal surgery. This vessel can be used, carefully, for venipuncture for blood sampling in lizards, although the preferred vessel is the ventral tail vein. For intravenous use, the cephalic vein may be accessed on the cranial aspect of the antebrachium, via a cut-down procedure, in the larger species.

Lymphatic system

The lymphatic system is similar to that of snakes, with no discrete lymph nodes.

Reproductive system

Male

The paired testes are situated cranial to the respective kidneys in those species which have abdominally positioned kidneys (Fig. 7.6). In those where the kidneys are more pelvic in position, the testes are located just caudal to the end of the lungs and liver, in the middle part of the coelomic cavity. They are supplied by several arteries each and drained by several veins. Both are very tightly adhered to their vascular supply, the left testicle being separated from the left renal vein (into which the left testicular veins drain) by the left adrenal gland. The right testicle is tightly attached to its right renal vein which separates it from the right adrenal gland. This positioning so close to such vital structures makes castrating aggressive lizards a difficult operation. The testes enlarge during the breeding season and regress out of it. Each testis drains into a vas deferens which has a tightly coiled course over the ventral surface of the respective kidney before emptying into the urodeum portion of the cloaca. Some species, such as the Chameleonidae, have a pronounced epididymis extending caudally from each testicle.

The male lizard has paired penises, as with the snake, known as hemipenes. These lie in the base of the tail structure, either side of midline, and function as with the snake family. At rest they are inverted sacs in the tail base. During copulation, one will engorge with blood and evert itself, creating a groove along its dorsal surface. Into this groove sperm and spermatic fluid will drop from the cloaca, and the hemipene will guide this into the female lizard's cloaca.

Female

The female lizard has much the same anatomy as that described for the snake.

Egg-producing physiology

Reproductive physiology in the female lizard is broadly similar to that of the avian patient. Some species, such as some of the Chameleonidae, are *ovoviviparous*. That is, they produce live young instead of laying eggs, although the *eggs are produced* internally. Some species are viviparous, in which a form of placenta or thin-walled egg structure allows the foetus to develop and live young are produced. Many other species are oviparous, i.e. they lay eggs. One or two species are *parthenogenic*: that is the females produce entire females with no need for a male lizard – some species of *Lacerta* and *Hemidactylus* (geckos) are capable of this.

Reptile eggs are generally soft shelled and more leathery than those of their avian cousins. Sexual maturity varies according to the species, green iguanas, for example, reaching it at 2–3 years.

Sex determination and identification

Sex determination is largely dependent on chromosomes. However, geckos as a family are temperature dependent, with 99% of eggs incubated between 26.7–29.4°C being female whereas if the temperature was greater than 32.2°C, 90% of the offspring would be male.

Sex may be identified by surgical probing as mentioned above. This is often the only method available for some species such as the beaded lizard, some monitors and the gila monster. However, in most other species there are external physical differences. These include the prominent pre-femoral pores of males that are seen on the caudoventral aspect of the thigh of iguanids (see Fig. 7.6). Some male lizards have a series of pre-anal pores just cranial to the vent. Males have wider tail bases than the females to house the large hemipenes (Fig. 7.7). Some males have greater ornamentation (Fig. 7.8). Male green iguanas and plumed basilisks have larger crests, male Jackson's chameleons have horns, male

water dragons have larger crest spines and many male geckos have a wider vent size and hemipenal bulge.

Skin

Lizard skin is much the same as that of snakes. The scales in most cases are much smaller than the snake equivalent.

Special cutaneous adaptations in lizards

There are some specialised skin glands and structures in lizards. The males of certain species, such as the green iguana, have secretory glands or pores. The green iguana's are on the ventrocaudal aspect of the femoral area. Some geckos have precloacal pores.

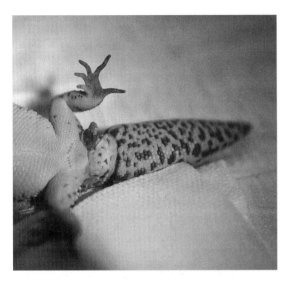

Fig. 7.7 Eversion of a hemipene in a male leopard gecko to remove a hemipenal plug (accumulation of dried secretion).

Many lizards have large numbers of chromatophores in their skins. These are connected to neural networks, allowing them to alter the colour they produce according to external stimuli and mood. This ability is seen in the chameleons, and, to a lesser extent, in green iguanas and many other species.

Unlike snakes, lizards have a tympanum, located ventrocaudal to the eye, and a middle ear.

Many males will have large amounts of ornamentation on their body surface for display purposes. Examples include the male green iguana which often has large coloured scales on the head and a bluish sheen to the head and neck colouring. Others, such as male anoles, have extendable chin flaps which are often brightly coloured and can be 'flashed' in display. Some males such as the male plumed basilisks, have larger nuchal crests than the female.

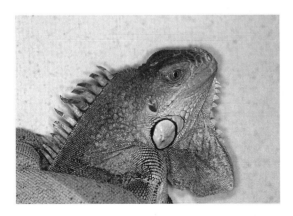

Fig. 7.8 Greater ornamentation: more spines and larger dewflaps as well as brighter colouration distinguish the male green iguana.

Many lizards, such as the green iguana have a parietal eye (Plate 7.3). This is a special adaptation on the very top of the skull midway between the eyes. It is connected directly, via neural pathways, to the pineal gland in the brain and it is responsible for informing the lizard about light intensity and daytime lengths. These in turn influence feeding and reproductive behaviour. In the tuatara, which is found in New Zealand, a primaeval lizard in its own class of the reptile family, this parietal eye actually has a vestigial lens within it.

CHELONIA (TORTOISES, TURTLES AND TERRAPINS)

Musculoskeletal system

Chelonia have a rigid upper and lower jaw structure similar to that of the lizard family, but unlike lizards they have no teeth. Instead, the maxillae and mandibles are edged with tough keratin to form a horny beak, similar to that seen in birds. The skull articulates with the atlantal cervical vertebra via a single occipital condyle, similar to birds and other reptiles. There are two strong muscles attached to the back of the chelonian skull, connecting it to the point of fusion of the cervical vertebrae with the shell. These are responsible for the retraction of the head in *Cryptodira*, those species which can pull their heads back into the shell.

There are some turtles (the side necked or *Pleurodira* turtles) which, as their name suggests, fold their head sideways into the shell, rather than fully retracting it in a craniocaudal manner. The thoracic vertebrae are fused with the dorsal shell, becoming flattened and elongated. The same is true of the lumbar and sacral vertebrae. The coccygeal vertebrae emerge distally to form the mobile tail.

Chelonia are distinguished from other animals by the presence of their shell. This structure is composed of fused *living* dermal bone covered by keratinised epidermis. It therefore can feel sensations and pain and so should never be used to tether tortoises to ropes or chains. The shell is composed of an upper section, known as the *carapace* (Fig. 7.9), and a lower, flatter ventral section, known as the *plastron* (Fig. 7.10). These two sections of the shell are connected either side between the fore- and hind limbs by the pillars of the shell. The carapace is a fusion of dermal bone, ribs, thoracic and lumbar vertebrae.

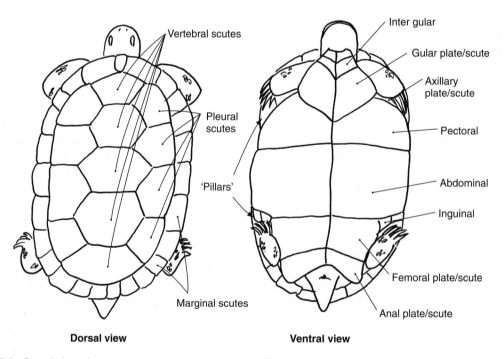

Dorsal view

Fig. 7.9   Dorsal view of carapace.

Ventral view

Fig. 7.10   Ventral view of plastron.

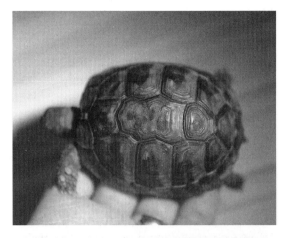

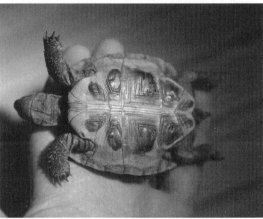

Fig. 7.11 Dorsal and ventral view of female tortoise.

The *scutes* (the individual segments of the shell epidermis) are given specific names (Fig. 7.11). They do not overlie directly the bone sections of the shell, there is some overlap. Some tortoises, such as the box turtle (*Terrapene carolina*), possess a hinge to the plastron allowing them to close themselves into their shells even further. Some of the Mediterranean species of tortoise such as the spur-thighed tortoise (*Testudo graeca*) can have caudal plastral hinges. This can be particularly useful in females, when they can increase the caudal exit space of the shell for egg laying.

Another unusual feature of Chelonia is that the scapulae are to be found on the inside of the shell, i.e. *inside* the ribcage, due to the shell structure. This is unique in the animal world. In addition the elbow joint is effectively rotated through nearly 180 degrees to cause the twisted forelimb so characteristic of tortoises.

The fore- and hind limbs are supplied with extensive muscles making them extremely strong for their size.

Respiratory system (Fig. 7.12)

Upper respiratory system

Chelonia have paired nostrils leading to the rostral portion of the oral cavity. As with other reptiles (excepting the crocodylians) there is no hard palate. The entrance to the trachea is guarded by the glottis, which, as with lizards and snakes, is closed at rest. It opens into the trachea, which has complete cartilaginous rings, and bifurcates relatively far cranially, often in the neck area, allowing the chelonian to breathe easily even when the neck is withdrawn deep into the shell.

Lower respiratory system

The two bronchi supply two lungs. These structures are situated in the dorsal aspect of the coelomic cavity against the inside of the carapace, and above the liver and digestive system. Between the lungs and the rest of the body organs there is a membrane but no true diaphragm. The lungs are sponge-like in structure and contain smooth-muscle and elastic fibres, forming essentially a non-collapsible structure. In some aquatic species the lungs have air sacs that act to increase buoyancy.

Respiration is aided by movement of the limbs and neck which act to pump the air into and out of the confined lungs. In addition, there are muscles attached to the membrane that separates the lungs from the rest of the viscera. In breathing, these contract and relax. Many chelonians can survive without breathing for several hours if necessary. The stimulus for respiration is, as with other reptiles, a fall in blood partial pressure of oxygen.

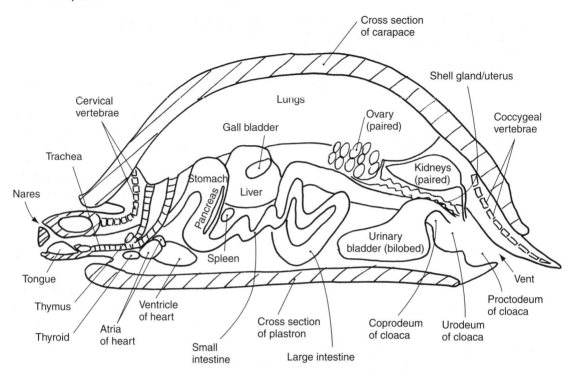

Fig. 7.12 Section through the midline of a female tortoise.

Digestive system

Oral cavity

The tongue is relatively tightly attached, but is fleshy in structure with the glottis at its base. Salivary glands secrete mucus only when eating to lubricate food. The pharynx is wide and passes into a distensible smooth-muscle covered oesophagus. Many of the aquatic turtles have caudally curved spines present in the caudal pharynx and oesophagus, which are thought to aid in swallowing slippery prey such as fish.

Stomach, associated organs and intestine

The stomach sits on the left side ventrally in the mid-coelomic cavity. It has a strong cardiac sphincter, making vomiting in the healthy chelonian rare. The stomach leads to the duodenum and a short but highly coiled small intestine. At the junction of the small and large intestine lies the

caecum which is often a rounded bag-like object. The large intestine itself has a large diameter and, for the herbivorous chelonia such as tortoises, is the principle site of fermentation. It then narrows to form the rectum. Next come the coprodeum, the urodeum and then the proctodeum of the cloaca, and finally the vent.

The liver is a bilobed structure situated transversely across the mid-section of the coelomic cavity, dorsal to the digestive system, and ventral to the lungs. There is a gall bladder to the right of the midline.

Urinary system

The paired kidneys are situated caudally within the shell, tightly adhered to the ventral surface of the inside of the carapace and caudal to the acetabulae of the pelvis. There is a difference in the marine species where the kidneys are situated cranial to the acetabulae. Two ureters empty into a urogenital sinus, a common chamber for the opening of the urinary and reproductive systems, which also connects with the urinary bladder. The latter organ is a large, bilobed, thin-walled structure which has some ability to reabsorb water. The urogenital sinus empties into the urodeum portion of the cloaca.

Cardiovascular system

Heart

As with lizards and snakes, the chelonian heart is a three-chambered organ situated within the pericardial sac. The two cranial vena cavae and one caudal vena cava merge to form the sinus venosus, which enters the right atrium.

Blood vessels

Paired aortae give rise to the carotid arteries that supply the head and neck. They then curve dorsally to fuse into the abdominal aorta. Just before fusing, the left aortic arch gives rise to arteries supplying the digestive tract, and the right aortic arch produces the brachiocephalic trunk that supplies the head and forelimbs. The abdominal aorta then courses down the ventral aspect of the vertebrae, supplying the shell and dorsal structures via intercostal arteries. The shell itself has a blood supply arising from cranially placed subclavian and caudally placed iliac arteries which anastomose widely.

The venous return of blood follows a similar pattern to lizards and snakes. Another bypass system exists whereby blood from the caudal vessels may cross from one side of the body to the other via transverse pelvic veins. From these, the blood may enter the paired abdominal veins which run along the floor of the ceolomic cavity. It is these latter vessels which must be carefully negotiated when performing abdominal surgery in chelonians.

Lymphatic system

The lymphatic system is essentially the same as in the snake and the lizard. The spleen is situated close to the caecum.

Reproductive system

Male

The testes are internal and often yellow cream coloured oval organs cranial to the kidneys. As with the liver, there may also be some dark pigmentation to the testes. The testes empty into the associated epididymal organs that overlie their surface. The sperm then enter the vas deferens, which courses over the ventral surface of the kidneys, and enters the urogenital sinus adjacent to the urodeum portion of the cloaca.

The phallus is a large fleshy organ, and, unlike snakes and lizards, there is only one of them. It lies on the ventral aspect of the cloaca at rest. When engorged, the free caudal end of the phallus is projected through the vent and curves cranially. In so doing a dorsal shallow seminal groove is formed to guide sperm into the female's vent.

Female

Paired ovaries are suspended from the mid-dorsal aspect of the coelomic cavity. They shed their ova into the infundibulum portion of the oviduct. This is connected to similar structures as in the snake and lizard families, including a magnum and a uterus. This finally connects to the smooth-muscle lined vagina which is responsible for keeping the oviduct closed to the outside world until egg laying occurs. The oviducts empty into the urogenital sinus and then into the urodeum portion of the cloaca.

Reproductive physiology

Folliculogenesis is stimulated by the time of year. In those chelonians such as the Mediterranean species of tortoise, hibernation is an important factor. This period is necessary for the preprogramming of the thyroid gland and the reproductive cycle. Two bouts of egg production can occur per year. On average 10–30 eggs are laid each year, depending on the species. Most Mediterranean tortoise species do not become sexually mature until they are 7–10 years of age.

The female tortoise will start to form fertile eggs after a successful mating. These are carried in her reproductive system for a period of time varying anywhere from 4 weeks to 3–4 years which means that it is possible for Mediterranean species to carry eggs through hibernation. The female can also store the sperm from a successful mating for long periods of time, eventually allowing fertilisation to occur many months to years after exposure to the male, a factor which makes identification of the father sometimes rather difficult!

Sex determination and identification

As with many reptiles, tortoise sex determination depends on the temperature at which the eggs were incubated. Spur-thighed tortoises (*Testudo graeca*) will produce males if the eggs are kept at 29.5°C and females if kept at 31.5°C. It seems that this fact can be applied to a large number of other tortoise species, with males being predominantly produced at the lower temperatures, and females at the higher ones. If the temperature range is kept from 28–31°C, a mixture of sexes is likely to be achieved.

Male Chelonia have longer tails, the vent being found on the tail caudal to the edge of the carapace, in order to house the single phallus. Males of many Mediterranean species of tortoise and turtles possess a dished plastron, and a narrower angle to the caudal plastron in front of the cloaca than the egg bearing female. Some female Mediterranean species have a hinge to the caudal part of the plastron to allow easier egg laying. The male of the box turtle (*Terrapene carolina*) has red coloured irises whereas the female has yellow/brown ones. The female leopard (*Geochelone pardalis*) and Indian starred tortoises (*Geochelone elegans*) have longer hind limb claws for digging than the males. The male red-eared terrapin (*Trachemys scripta elegans*), has longer forelimb claws than the females. Some males, such as the Horsfield's tortoise (*Testudo horsefieldii*), have a large, hooked scale at the tip of their tails. In some species there is a size difference between the sexes, the female of the Indian starred tortoise and the red-eared terrapin species is larger than the male when full grown, but the reverse is true of the red-footed tortoise (*Geochelone carbonaria*).

Skin

The skin covering the head, neck, limbs and tail of the chelonian is much the same as that of snakes and lizards. Many species of tortoise have enlarged scales over their forelimbs, and some have horny spurs on their hind limbs. The skin is particularly tightly adhered to the underlying bony structures over the distal limbs and the head.

Tortoises and most other Chelonia have visible auditory membranes covering the entrance to the middle ear. These lie caudoventral to the eyes at the rear of the skull.

The shell is formed from the fusion of islands of bone produced within the chelonian's dermal layer the skin, rather than from the limbs or ribs. The overlying epidermis is highly keratinised and pigmented. The lines joining individual scutes on the shell are not directly above the corresponding suture lines in the bony part of the shell. There is some considerable overlap which reinforces the structure.

CROCODYLIA (CROCODILES, ALLIGATORS, CAIMANS, AND GHARIALS)

Musculoskeletal system

The body plan for the Crocodylia is not dissimilar to that of the Sauria. The basic structure is a quadruped reptile, with an elongated tail, but instead of the short- to medium-length head, the crocodylians have elongated jaws. This is particularly accentuated in the long thin jaws of the fish eating gharial family.

The teeth are continually replaced and are held in crude sockets. One of the distinguishing features between the more bad-tempered crocodiles and the alligator family is that the fourth mandibular tooth on either side is visible in the crocodiles. In the alligator subfamily the tooth is hidden in a maxillary pocket.

The articulation point of the upper and lower jaws is located at the rear of the skull, giving more room for teeth and allowing a larger gape. The jaws are powered by strong temporal and pterygoid muscles, allowing immense crushing forces to be applied. Interestingly though, the muscles responsible for opening the jaws are relatively weak, hence once closed and taped shut a crocodilian cannot easily open its mouth again.

There are eight pairs of ribs arising from the thoracic vertebrae, with additional dermal bones embedded in the ventral body wall known as *gastralia* or floating ribs. There are also thickened transverse processes of the sacral vertebrae which float freely alongside the respective vertebral bodies and have also been called ribs. The femur is proportionally longer than that of the saurians, leading to a raised appearance to the crocodylian hindquarters.

Respiratory system

Upper respiratory system

The nares of the Crocodylia are frequently protected by lateral skin flaps which can be contracted medially to close them when submerged. The nasal passages have excellent neural endings in the ethmoid/olfactory chamber area allowing an acute sense of smell. The crocodiles have a true hard palate that separates the oral and nasal passages. The internal nostrils open caudally, therefore the glottis guarding the trachea is also situated caudally.

The entrance to the larynx is guarded by the glottis but also by gular and a basihylar fold which originate in, respectively, the floor and roof of the oropharynx and can close access to the glottis from the mouth when a crocodilian is submerged. This allows them to drag prey underwater at the same time preventing any water from entering the caudal aspect of the pharynx. Providing its nostrils are above water, the crocodilian can still draw air in through the nasal passages.

The trachea is composed of complete cartilage rings, similar to Chelonia and birds.

Lower respiratory system

The trachea bifurcates within the 'chest' into two primary bronchi, each supplying a well-formed lung structure. The lungs are basic in design, and do not contain well-defined lobules, as do their mammalian counterparts, although they are very well vascularised. There are air sacs more caudally which can be inflated to provide some buoyancy. More importantly, they can function as a gas reserve, allowing them to remain submerged for up to 1–2 hours before anaerobic respiration takes over. The lungs are also different from other reptiles in that there is a muscular, crude diaphragmatic structure separating the dorsally-situated lung fields from the ventrally-situated heart and digestive system. The diaphragm as well as the intercostal muscles are important for respiration in crocodylians.

Digestive system

Oral cavity

The crocodylian tongue is large and fleshy, but immobile. Caudally, the floor of the mouth forms a transverse fold, as does the palate above. This shuts the oropharynx off completely from the glottis and nasopharynx.

Stomach, associated organs and intestines

The crocodilian stomach is large and divided into two areas, known as the *body* and the *pars pylorus*. The body area is heavily populated by mucus-secreting glands and surrounded by a thick band of smooth muscle. It is in this area that stones swallowed by the crocodilian may be found, and therefore this area seems to be responsible for grinding and massaging food into smaller pieces, similar to the action of the avian gizzard. The pars pylorus has acid and pepsin secreting glands and empties into the small intestine through the well-developed pyloric sphincter.

The small intestine meets the large intestine at the ileocaecal sphincter. The large intestine empties into the coprodeum portion of the cloaca, which opens into the urodeum, then the proctodeum before ending at the vent to the outside world.

Urinary system

There are paired kidneys located in the caudal abdomen, and extending into the pelvis. The aquatic crocodile kidney excretes waste protein nitrogen as ammonia rather than as the more usual reptilian uric acid, although the latter can also be produced, particularly when the animal is dehydrated. Osmoregulation, the maintenance of the electrolyte and water balance within the body, is not solely performed by the kidneys, as with many other reptiles. Instead, there are salt-secreting glands in the mouth which aid excretion of excess sodium as sodium chloride. There are no truly marine crocodilians, although the salt water crocodile and the American crocodile will spend time in brackish water and will venture out into the sea.

The oral salt-secreting glands of the alligator subfamily are not as highly developed, reflecting their more freshwater habitat. The kidneys empty through the ureters which travel into the urodeum portion of the cloaca.

Cardiovascular system

Heart

The crocodilian heart is different from that of other reptiles in that it has four chambers, similar to the mammalian model. There is however a small 'hole in the heart' between the two ventricles, known as the *foramen of Panizza*, which allows some mixing of oxygenated and deoxygenated blood.

The rate of mixing is dependent on the pressures within the left and right ventricles. While the animal is breathing, the left ventricle has higher pressure and so blood moves from the oxygenated side to the deoxygenated side. More important for the crocodilian is what happens when he is submerged and not breathing. The increased pulmonary resistance so produced forces blood from the right ventricle to the left and out through the abdominal aorta, decreasing the blood flow to the non-functional lungs and sending it back around the body. The left ventricle blood, still returning from the lungs and so still relatively well oxy-genated, is diverted through the brachicephalic trunk to the head and heart muscle which need more oxygen to keep functioning. This allows the crocodilian to function in conditions of reduced oxygen and anaerobic metabolism for up to 6 hours!

Blood vessels

The basic structure of the blood vascular system is similar to the lizard's. There are paired aortae from the right and left ventricles which fuse to form a single abdominal aorta after giving off the brachicephalic trunk which supplies the head and forelimbs.

The venous system has many parallels with the Sauria. There is an hepatoportal system supplying the liver directly from the intestines and a renal-portal system wherein the blood returning from the hind limbs and tail enters a venous circle around the kidneys.

There is a large venous sinus caudal to the occiput of the skull on either side of the midline which may be used for venipuncture. Alternatively, the ventral tail vein may be used for blood sampling purposes.

Lymphatic system

The lymphatic system parallels the saurian system.

Reproductive system

Male

The testes are long, thin organs situated medial to their respective kidneys either side of the caudal vena cava. The vasa deferentia travel to the urodeum portion of the cloaca. The testes enlarge during the reproductive season.

On the ventral aspect of the cloaca lies the phallus. This is a fibrous organ which has little erectile tissue, but once everted forms a dorsal groove into which the semen is deposited. There are two accessory ducts entering this groove which supply seminal fluids from the caudal kidney area.

Female

The paired ovaries are also to be found medial to their respective kidneys. Each ovary is slightly flattened and has a central medullary area which is supplied with nerves and blood vessels. The rest of the reproductive system consists of the fimbria or ostium which catches the ova, then there is a muscular portion followed by the isthmus and the shell gland or uterus. The paired oviducts open into the urodeum of the cloaca, adjacent to the clitoris.

Reproductive physiology

Follicular activity is triggered by increasing day length in March–May, there being one cycle per year. An average clutch of follicles varies from 20–80 per cycle.

Sex determination and identification

This varies with species. In the case of alligators and caimans, the lower incubation temperatures (from 28–31°C) produce all females. An intermediate temperature (from 31–32°C) produces males and females and a higher temperature (from 32–34°C) produces all males. In the case of crocodiles, temperatures at the lower end of the range (from 28–31°C) also produce all females. Intermediate temperatures (from 31–33°C) produce some females but a predominance of males. For higher temperatures (from 33–34°C), predominantly female crocodiles, with some males, are produced.

The best method of sex identification is by manual palpation of the ventral surface of the cloaca for the presence of the phallus. This is an obvious structure if present, as otherwise the cloaca is completely smooth walled. The crocodilian involved must be in dorsal recumbency and adequately restrained in order to perform this!

Skin

The epidermis and dermis of Crocodylia is composed of thickened scales which are joined together like a patchwork quilt by elastic tissue.

The skin is tightly attached to underlying bone over the feet and the skull. The skin covering the dorsum has layers of dermal bone present within it, making this area extremely thick and impossible to penetrate for injections. The caimans have areas of bone in the skin covering their ventral surface as well.

Specialised skin areas

Within the majority of the scales of the crocodile subfamily are present *integumentory sense organs* (ISO). These are absent in the alligator subfamily. Their function is to determine underwater pressure sensations which can be used to locate prey whilst submerged.

Overview of reptilian haematology

The cells found in the reptilian bloodstream broadly mirror those seen in mammals. There are however a few important differences:

- The reptilian (and amphibian) erythrocyte is oval in shape rather than biconcave and has a nucleus even when fully matured.
- The reptile, like the avian patient, has a slightly different version of the mammalian neutrophil, known as the *heterophil*. This white blood cell has a bilobed nucleus, like the neutrophil, and contains cytoplasmic granules, but these stain a variety of colours with Romanowsky stains, rather than remaining neutral as seen in neutrophils. The heterophil performs similar functions to the neutrophil, being a first line of defence for infection. However, although its numbers *may* be increased during infections, they may stay the same, in which case the only tell-tale sign of an inflammatory process occurring is vacuolation and degranulation of the cell (the so-called 'toxic' cell). This makes cytological examination more important than cell counts in reptiles.
- An additional mononuclear cell is the *azurophil*. It stains a blue red colour and is a large, single nucleated cell with moderate cytoplasm present. It is found normally in small

numbers, but if elevated in lizards and chelonia, it suggests an inflammatory/infectious process. It is particularly associated with chronic granuloma formation.

- Eosinophils and basophils are present in most species, basophils being common in turtles. Basophils generally stain blue, and are small spherical cells with a non-lobed nucleus. The eosinophil is a larger spherical cell with eosinophilic cytoplasmic granules and a mildly-lobed to elongated nucleus. However, in the green iguana they often stain blue!
- Lymphocytes may vary with the season showing a decrease in the 'winter'/colder months in tropical species. Unlike mammals, the B-lymphocyte can change into the plasma cell form within the bloodstream during chronic or severe infections of reptiles. Hence, the eccentrically placed nucleus and pale staining 'clock-face' cytoplasm of the plasma cell may be seen in blood smears of reptiles.
- The thrombocytes (platelets) of reptiles, like avian species, are also nucleated.

Most importantly, when collecting blood samples from reptiles, it is better to do so into heparinised containers for haematology, rather than potassium EDTA tubes used in birds and mammals. This is because the blood cells, particularly erythrocytes, of many species (particularly the Chelonia) will rupture in potassium EDTA. An air-dried smear for staining made at the time of sampling is also useful, as heparin interferes with the Romanowsky stains.

AMPHIBIANS

Musculoskeletal system

The body plan of amphibia in general varies greatly within the family from the classic lizard shape of the salamanders and newts, through to the tail-less quadruped form of the anurans (frogs and toads) through to the worm-like caecilians.

In the case of the anurans and the salamanders, the skeletal structure is very basic but similar to the saurian model described above. The main differences lie in the anurans which have long femurs, tibias and fibulas, and metatarsals which are developed into the well-muscled hind limbs. There is a basic spinal column of cuboid vertebral bodies joining to the primitive pelvis caudally and the single occipital condyle of the skull cranially.

The skull possesses a mandible and maxilla with, in many cases, simple peg-like, open-rooted and continually replaced teeth. The eye sockets are large in anurans, as is the well developed eardrum that leads to the middle ear. Sight is mainly based on movement rather than sharp focus, but the sense of hearing is very good, although low frequency sounds are transmitted through the bones of the forelimbs, and high frequency ones through the actual eardrum.

The majority of anurans have five digits on the forelimbs and four on the hind limbs. Many salamanders and newts have four digits on their forelimbs and four or five digits on their hind limbs. Many salamanders will show autotomy or tail shedding when roughly handled as with many saurians.

Many amphibians possess vestigial rib structures, and the majority also have a sternum. The pectoral and pelvic girdles are fused to the spine, giving increased rigidity to the body structure.

The caecilians have a much simpler body plan with few if any bones. Their body plan is more worm-like, although they are amphibians rather than insects, but they do possess jaws, a primitive skull and a fibrocartilaginous spinal column. They also have small eyes and nostrils in the head.

Respiratory system

In aquatic amphibians such as the primitive *axolotl*, gills are still present. Indeed, as an amphibian metamorphoses through from egg to larval or tadpole form it will also have gills, although these may be lost as the adult form is reached.

Terrestrial amphibians, such as many of the anurans, have an internal lung structure. This is often no more than a simple air sac structure. There are no internal alveolar areas to this lung, although it may be folded to increase its surface area. No diaphragm is present, giving a continuous body cavity or coelom, hence respiration for those amphibians possessing lungs occurs due to intercostal muscle and limb movements pulling the chest wall up and outwards.

Many amphibians will use the skin surface for gaseous exchange, whether they possess an internal lung structure or not. Indeed the skin is often solely used for gas exchange during periods of low oxygen requirement, such as during hibernation. For other skin breathers, such as the plethodontid salamanders, other adaptations, such as increasing the skin's surface area by having folds of skin, or by having 'hairs' on their surface (for example, the African hairy frog), or reducing oxygen demands/metabolic rates, are necessary.

Digestive system

Most adult amphibians are carnivorous, and their digestive systems are adapted to this diet. The majority possess a tongue which can be projected at high speed towards their prey. It is covered in fine sticky cilia, as in many anurans, enabling it to capture flying prey. The salamanders, newts and most anurans have vestigial peg-like teeth. There are frequently cilia within the oral cavity and oesophagus, which aid in the propelling of food into the stomach. Terrestrial amphibians also have mucus-secreting salivary glands to aid in the swallowing of prey.

The stomach is simple in nature, possesses mucus-secreting glands and, in the majority of cases, combined acid- and pepsinogen-secreting glands. The small intestine is short, and little defines its finish and the start of the rectum which empties into the cloaca.

The liver is frequently dark coloured due to melanin pigmentation for protection from ultraviolet light, necessary due to the thin nature of amphibian skin.

Urinary system

As with the reptile family, amphibians cannot concentrate urine beyond plasma tonicity. The main excretory product of aquatic amphibians such as caecilians and aquatic newts and the axolotl, is ammonia. This is actually excreted, as with fish, through the gills if present, and the skin if not, rather than the kidneys.

In terrestrial amphibians, urea is the main waste product of nitrogen metabolism and this is excreted through a primitive paired kidney structure. The cloaca of these species (chiefly the anuran toad family) may also have a pocket forming a primitive bladder. One or two amphibians can produce uric acid. The kidneys empty into ureters which travel to the urodeum portion of the cloaca, before either refluxing into the bladder (if present) or emptying through the vent.

Cardiovascular system

Heart

The circulatory system changes dramatically during the metamorphosis of the amphibian. At the larval stage the circulatory system is more fish-like, with a two chambered heart possessing only one atrium and one ventricle. When the adult form is achieved the heart has divided itself into three chambers by producing an intra-atrial septum, and also rerouted its circulation away from the gill arches of the larvae to the adult respiration organ (the skin, lungs or again gill arches).

Blood vessels

As far as the more peripheral vascular system is concerned, the amphibians differ from the reptiles in that the caudal body drainage goes through the hepatic portal system rather than the renal portal system. This is important for the administration of hepatically metabolised drugs or hepatotoxic drugs in the caudal half of an amphibian.

Lymphatic system

There is a large lymphatic drainage system, with paired dorsal lymph sacs in anurans lying cranial to the hind limbs laterodorsally. These help propel lymph fluid as well as draining it via lymph hearts back to the true heart. They may also play a role in electrolyte balance through the skin overlying them.

Reproductive system

There are paired internal testes or ovaries depending on the sex. There is some variation in the size of the gonads during the reproductive season, and basic hormones resembling the activity of FSH and LH are produced.

In the female there are paired oviducts which are responsible for producing the jellylike material that coats the ova. Most amphibians fertilise their eggs outside the body, but one or two species of anuran, and the caecilians, do have a form of phallus for internal fertilisation. Indeed some caecilians are viviparous and actually secrete a uterine milk to nourish the foetuses within the oviduct.

When hatched, the amphibian then metamorphoses through a series of changes, often known as *instars*, one of which we all know as the 'tadpole' of the anurans which has external gills and a tail and no legs initially. The stimuli for the metamorphosis seem to come from various external sources, such as environmental iodine levels, as well as internal hormonal influences from the thyroid gland.

Skin

The terrestrial amphibian has a thin stratum corneum which provides extra cutaneous protection above that seen in aquatic species. It also reduces water loss from the skin. The skin is shed regularly, similarly to a snake, and is frequently then eaten by the amphibian. The skin contains many glands which secrete oils and mucus in to further protect against water loss, but amphibians always have to have access to damp conditions or free water to survive.

Many of the toad family have poison glands located in their parotid glands which are used as a form of protection. A similar ploy is used in the poison arrow tree frogs which secrete neurotoxins onto the surface of their skin.

Some anurans, such as the midwife toad *Xenopus laevis*, have claws, but most have very fragile skin, which, as mentioned above, may have gas exchange as well as water and electrolyte exchange capabilities.

Some male amphibians can be identified by skin colour or ornamentation. The male great crested newt has a larger crest than the female, for example, and many male frogs and toads have a swelling in the 'thumb' area of the hand which contains scent glands. Male caecilians often have a phallus in the cloaca.

Chapter 8

Reptile and Amphibian Housing, Husbandry and Rearing

There are many good books available on the husbandry of reptiles and amphibians, and some are listed at the end of this chapter. This chapter will therefore provide only a brief overview of the main points in housing and caring for reptiles and amphibians.

Vivarium requirements

Dimensions and construction

Vivarium designs vary, as does their construction material. The main aim though is to ensure that they are durable, easily cleaned for hygiene reasons and that they provide enough space for the captive reptile to demonstrate normal behaviour (Plate 8.1). Strict cage dimensions are therefore difficult to quantify, as each situation should be judged on its own merits. However some general principles apply (Fig. 8.1).

For species which are more arboreal (tree climbing) in nature, such as the green iguana, and many snakes, such as the boa constrictor and Burmese python, the emphasis in cage design should be more on vertical height rather than horizontal space. For species such as the tortoise family however, the provision of too much vertical space is pointless, as they are not renowned for their tree-climbing tendencies! Horizontal space is thus more important.

Cage materials commonly used include perspex, reinforced glass and fibreglass (Figs 8.2 and 8.3). Wood should be avoided unless it is sealed to prevent moisture damage and rotting. Glass and clear perspex are useful when showing off a collection, but care should be taken as many reptiles cannot see the tank sides, and so may continually rub their snouts along the inside of

the vivarium, causing severe abrasions which can become infected. Often the provision of a tape strip on the outside of the glass at reptile level allows them to appreciate that a barrier exists and prevents this problem.

Heating

Reptiles are ectothermic by nature – that is they rely on the environment to provide sufficient heat to warm them to their *preferred body temperature* (PBT). To do this the reptile must be provided with a preferred optimum temperature zone (POTZ) within which it may position itself in order to maintain its PBT. This necessitates the provision of some form of artificial heating within the tank, or vivarium, as it is more commonly known.

Two main forms of heating are advised. A background, continuous heat source is important to raise the vivarium temperature above the background room temperature. This is often provided in the form of a radiant heat mat. This is a mat which emits heat continuously, and is placed on the *outside* of the vivarium, usually on the back wall of the tank (Fig. 8.1). It then radiates heat through the tank wall. Placing it on the outside of the tank avoids the possibility of the reptile chewing, urinating or defaecating on it, so increasing hygiene and safety. The size of the available mats vary, but in general a rough rule is that one third to one half of the longest side of the tank should be covered with the mat. Some form of insulation on the outside of the mat, increasing reflection of heat into the vivarium, is also useful.

In addition, the vivarium requires a focal hot spot, which may be provided in the form of a ceramic or infra-red heat bulb. This should be suspended from the ceiling of the vivarium, and should be protected from the reptile to avoid the

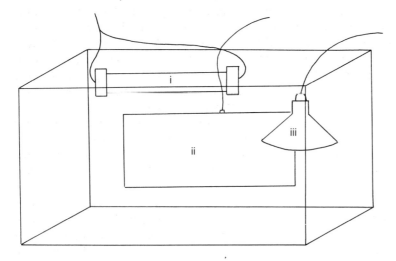

Fig. 8.1 Basic diagrammatic representation of a vivarium: (i) ultraviolet light source (on inside of tank as glass filters out UV light); (ii) radiant heat mat, usually placed on outside of tank for hygiene reasons; (iii) focal heat source such as a heat lamp to provide a temperature gradient.

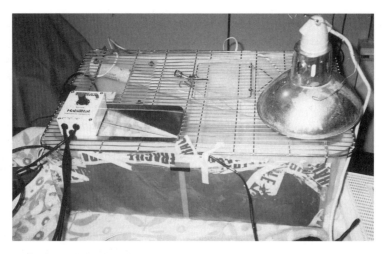

Fig. 8.2 Basic layout of traditional plastic tank.

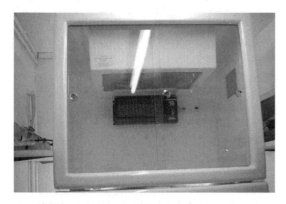

Fig. 8.3 More sophisticated tank system made of moulded fibreglass.

risk of burns. The bulb should be attached to the mains via a thermostat, which will allow maximum and minimum tank temperatures to be set. The importance of a focal heat source is that it provides a temperature gradient, allowing the reptile to bask underneath the heat source or to escape to a cooler end of the tank when overheated. The reptile can then maintain its PBT by positioning itself at different points in the tank during the course of the day.

The temperatures required for different species of reptile will naturally differ depending on the part of the world from which they originate. Mediterranean tortoises may cope adequately outside in the warmer British summers, but leopard geckos will require more desert-like temperatures for normal homeostasis systems to work properly. A list of some species and their temperature requirements is given in Table 8.1.

Humidity

Humidity can also be important. Many species of reptile come from dry desert regions, but equally many originate in tropical rain forests. Therefore their tolerance of water moisture in their environment will vary. A water dragon, basilisk or garter snake, all used to living near or in water, will require a 75–90% humidity level. This may be difficult to maintain in a heated environment, as the hotter the air the more water droplets the air can hold, and so the relative humidity levels drop. Thus, spraying the enclosures frequently, using a hand-held plant mister, with previously boiled and then cooled water is useful. Alternatively, the provision of water baths, or damp substrate within the tank can be used to increase humidity. Care should be taken over hygiene levels though, as a too damp and soiled substrate can lead to skin infections such as blister disease, a common problem in garter snakes. In the case of reptiles from more arid climates, such as the Mediterranean tortoises, leopard geckos and bearded dragons, a relative humidity of between 25–50% is often adequate. This is around the normal level of the average centrally heated home.

Lighting

Lighting is particularly important for the growing juveniles of many species. In the wild, many of these reptiles live in parts of the world where the intensity of the sun's ultraviolet rays is high. These ultraviolet rays stimulate a number of functions in the reptile, often encouraging mating at certain times of year, and may act as a general appetite stimulus. This seems to be the role of the A section of the ultraviolet waveband.

The B waveband of the ultraviolet spectrum is important in all species in encouraging the production of vitamin D_3 from precursors in the reptile's skin. Vitamin D_3 is intimately involved in the metabolism of calcium and bone growth within the juvenile reptile. A lack of ultraviolet light therefore can be responsible for the presence of metabolic bone disease in several species, particularly the green iguana and the Mediterranean tortoises (see section on reptile and amphibian diseases p. 171).

Artificial ultraviolet lighting is therefore important in these species, and should be provided on the *inside* of the vivarium. This is because glass and perspex will filter out the UV rays if the light is placed on the outside of the tank. In addition, the light source should be positioned close to the reptile, i.e. within 30–45 cm. This is because the intensity of these artificial lights is relatively low, and the inverse square rule tells us that the intensity of the light diminishes with the square of the distance from its source (e.g. the intensity at 2 m from the source is a quarter of that 1 m from its source).

Some species are not so susceptible to ultraviolet deprivation, including more nocturnal species such as the leopard gecko and many snakes. The theory is that these species gain sufficient preformed vitamin D_3 in their diets to cope. This is important if the owner is not feeding them correctly, as metabolic bone disease may then be seen.

Cage 'furniture' and environmental enrichment

Many reptiles are relatively poorly adapted to captivity, being wild animals in a confined space, and so it is important to ensure that their environment adequately caters for their requirements.

As previously mentioned, many arboreal species, such as the green iguana and members of

Table 8.1 Preferred optimum temperature zones for selected species of reptile.

Species	Temperature range (°C)
Mediterranean tortoises	20–27
Green iguana	25–32
Leopard gecko	25–34
Water dragon	24–30
Bearded dragon	25–32
Corn snake	23–30
Burmese python	25–30

the python family, enjoy exploring vertical space. They should therefore be provided with branches and ramps up which they may climb. It is often useful to provide an elevated basking spot which they can lie out on near to the focal heat source.

In the case of ground-dwelling species, the provision of some form of floor furniture is important. Tortoises are in general best kept singly, except when breeding of course, or in the case of small hatchlings which prefer to be in groups. In these cases the provision of visual barricades which they can hide behind and so get out of view of one another is useful.

All reptiles should be provided with a hide. This is an area to which they can escape to digest food in peace, and to escape the view of other reptiles, predators and nosey humans! This is important particularly for many snakes which will often refuse to eat their prey in the open, but rather prefer to take it back into the hide area away from view. The size of these areas does not need to be that large, in the case of most species a space 2–2.5 × the size of the reptile housed is sufficient.

Flooring

The substrate of the vivarium, or floor covering, is important. It is vital that any substrate used is non-toxic to the reptiles housed and is easily cleaned. In many cases the provision of newspaper, or unbleached household paper is perfectly sufficient, although possibly not so aesthetically pleasing, as more naturalistic substrates. Care should be taken with smaller reptiles with newspaper, as the ink from the newsprint may prove irritant.

Other substrates used commonly include bark chippings, sand, coral and peat. Bark chippings are a good choice for deep litter situations, particularly when providing enough substrate for a pregnant female to dig a nest in which to lay eggs. However, the chips should not be of cedar as the resins from this can be irritant. It is also more difficult to monitor the cleanliness of bark chippings as faeces and urine may fall into the substrate and so avoid detection.

Sand is useful for desert species such as leopard geckos, collared lizards, sand boas etc., but care should be taken with any reptile on this substrate as if the diet contains mineral deficiencies, or there is intestinal parastism present, many species will consume the sand and may suffer intestinal blockages.

Peat can be useful for species requiring damper conditions such as water dragons, red-footed tortoises etc., but care again should be taken with the hygiene of this substrate, as waste materials may build up unnoticed. Coral is not advised as a substrate for ecological reasons as well as the tendency for reptiles to eat the substrate and suffer gut impactions.

Aquatic species and amphibians

Species requiring fresh water to bathe or live in include all amphibians, red-eared terrapins, soft-shelled turtles, water and garter snakes. Some, such as the terrapins and turtles, require large areas of free water, some, such as frogs and toads, a small area but damp environmental conditions (Fig. 8.4).

In the case of freshwater species, tap water may be used, but it should be conditioned first, that is the water must first be dechlorinated. This may be done by standing it in an open container for 24 hours prior to use or by using any commercial dechlorinating tablets available from aquarists. In addition, the tap water should be allowed to come up to room temperature before being introduced to avoid cold shocking the reptile or amphibian.

Where large areas of water are provided, it is important to keep them clean. It is advisable for terrapins and soft-shelled turtles that their habitat provides an area in which they can immerse themselves completely in water, and an area into which they can pull themselves out to bask and dry themselves off, preferably with a focal heat source above it. It is often advisable to remove them from the water and place them in a separate dry or water-containing feeding tank. This is because they are extremely messy eaters and will quickly contaminate their water with food. The food acts as a substrate for bacteria, and this can increase the risk of shell infections and septicaemia. An alternative would be a powerful water filtration device placed in the tank to cope with the large volumes of organic debris produced. Even if a

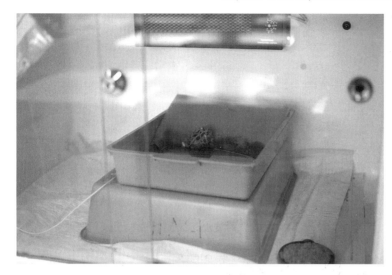

Fig. 8.4 Example of hospital tank provision for an amphibian, in this case an Argentinian horned frog.

feeding tank is provided, regular water changes or filtration is required, as they will of course still urinate and defaecate in their water.

Many anurids, such as White's tree frogs and fire-bellied toads, will appreciate a small amount of free water, but the rest of their vivarium should be well-supplied with moisture-retaining substrate such as mosses or peat substitute mulches. These retain moisture and increase the humidity of the tank, ensuring protection of the sensitive amphibian's skin. Other amphibians, such as newts and salamanders, require more access to free fresh water and precautions similar to those mentioned for freshwater turtles and terrapins should be taken. In addition, for all these species, the construction of the vivarium should ensure that it is waterproof!

Egg incubation of reptiles

It is necessary for successful egg incubation to use an incubator. The basic components of a reptile egg incubator are as follows: the basic requirement is for a plastic, perspex or toughened glass tank, with a plastic lid containing aeration holes that can be covered to regulate humidity and temperature. Nesting substrate is placed into small open containers within the above tank, and the eggs are placed in slight depressions within the substrate. A useful substrate is the loft insulating

material vermiculite. Alternatives include damp sand, sphagnum moss or even peat. When the eggs are retrieved from the nest site particular care should be taken to maintain the same position of the egg in the incubator. The eggs should not be turned or touched during the incubation process as this can cause significant foetal mortality.

The tank requires a source of humidity and heat production. There are two methods for providing these. The containers containing the eggs and substrate may be placed onto a wire mesh which divides the tank into a top and a bottom compartment. The bottom compartment may then be three quarters filled with filtered water, and a thermostatically controlled water heater placed into it. This technique will provide heat and moisture, and is good for the higher-moisture-requiring species, such as the water or garter snakes which need an average 80% humidity.

An alternative set-up is to attach a thermostatically-controlled radiant heat mat to the outside of the tank. The tank is then completely filled with the substrate, which is kept moist by regular misting with a plant sprayer, and by placing shallow containers of filtered and previously boiled water in amongst the eggs. This provides a drier atmosphere, more suitable for the desert dwelling species.

Care should be taken not to allow the humidity to drop below 50%, as reptile eggs are porous and excessively dry conditions will dehydrate the foetus inside and lead to high levels of mortality. Equally, excessive levels of humidity will lead to an increased risk of fungal infection of the shell and contents and again higher mortality rates. It is therefore important to have both a thermometer and a humidity gauge within the incubator, and both should be monitored regularly.

Temperatures for incubation of reptile eggs vary from 26–32°C with an average incubation period in snakes of 45–70 days. Incubation periods vary from 45–70 days in smaller lizards to 90–130 days for iguanas and larger lizards.

For chelonians, the colder, northerly climes of the United Kingdom mean the incubation of eggs in an outside environment is not possible because of the high incubation temperatures required. It is therefore necessary to remove the eggs from wherever they have been laid by the female and transfer them to a purpose-built incubator for hatching. Once laid the eggs will hatch for most tortoise species in 8–12 weeks depending on the temperature at which they are incubated.

Further reading

Beynon, P.H., Lawton, M.P.C. and Cooper, J.E., eds (1992) *Manual of Reptiles*. BSAVA, Cheltenham.

Cooper, J.E. and Jackson, O.F., eds (1981) *Diseases of the Reptilia, Volumes 1 and 2*. Academic Press Ltd., London.

Frye, F. (1991) *Biomedical and Surgical Aspects of Captive Reptile Husbandry, Volume 1 and 2*. Kreigar Publishing, Malabar, Florida.

Mader, D., ed (1996) *Reptile Medicine and Surgery*. W.B. Saunders, Philadelphia.

Chapter 9

Reptile and Amphibian Handling and Chemical Restraint

Handling the reptilian patient

Is there a need to restrain the reptilian patient?

Reptiles are less easily stressed than their avian cousins, and so restraint may be performed without as much risk in the case of the debilitated animal. However, it is still worthwhile considering factors that may make restraint dangerous to animal and nurse alike.

- Is the patient in respiratory distress? For example, consider pneumonic cases, where mouth breathing and excessive oral mucus may be present and where excessive manual manipulation can be dangerous.
- Is the species of reptile a fragile one? Day geckos are extremely delicate and prone to shedding their tails when handled. Similarly some species such as green iguanas are prone to conditions such as metabolic bone disease wherein their skeleton becomes fragile and spontaneous fractures occur.
- Is the species an aggressive one? Some are naturally so, e.g. snapping turtles, tokay geckos and rock pythons.
- Does the reptile patient require medication or physical examination, in which case restraint is essential.

It should be noted that many species of reptile have a normal bacterial flora in their digestive systems which frequently includes species such as the Salmonella family. These bacteria are found in abundance all over the body of the reptile. Personal hygiene is therefore very important when handling these patients to prevent zoonotic diseases.

The need for restraint therefore needs to be considered carefully before physical attempts are made.

Techniques and equipment involved in restraining reptile patients

Because of the variety of reptile species and their diversity, this section is easier considered under specific Orders of reptile.

Sauria

This Order includes the members of the lizard family such as geckos, iguanas, chameleons and agamas.

Lizards come in many different shapes and sizes, from the four-foot-long adult green iguana to the 4–5 inch-long green anole. They all have the same structural format, with four limbs (although these may be vestigial in the case of the slow-worm for example) and a tail. Their main danger areas to the handler are their claws and teeth, and in some species, such as iguanas, their tails – which can lash out in a whip-like fashion.

Geckos other than tokay geckos are generally docile as are lizards such as bearded dragons. Others, such as green iguanas, may be extremely aggressive, particularly sexually mature males. They may also be more aggressive towards female owners and handlers as they are able to detect pheromones secreted during the menstrual cycle.

They are best restrained by grasping around the shoulders (the pectoral girdle) with one hand, from the dorsal aspect, so controlling one fore-limb with forefinger and the thumb and the other between middle and fourth finger. The other hand is used to grasp the pelvic girdle from the dorsal aspect, controlling one limb with the thumb and forefinger, the other again between middle and fourth finger. The handler may then hold

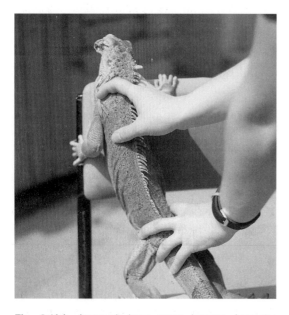

Fig. 9.1(a) Approach large green iguanas from the dorsal aspect with two hands, one over the shoulder area and one over the pelvic area.

the lizard in a vertical manner, with head uppermost, placing the tail underneath his or her arm (Figs 9.1a and 9.1b). It is then possible to present the head and feet of the lizard away from the handler to avoid injury. The handler should allow some flexibility as the lizard may struggle and overly rigid restraint could damage the spine.

Some of the more aggressive iguanas may need to be pinned down first. Here, as with avian patients, the use of a thick towel to control the tail and claws is useful. Gauntlets may be necessary for particularly aggressive large lizards or for those which may have a poisonous bite (the gila monster and the beaded lizard). It is important to ensure that you do not use too much force when restraining the lizard, as those with skeletal problems, such as metabolic bone disease, may be seriously injured. In addition, lizards, like other reptiles, do not have a diaphragm and so over zealous restraint will lead to the digestive system pushing onto the lungs and increasing inspiratory effort.

Day geckos and other fragile species are best examined in a clear plastic container. Other geckos have easily damaged skin and latex gloves and soft cloths should be used for examination. When handling small lizards, they may be cupped

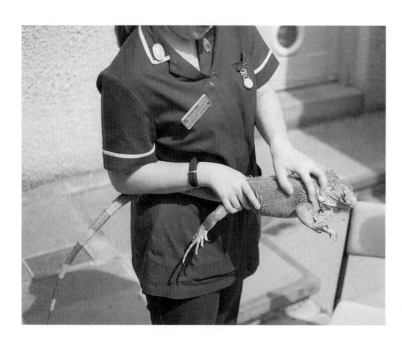

Fig. 9.1(b) The iguana may then be firmly but gently controlled. Tucking the tail underneath the arm prevents eye injuries.

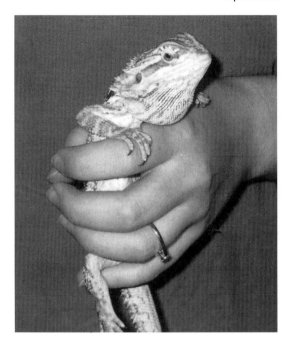

Fig. 9.2 Docile species such as the bearded dragon, *Pogona vitticeps*, may be cupped in the hand for routine examination.

in the hand (Fig. 9.2, Plate 9.1) and their heads controlled by holding between the index finger and thumb to prevent biting.

It is important that lizards are never restrained by their tails. Many will shed their tails at this time, but not all of them will regrow. Green iguanas for example will only regrow their tails as juveniles (less than 2.5–3 years of age). Once they are older than this, they will be left tail-less.

Vago-vagal reflex

The vago-vagal reflex can be used to place members of the lizard family into a trance-like state. The eyelids are closed and gentle digital pressure is applied to both eyeballs. This stimulates the autonomic parasympathetic nervous system resulting in a reduction in heart rate, blood pressure and respiration rate. Providing there are no loud noises or environmental stimulation, after 1–2 minutes the lizard may be placed on its side, front, back etc. allowing radiography to be performed without using physical or chemical restraint. A loud noise or physical stimulation will immediately revert the lizard to its normal wakeful state.

Serpentes

The Serpentes are the snake family, which includes a wide range of sizes from the enormous anacondas and Burmese pythons, which may achieve lengths of up to 30 feet or more, down to the thread snake family which may be a few tens of centimetres long. They are all characterised by their elongated form and absence of limbs. The danger areas for the handler are their teeth (and in the case of the more poisonous species such as the viper family their fang teeth), and, in the case of the constrictor and python family, their ability to asphyxiate their prey by winding themselves around the victim's chest and neck.

With this in mind, the following restraint techniques may be employed. Non-venomous snakes can be restrained by controlling the head initially. This is done by placing the thumb over the occiput and curling the fingers under the chin (Plate 9.2). Reptiles, like birds, have only the one occipital condyle so it is important to stabilise the occipitoatlantal joint. It is also important to support the rest of the snake's body so that not all of the weight of the snake is suspended from the head. Allow the smaller species to coil around the handler's arm, so the snake is supporting itself (Fig. 9.3).

In the larger species (longer than 10 feet) it is necessary to support the body length at regular intervals. This often requires several handlers. Indeed, it is *vital* to adopt a safe operating practice with the larger, constricting species of snake. A 'buddy system' should be operated, as with scuba diving, wherein any snake longer than 5–6 feet in length should only be handled by two or more people. This ensures that if the snake were to enwrap one handler, the other could disentangle him or her by unwinding from the tail end first. Above all it is important not to grip the snake too hard as this will cause bruising and the release of myoglobin from muscle cells. This will lodge in the kidneys, causing damage to the filtration membranes.

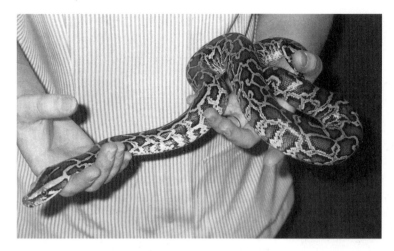

Fig. 9.3 Allowing the snake to coil itself around the handler's hand and arms is preferable to over-zealous restraint in non-aggressive species such as this small Burmese python.

Poisonous snakes (such as the viper family, rattlesnakes etc.) or very aggressive species (such as anacondas, reticulated and rock pythons) may be restrained initially using snake hooks. These are 1.5–2 ft steel rods with a blunt shepherds hook on the end. They are used to loop under the body of a snake to move it at arms length into a container. The hook may also be used to trap the head flat against the floor before grasping it with the hand. Once the head is controlled safely the snake is rendered harmless. Exceptions include the spitting cobra family where handlers should wear plastic goggles, or a plastic face visor as they can spit poison into the prey or assailant's eyes and mucus membranes causing blindness and paralysis.

Chelonia

The Chelonia include all land tortoises, terrapins and aquatic turtles.

Chelonia vary in size from the small Egyptian tortoises weighing a few hundred grams all the way up to adult leopard tortoises at 40 kg and the Galapagean tortoise family which can weigh several hundred kilograms. The majority of Chelonia are harmless, although surprisingly strong. The exceptions include the snapping turtle and the alligator snapping turtle, both of which can give a serious bite. Most of the soft-shelled terrapins have mobile necks and can also bite. Even red-eared terrapins may give a nasty nip!

For the mild-tempered Mediterranean species, the tortoise may be held with both hands, one on either side of the main part of the shell behind the front legs (Plate 9.3). To keep the tortoise still for examination, it may be placed onto a cylinder or stack of tins, raising its legs clear of the table as it balances on the centre of the underside of the shell (plastron) (Plate 9.4).

For aggressive species it is essential that you hold the shell on both sides behind and above the rear legs to avoid being bitten. Chemical restraint is necessary in order to examine the head region in these species.

For the soft-shelled and aquatic species, soft cloths and latex gloves may have to be used to prevent damaging the shell.

Crocodylia

The Crocodylia include fresh- and salt-water crocodiles, alligators, fish-eating gharials, and caimans. Their dangers to the handler lie in their impressively arrayed jaws and often their sheer size – an adult bull Nile crocodile may weigh many hundreds of kilograms and may live for up to 50 years or more.

Small specimens may be restrained by grasping the base of the tail in one hand whilst the other is placed behind the head. For slightly bigger specimens, a rope halter or noose may be tied around the snout so securing it closed. All of the major muscles in the crocodylian jaws are involved in closing not opening them, hence relatively fine rope or tape can be used to keep the mouth closed. The rest of the animal is restrained by pinning it to the ground.

Always approach crocodylians from head on, as their binocular vision is poor (although the alligator family does have some). Care should be taken when close to the crocodylian for head and tail movements both are directed at the assailant at the same time!

Much larger crocodiles require teams of people, with nets and snout snares in order to quickly clamp the jaws closed and to restrain the dangerous thrashing tail. Chemical immobilisation via dart guns is another option to be seriously considered.

Principles of chemical restraint

Chemical restraint is necessary for many procedures in reptile medicine, ranging from minor procedures such as extracting the head of a leopard tortoise or box turtle from its shell, to enabling a jugular blood sample to be taken or to carrying out coeliotomy procedures because of egg-binding. Before any anaesthetic or sedative is administered, an assessment of the reptile patient's health should be made. Considerations include:

- Is sedation or anaesthesia necessary for the procedure required?
- Is the reptile suffering from respiratory disease or septicaemia?
- Is the reptile's health likely to be made worse by sedation or anaesthesia?

Before discussing the administration of chemical restraint it is important to understand the reptilian respiratory system.

Overview of reptilian respiratory anatomy and physiology

The reptilian patient has a number of variations on the basic mammalian respiratory system.

The reptile patient has a glottis similar to the avian patient, which lies at the base of the tongue. This is more rostral in snakes and lizards and more caudal in chelonia (Figs 9.4a,b). At rest the glottis is permanently closed, opening briefly during inspiration and expiration. In crocodiles the glottis is obscured by the basihyal valve which is a fold of the epiglottis. This fold has to be deflected before they can be intubated (Bennett, 1998).

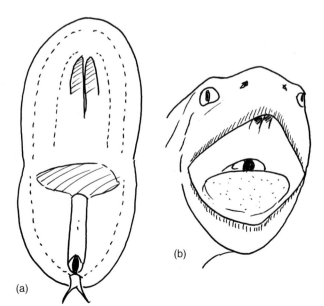

(a)

(b)

Fig. 9.4 Intraoral views of (a) Snake, showing 6 rows of teeth, and the glottal tube with the entrance to the trachea located rostrally, just behind the tongue sheath. (b) Tortoise, showing large fleshy tongue, at the base of which is the glottis.

The trachea varies between orders. In Chelonia and Crocodylia complete cartilagenous rings similar to those of the avian patient are found, with chelonians having a very short trachea. In some species this trachea bifurcates into two bronchi in the neck. Serpentes and Sauria have incomplete rings, such as those of the cat and dog, with Serpentes having a very long trachea.

The lungs of serpent and saurian species are simple and elastic in nature. The left lung of most serpents is absent, or vestigial in the case of members of the boiid family. The right lung of snakes frequently ends in an air sac. Chelonian species have a more complicated lung structure, and the paired lungs sit dorsally inside the carapace of the shell. Crocodylian lungs are similar to mammalian lungs and are paired.

No reptile has a diaphragm, although crocodylian species have a pseudodiaphragm which changes position with the movements of the liver and gut so pushing air in and out of the lungs. Most reptiles use intercostal muscles to move the ribcage in and out in a manner similar to birds. The exception to this is members of the order Chelonia. These species need to move their limbs, neck and head into and out of the shell in order to bring air into and out of the lungs.

Some species can survive in oxygen deprived atmospheres for prolonged periods – chelonian species may survive for 24 hours or more, and even green iguanas may survive for 4–5 hours. This makes induction of anaesthesia via inhalation of a gaseous anaesthetic agent almost impossible in these animals.

Pre-anaesthetic preparation

Weight measurement

This is important for accuracy as some species of reptile may be very small. Scales accurate to 1 g are therefore advised for smaller reptiles to ensure correct dosage.

Blood testing

It may be advisable to test biochemical and haematological parameters prior to administering chemical immobilising drugs. Blood samples can be taken from:

- Jugular vein in Chelonia
- Dorsal tail vein in Chelonia
- Ventral tail vein in Serpentes, Crocodylia and Sauria
- Palatine vein or cardiac puncture in Serpentes (although they frequently need to be sedated or anaesthetised to collect blood from these routes).

Fasting

Fasting is necessary in Serpentes to prevent regurgitation and pressure on the lungs or heart. It is advisable to ensure that no prey has been offered in the two days prior to anaesthesia. Other reptiles require less fasting. For example, chelonians rarely if ever regurgitate. However, it is important not to feed live prey to insectivores such as leopard geckos 24 hours prior to an anaesthetic as the prey may still be alive when the reptile is anaesthetised.

Pre-anaesthetic medications

The premedications are the same drugs used in cats and dogs to provide cardiopulmonary and central nervous system stabilisation, a smooth anaesthetic induction, muscle relaxation, analgesia and a degree of sedation.

Antimuscarinic medications

Atropine (0.01–0.04 mg/kg intramuscularly) or glycopyrrolate (0.01 mg/kg intramuscularly) may be used to reduce oral secretion and reduce bradycardia, however these problems are not usually of concern in reptile patients. Indeed, antimuscarinics may increase the thickness of mucus secretions, leading to more rapid blocking of the airways.

Tranquilisers

Acepromazine (0.1–0.5 mg/kg intramuscularly) may be given one hour before anaesthetic induction to reduce the levels of anaesthetic required, as can diazepam (0.22–0.62 mg/kg intramuscularly in alligators) and midazolam (2 mg/kg intramuscularly in turtles) (Bennett, 1998).

Alpha-2 adrenoceptor stimulants

Xylazine at 1 mg/kg can be used 30 minutes prior to ketamine in crocodylians to reduce the dose of ketamine needed. Medetomidine, used at doses of 100–150 µg/kg, markedly reduces the dose of ketamine required in chelonians, and has the advantage of being reversible with atipamezole at 500–750 µg/kg.

Opioids

Butorphanol (at 0.4 mg/kg intramuscularly) can be administered 20 minutes before anaesthesia so providing analgesia and reducing anaesthetic required, and may be combined with midazolam at 2 mg/kg.

Fluids

Fluid therapy is, as with avian patients, very important, and correction of fluid deficits should be attempted prior to surgery. Maintenance levels in reptile patients have been quoted as 25–30 ml/kg/day (pages 178–9).

Induction of anaesthesia

It should be noted that reptiles should never be immobilised by chilling or cooling them down. This does not provide analgesia and has serious welfare implications.

Injectable agents

Table 9.1 describes the advantages and disadvantages of injectable anaesthetic agents.

Dissociative anaesthetics

Ketamine: ketamine has been widely used in reptile patients. The effects produced vary depending on the species and dosage. Recommended levels range from 22–44 mg/kg intramuscularly for sedation to 55–88 mg/kg intramuscularly for surgical anaesthesia. Lower levels are needed if combined with a premedicant such as midazolam or medetomidine (Bennett, 1996).

Table 9.1 Advantages and disadvantages of injectable anaesthetics.

Advantages	Disadvantages
Ease of administration	Recovery often dependent on organ metabolism
Prevention of breath-holding on induction	Difficult to reverse rapidly
Reduced costs	Often prolonged recovery times
Easy to administer	Muscle necrosis at site of injection
Low risk to anaesthetist	

Effects are seen in 10–30 minutes but may take anything up to 4 days to wear off, particularly at low environmental temperatures. Its main use is therefore at the lower dose range, to allow sedation, facilitate intubation and maintenance of gaseous anaesthesia in species such as chelonians that hold their breath during gaseous induction.

It is however frequently painful on administration. Also, because ketamine is excreted by the kidneys, it is recommended that it is administered in the cranial half of the body. This is because, in reptiles, blood from the caudal half of the body travels to the kidneys *before* returning to the heart and the anaesthetic may thus be excreted before it has a chance to work.

Steroid anaesthetics

Alphaxalone/alphadolone: this combination allows intubation within 3–5 minutes when administered intravenously. It may be administered intramuscularly, but induction takes longer via this route (25–40 minutes). If used alone, it will provide anaesthesia for from 15–35 minutes at a dose of 6–9 mg/kg for intravenous administration, or 9–15 mg/kg if given intramuscularly. Although recovery time is quicker than for ketamine, it may still take 1–4 hours for full recovery to occur. It can be very useful in chelonians and in general has a wide safety margin.

Other injectable anaesthetics

Propofol: propofol produces rapid induction and recovery, and is becoming the induction agent of choice in many practices specialising in reptile medicine and surgery. Its advantages also include a short elimination half-life and minimal organ metabolism, making it particularly safe to use in debilitated reptiles which frequently have some degree of liver damage.

Its main disadvantage is that it requires intravenous access, although use of the intraosseous route has been shown to be successful in green iguanas at a dose of 10 mg/kg. As with cats and dogs, propofol also produces a transient period of apnoea and some cardiac depression. In this situation intubation and positive pressure ventilation is necessary.

Doses of 10–15 mg/kg in chelonians given via the dorsal coccygeal (tail) vein have successfully induced anaesthesia in under one minute. This allows intubation and maintenance on a gaseous anaesthetic if required. Alternatively, propofol can be used alone providing a period of anaesthesia of 20–30 minutes.

Depolarising muscle relaxants

Succinylcholine: this is a neuromuscular blocking agent and produces immobilisation without providing analgesia. Therefore it should only be used to aid the administration of another form of anaesthetic or for transportation, and not as a sole source of anaesthesia. Recovery is dependent on liver metabolism and its use in animals with possible liver disease should be avoided.

It can be used in large Chelonia (such as the giant Galapagoas species) at doses of 0.5–1 mg/kg intramuscularly and will allow intubation and conversion to gaseous anaesthesia. Crocodilians can be immobilised with 3–5 mg/kg intramuscularly, with immobilisation occurring within 4 minutes and recovery in 7–9 hours. Respiration usually continues without assistance at these doses, but is important to have assisted ventilation facilities to hand as paralysis of the muscles of respiration can easily occur.

Gaseous agents

The gaseous anaesthetics used for induction will be discussed in the next section on maintenance of anaesthesia, however a table listing their advantages and disadvantages is presented below.

Table 9.2 Advantages and disadvantages of gaseous anaesthetic.

Advantages	Disadvantages
Ease of administration via face-mask/ induction chamber	Breath-holding (Chelonia particularly)
Pain free	Environmental pollution
Minimial tissue trauma	Health risk to anaesthetist
	Risk with dangerous reptiles during handling

Maintenance of anaesthesia

Injectable agents

Dissociative anaesthetics

Ketamine: ketamine may be used on its own for anaesthesia at doses of 55–88 mg/kg intramuscularly. It is worthwhile noting though that as the dosages get higher the recovery time also increases, and in some cases it can be as long as several days. It should be noted that doses above 110 mg/kg will cause respiratory arrest and bradycardia.

Ketamine may be combined with other injectable agents to provide surgical anaesthesia. Examples of these combinations include:

- Midazolam at 2 mg/kg intramuscularly with 40 mg/kg ketamine in turtles (Bennett, 1996)
- Xylazine at 1 mg/kg intramuscularly, given 30 minutes prior to 20 mg/kg ketamine in large crocodiles (Lawton, 1992)
- Medetomidine at 100 µg/kg intramuscularly with 50 mg/kg ketamine in kingsnakes (Malley, 1997).

Other injectable anaesthetics

Propofol: propofol may be used to give 20–30 minutes of anaesthesia after administration, allowing minor procedures such as wound repair, intraosseous or intravenous catheter placement or oesophagostomy tube placement to be carried out.

It may be topped up at 1 mg/kg/min intravenously or intraosseously, but apnoea is extremely common and intubation and ventilation with 100% oxygen is frequently required.

Alphaxalone/alphadolone: this injectable combination can be used for induction and also for short periods of anaesthesia (average 25 minutes) at 6–9 mg/kg intravenously. Intramuscular doses may be given but onset of anaesthesia may take 20–30 minutes. Its disadvantages include a prolonged recovery time (1–4 hours), the need for relatively large doses and the need to intubate many reptiles due to relaxation of the muscles which keep the glottis open to allow breathing.

Gaseous agents (see also Table 9.2)

Halothane

Halothane is the anaesthetic gas most widely available in general practice and can be used in reptile anaesthesia, both for maintenance and induction. Face-mask or induction chambers can be used for induction at levels of 4–5%, although certain species, such as Chelonia, can hold their breath for long periods making gaseous induction difficult. Maintenance can be achieved at 1–2.5%. Disadvantages of halothane are:

- It can induce myocardial hypoxia and dysrhythmias
- 15–20% of halothane is metabolised by the liver before recovery can occur. As many diseased reptiles have dysfunctional or impaired livers, this makes its use limited.
- It can excite reptiles in the early stages of anaesthesia
- Cardiac arrest and apnoea frequently occur simultaneously, reducing available resuscitation response times.

Isoflurane

Isoflurane is the gaseous maintenance anaesthetic of choice. Although more expensive than halothane, isoflurane is minimally metabolised in the body (0.3%) and has a very low blood–gas partition coefficient (1.4 compared with 2.3 for halothane in human trials). This means that it has a very low solubility in blood, so as soon as isoflurane administration is stopped the reptile starts to recover, excreting it from the lungs. In addition it has lower fat solubility than halothane and so excretion from the body is quicker still. Isoflurane still has excellent muscle relaxing properties and is a good analgesic. Apnoea *precedes* cardiac arrest, unlike the case with halothane anaesthesia.

It can be used to induce anaesthesia by face-mask application or, in those species not exhibiting breath-holding capabilities at levels of 4–5%, by induction chamber. It is also possible to adapt the cases of 20 ml and 60 ml syringes to form long thin face-masks to induce snakes. Isoflurane can then be used to maintain anaesthesia, preferably via endotracheal tube, at levels from 2–3% depending on the procedure.

A summary of the advantages of isoflurane over halothane may been seen in Table 9.3.

Nitrous oxide

Nitrous oxide can be used in conjunction with halothane or isoflurane, reducing the percentage of gaseous anaesthetic required for induction and maintenance of anaesthesia. Its other advantages include good muscle relaxation and excellent analgesic properties, making it useful in orthopaedic procedures.

Disadvantages of nitrous include its tendency to accumulate in hollow organs. This may prove a problem for herbivorous reptiles as they often have capacious hind guts and nitrous oxide can accumulate there. Nitrous oxide also requires

Table 9.3 Comparison of halothane and isoflurane gaseous anaesthetics.

Halothane	Isoflurane
Organ metabolism required for recovery	Minimal organ metabolism required for recovery
Induces cardiac arrhthymias	Relatively few arrhthymias induced
Cardiac arrest and respiratory arrest coincide	Respiratory arrest precedes cardiac arrest
Good analgesia	Good analgesia
Blood gas partition coefficient 2.3	Blood gas partition coefficient 1.4
Highly fat soluble	Lower fat solubility than halothane

some organ metabolism for full excretion and so may be a problem in a seriously diseased patient.

Aspects of gaseous anaesthesia maintenance for reptiles

Inhalant gaseous anaesthesia is becoming the main method of anaesthetising reptiles for prolonged procedures. The reptile patient should preferably be intubated to allow the inhalant anaesthetic to be delivered in a controlled manner.

Intubation

Intubation is straightforward in reptiles as they do not have an epiglottis and the glottis, which acts as the entrance to the trachea, is relatively cranial in the majority of species. It is useful to note that the glottis is kept closed at rest, so the operator must wait for inspiration to occur to allow intubation. Reptiles produce little or no saliva when at rest or not eating, so blockage of the tube is uncommon.

In Serpentes, the glottis sits rostrally on the floor of the mouth just caudal to the tongue sheath and is easily visible when the mouth is opened (Fig. 9.4a). Intubation may be performed in the conscious patient if necessary, as reptiles do not have a cough reflex. The mouth is opened with a wooden or plastic tongue depressor and the endotracheal tube inserted during inspiration. Alternatively, an induction agent may be given and then intubation attempted.

In Chelonia, the glottis sits slightly more caudally at the base of the tongue (Fig. 9.4b). The trachea is very short and the endotracheal tube should only be inserted a few centimetres otherwise there is a risk that only one or the other of the bronchi will be intubated, leading to only one lung receiving the anaesthetic. An induction agent such as ketamine or propofol is advised for chelonians prior to intubation due to their ability to breath-hold and difficulty in extracting the head from the shell.

Sauria vary depending on the species of lizard, most having just a glottis guarding the entrance to the trachea (Fig. 9.5). Some species possess vocal

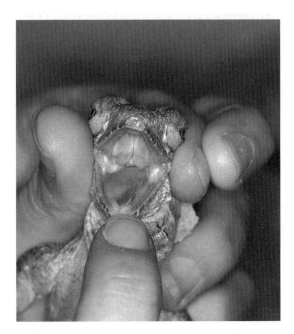

Fig. 9.5   Intraoral view of a spiny-tailed iguana showing fleshy tongue. Glottis is caudal to this structure.

folds, notably some species of gecko (Porter, 1972). Some may be intubated consciously, but most are better induced with an injectable preparation or by face-mask using gas. Some species may be too small for intubation. Plate 9.5 shows an intubate green iguana.

Crocodylia have a basihyal fold (Bennett, 1998) which acts as an epiglottis and needs to be depressed prior to intubation. Because they are potentially dangerous, these species require some form of injectable chemical sedation or induction prior to intubation.

Intermittent positive pressure ventilation (IPPV)

If intubation is performed on a conscious patient, anaesthesia may be induced, even in breath-holding species, by using positive pressure ventilation. This has some advantages as it leads to rapid post-operative recovery.

Many species require positive pressure ventilation during the course of an anaesthetic. Chelonia for example are frequently placed in dorsal recumbency during intracoelomic surgery. As they

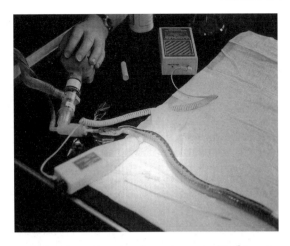

Fig. 9.6 Manual bagging of a garter snake. Note Doppler probe to monitor heart sounds, and Mapleson C circuit for smaller species.

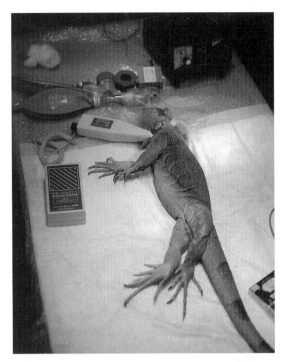

Fig. 9.7 Mechanical IPPV using a ventilator in a green iguana. Note again Doppler probe and cranial position of the heart in iguanids.

have no diaphragm, and the lungs are situated dorsally, the weight of the digestive contents pressing on the lungs will reduce inspiration and slowly lead to hypoxia. This is in addition to the fact that most inspiratory effort is induced by movement of the chelonian limbs, which are hopefully immobile during anaesthesia! Also, if a neuromuscular blocking agent such as succinylcholine has been used, positive pressure ventilation may be needed as respiratory muscle paralysis may occur.

The aim of IPPV is to inflate the lungs with an oxygen and anaesthetic mixture enough for an adequately oxygenated state to be maintained and for the animal to remain anaesthetised. To this end it is sufficient to ventilate most reptiles two–six times a minute and no more, at a pressure of 10–15 cm water (100–150 mm mercury). As with birds, a ventilator unit makes life much easier, but, with experience, manual 'bagging' of the patient with enough pressure just to inflate the lungs and no more can be achieved (Figs 9.6 and 9.7). A rough guide is to inflate the first two fifths of the reptile's body at each cycle (Malley, 1997).

Anaesthetic circuits

For species weighing less than 5 kg, a non-rebreathing system with oxygen flow at twice the minute volume is suggested (Bennett, 1998). This approximates to 300–500 ml/kg/minute for most species. Ayres T pieces, modified Bain circuits and Mapleson C circuits may all be used.

Additional supportive therapy

Recumbency

Many chelonians are placed in dorsal recumbency for intracoelomic surgery. Other groups of reptiles may also be placed in this position for similar techniques. The use of foam wedges, or positional polystyrene-filled vacuum bags, is essential to maintain stability.

Snakes may become extremely flaccid during surgery. In order to provide stability they may be strapped to a long board or wedged in place with foam wedges or vacuum bags. In any case, it is important to keep the body wall of non-chelonian species free of constraint and to use IPPV if necessary.

Maintenance of body temperature

Maintaining body temperature is important for successful recovery. Body temperature can be monitored using a cloacal probe attached to a digital thermometer. Reptiles should be maintained as near to their PBT (preferred body temperature) as possible (pages 127–8) which lies in the range 22–30°C for most species. This can be done by placing the reptile onto a circulating water heating pad during anaesthesia and room temperature should be kept up to reduce heat losses. Warmed subcutaneous or intracoelomic fluids can be given during and after surgery.

Hot water bottles, or hot-water-filled latex gloves may also be used, but must be wrapped in towelling to prevent direct contact with the reptile. Care should be taken when these cool down, as they may then draw heat *away* from the patient rather than provide it. The use of clear drapes will also help to keep heat in as will the utilisation of light sources for surgery, many of which radiate heat.

Fluid therapy

Fluid therapy is covered in more detail from page 175. However it should be noted that, as with small mammals, post-operative fluid therapy may enhance the recovery rate and improve the patient's return to normal function. Recommended fluid volumes are 20–25 ml/kg every 24 hours across the species (Frye, 1991). They should not exceed 2–3% body weight in chelonians.

Monitoring anaesthesia

Table 9.4 shows the stages of anaesthesia seen in reptiles.

Monitoring the heart rate and rhythm can be extremely difficult with a conventional stethoscope as the reptilian scales interfere with sound transmission and the presence of the three-chambered heart reduces the clarity of the beat. Some of this can be overcome by placing a damp towel over the area to be auscultated, deadening the sound of the scales, but in many cases the best solution is to use a Doppler probe. This is an ultra-

Table 9.4 Stages of anaesthesia in reptiles (adapted from Bennet, 1998 and Malley, 1997).

Stage 1
— Limb movements reduced
— Righting reflex present (reptile will flip back onto its feet after being inverted)
— Snake tongue withdrawn after being grasped
— Responds to noxious stimuli
— Muscles are tense
— Writhing movements occur
— Vent stimulation reflex present
— Palpebral reflex present

Stage 2
— Righting reflex ceases
— Tongue withdrawal reflex much reduced
— No response to noxious stimuli
— Muscles start to relax
— Writhing movements cease
— Vent reflex reduced
— Palpebral reflex diminished

Stage 3
— Righting reflex ceased
— No voluntary motion
— Tongue withdrawal reflex totally absent
— No response to noxious stimuli
— Muscles totally relaxed
— Snakes: Bauchstreich reflex (where stroking of the ventral scales produces movement in the body wall) much reduced
— Laryngeal reflexes lost in alligators
— Chelonia still have a corneal reflex
— Vent reflex much reduced – loss of this indicates anaesthesia is too deep

Stage 4
— Extreme depression and death (Chelonia lose corneal reflexes just before entering this phase).

sound probe unit attached to a microphone which responds to fluid movement, converting it to sound (Fig. 9.8).

ECG leads may be attached to the patient to give an electrical trace of heart activity. To minimise the crushing effect of the alligator forceps on the leads, they may be attached to hypodermic needles which can then be attached to the patient. In snakes, ECGs can still be made, even in the absence of limbs. The leads are placed two heart lengths cranial and caudal to the heart. In some saurians, such as iguanas, skinks, chameleons and water dragons, the heart is situated far cranially so the forelimb leads are better placed cervically.

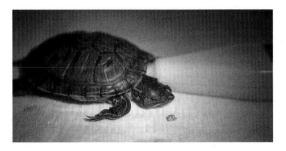

Fig. 9.8 Doppler probe monitoring of heart sounds in an anaesthetised red-eared terrapin.

Respiratory flow monitors are not very useful due to the need for IPPV in most reptile species Pulse oximeters are, however, useful, with reflector probes being used *per cloaca* or *per os* to measure the percentage saturation of the haemoglobin with oxygen.

Recovery and analgesia

Recovery

Reptiles often recover rapidly from isoflurane anaesthesia. But, if other injectable drugs were used, such as alphadalone/alphaxolone or ketamine, recovery may be prolonged. It is essential at this time to keep the reptile patient calm, stress free and at its optimum preferred body temperature. It may also be necessary to keep the patient intubated and on IPPV with oxygen, if high doses of the above agents have been used, until the reptile is once again breathing for itself. The use of doxapram at a dose of 5 mg/kg by intramuscular or intravenous injection is useful to help stimulate respiration. It should be noted, however, that the stimulus for reptiles to breathe is a falling blood partial pressure of oxygen, and not a rising partial pressure of carbon dioxide, so IPPV with 100% oxygen may actually inhibit respiration. IPPV with atmospheric air may therefore be preferable once any gaseous anaesthetic has been flushed from the airways.

Fluid therapy during this period will also help to speed recovery, especially from agents such as ketamine which are cleared through the kidneys. Once recovery is complete, the reptile should be

encouraged to eat, or, if anorectic, the patient should be assist fed, stomach tubed etc.

Analgesia

Analgesia is an important aspect of post-operative recovery. Reptiles which have been provided with analgesia have been shown to have a quicker return to normality, eating, normal behaviour etc. than those who have not.

Opioids

Butorphanol at 0.4 mg/kg intramuscularly, intravenously or subcutaneously and buprenorphine at 0.01 mg/kg intramuscularly have been recommended (Lawton, 1991; Bennett, 1998).

Non-steroidal anti-inflammatory drugs (NSAIDs)

NSAIDs also seem to be beneficial. The following have been recommended: carprofen at doses of 2–4 mg/kg intramuscularly initially, and then 1–2 mg/kg every 24–72 hours thereafter (Malley, 1997); meloxicam at 0.1–0.2 mg/kg orally every 24 hrs; ketoprofen at 2 mg/kg intramuscularly every 24 hours (Bennett, 1996); flunixin meglumine at 0.1–0.5 mg/kg intramuscularly every 24 hours (Lawton, 1992). It should be noted that all of these are potentially nephrotoxic and have gastrointestinal ulcerative side-effects, hence fluid therapy should be given and patients should be closely monitored for side-effects.

Overview of amphibian anaesthesia

Techniques and equipment involved in restraining amphibian patients

Examination of the amphibian patient should be performed at that species' optimum preferred body temperature, as with reptile patients. A rough guide is between 21–24°C, which is lower than the more usual 22–32°C reptile housing conditions.

The examination table should be covered with paper towels (unbleached) that have been soaked in dechlorinated water – preferably purified water. More purified water should be on stand-by to be applied to the amphibian patient to prevent dehydration during the examination.

Initially it is useful not to restrain the amphibian patient until the extent of any problem is assessed, as many have severe skin lesions which are extremely fragile. Once an initial assessment has been made, the patient may be restrained manually. First, it is advisable to put on a pair of non-powdered hypoallergenic latex gloves in order to minimise irritation to the amphibian's skin caused by either the handler's normal acidic skin environment or by the powder in many prepacked latex gloves. The wearing of gloves is also essential in species such as the toad family or the arrow tree frogs whose skin can produce irritant or even potentially deadly toxins which can be absorbed through unprotected human skin. It may also be necessary to wear goggles when handling some species of toad – the giant toad *Bufo marinus* can squirt a toxin from its parotid salivary glands over a distance of several feet.

When handling the amphibian patient the method of restraint will obviously depend on the animal's body shape. The elongated form of salamanders and newts will require similar restraint to that of a lizard, with one hand grasping the pectoral girdle from the dorsal aspect, index finger and thumb encircling one forelimb, second and third fingers the other, with the opposite hand grasping the pelvic girdle, again from the dorsal aspect in a similar manner. Some salamanders will shed their tails if roughly handled so care should be taken with these species.

Large anurans (members of the frog and toad family) can be restrained by cupping one hand around the pectoral girdle immediately behind the front limbs with the other hand positioned beneath the hind limbs. Care should be taken with some species which have poison glands in their skin, as mentioned above, and in the case of species such as the Argentinian horned frog care should be taken with their bite. This species will eat whole small rodents when adult and can inflict unpleasant bite wounds.

Aquatic urodeles should be examined only in water as removal causes skin damage. Some of the larger urodeles, such as the hellbender species (*Cryptobranchus* spp) can also inflict unpleasant bite wounds on handlers, so firm restraint is required.

Smaller species and aquatic species may be best examined in small glass jars.

Aspects of chemical restraint in amphibians

There are three main routes of administration of anaesthetic and sedative agents to amphibians: injections, inhalant gaseous anaesthetics and in-water methods.

In-water anaesthetic agents

There are two main medications for this route – MS-222 and benzocaine.

MS-222

This is tricaine methanesulphonate, an anaesthetic used commonly in fish restraint. It is a water soluble white powder. A range of 1–2 g/l water is required to anaesthetise most frogs and urodeles, but a solution of 3 g/l is required for most toads (Wright, 1996). A much reduced level of 0.5 g/l can be used for tadpole anaesthesia.

It is best to use the amphibian's own water to minimise environmental changes, and to place this into a plastic bag, or plastic-lined box. This is useful as many amphibians go through an excitated stage during anaesthesia, and the slight give in the plastic bags reduces skin damage. It is also important to ensure any anurans and other non-gilled amphibians can raise their nostrils above the water, otherwise they will drown.

Anaesthesia induction will take 20 minutes or so, with respiration rate reducing. Respiration may even stop, although cardiac function persists. During the induction period, the ventrum of the amphibian will redden and anurans will become excited, making leaping movements.

Initial anaesthesia is manifested by the inability of the amphibian to right itself, and loss of the corneal reflex, but with pain reflexes still intact. A deep plane of anaesthesia is when all of these are abolished and only the heart-beat can be seen as a sign of movement. The level of anaesthesia can be maintained by trickling the anaesthetic solution over the amphibian's body once the amphibian is removed from the solution. Reversal is achieved by trickling fresh, distilled, oxygenated water over the amphibian's skin.

Benzocaine

This is related to MS-222 and can be used to anaesthetise many adult amphibians at solutions of 0.2–0.3 mg/l water. It is more soluble in ethanol than in water and so is often dissolved in a small volume of this before it is added to the water. Recovery occurs some 60 minutes after rinsing the amphibian with benzocaine-free water.

It is worth noting that both anaesthetics are acidic in nature and hence will lower the pH of the water solution. It may be necessary to add a buffer solution to the water to correct this.

Injectable anaesthetic agents

Ketamine may be used, but is less preferable to MS-222. This is because relatively large volumes are required (75–100 mg/kg (Bennett, 1996)), and the anaesthetic takes a variable period to take effect – from 10 minutes to 1–2 hours. Injections may be made intramuscularly, intravenously into the midline ventral abdominal vein or subcutaneously.

Inhalant gaseous anaesthetic agents

Isoflurane

This may be used, either in an induction chamber at dose of 2.5–3%, or, in the larger species of toads, by dripping it directly onto the toad's skin.

Some of the larger species may also be intubated, but anaesthesia is often erratic, as alternative respiratory routes are available to amphibians (cutaneous or buccopharyngeal routes – i.e. the amphibian can breathe through its skin or oral membranes). Some of the more fragile species, such as the smaller urodeles or caecilians may actually suffer severe skin irritation during gas chamber induction due to the direct irritant effect of the anaesthetic on the skin.

Halothane

This anaesthetic has the same problems as isoflurane, but in both cases the larger anuran species may be anaesthetised by this method.

References

Bennet, R.A. (1996) Anaesthesia. In *Reptile Medicine and Surgery* (Mader, R., ed), pp. 241–247. W.B. Saunders, London.

Bennet, R.A. (1998) Reptile anaesthesia. *Seminars in Avian and Exotic Pet Medicine*, **January**, 30–40.

Frye, F. (1991) *Biomedical and Surgical Aspects of Captive Reptile Husbandry*. Krieger, Malabar, Florida.

Lawton, M.P.C. (1992) Anaesthesia. In *Manual of Reptiles*. BSAVA, Cheltenham.

Malley, D. (1997) Reptile anaesthesia and the practising veterinarian. *In Practice*, **July/August**, 351–368.

Porter, K.R. (1972) *Herpetology*. W.B. Saunders, Philadelphia.

Wright, K.M. (1996) Amphibian husbandry and medicine. In *Reptile Medicine and Surgery* (Mader, D., ed), pp. 436–458. W.B. Saunders, Philadelphia.

Further reading

Page, C.D. (1993) Current reptilian anaesthesia procedures. In *Zoo and Wildlife Medicine: Current Therapy 3* (Fowler, M., ed), pp. 140–143. W.B. Saunders, Philadelphia.

Chapter 10
Reptile and Amphibian Nutrition

Classification

Reptiles and amphibians may be classified in a number of different ways, one of which is according to their diet. Of the commonly seen species there are four main categories as defined by diet. These are:

- **Carnivores** are predominantly the members of the snake family, which will eat whole avian, amphibian or mammalian prey. To do this they have powerful crushing jaws. Some have poison fangs while others, such as the boa and python species, rely on suffocating their prey.
- **Herbivores** come from a variety of species, from the tortoise family, for example the Greek or spur-thighed tortoises, through to the lizard family, for example the green iguana.
- **Insectivores** are predominantly from the lizard family, for example the leopard geckos, collared lizards etc., and from the amphibians, for example the frogs, salamanders etc.
- **Omnivores** are from a variety of reptile species, and the term may be used to refer to reptiles which change their eating habits during the course of their life. For example, the bearded dragon starts off as an insectivore, but becomes more and more dependent on fruit and vegetable matter as it gets older.

In all of these cases, the individual species have become highly evolved to cope with certain types of food. We also know that many of these creatures in the wild have a changing food supply throughout the year, so what may form a staple diet in the summer does not necessarily apply come the winter.

General nutritional requirements

Water

As mentioned in the chapter on avian nutrition the most important thing about the water provided is its quality. Reptiles may defaecate in their water bowls and turtles and terrapins eat in their water. These habits cause pollution and leading to disease.

To prevent this, either the water must have a powerful filter system, or the terrapins/turtles fed in a separate feeding tank which may be cleaned out after feeding.

Vitamin and mineral supplements administered in the water will allow rapid bacterial growth over 24 hours, so bowl hygiene must be rigorous.

The amount of water consumed by individual reptiles and amphibians will depend on the diets being offered as well as on the species. On dry, insect-based diets water consumption will be much higher than for reptiles and amphibians which consume large amounts of fruit and vegetables. Even so a leopard gecko may only consume 5 ml of water in a 24-hour period.

Tap water contains chlorine, which may irritate the skin of sensitive aquatic species such as amphibians or soft-shelled turtles. It is advised that tap water be allowed to stand for 24 hours to let the chlorine escape and to allow it to come up to room temperature.

Renal disease as a result of chronic dehydration is common in captive reptile species. Many of these animals, for example green iguanas and water dragons, come from parts of the world which have high relative humidities – anywhere from 60–100%. If these species are kept in vivaria at their correct temperatures (high twenties to low thirties degrees centigrade) then the air can hold large amounts of water, consequently the relative humidity often drops at these temperatures. Combine this with the fact that many reptiles will not drink from water bowls, instead preferring to lick moisture from leaves or cage furniture, and we can see that chronic dehydration can occur. To prevent this, it is important not only to provide drinking bowls, but also to mist the cage, the reptile and the cage furniture several times daily. This is of course less necessary for desert-dwelling species, such as leopard geckos, pancake tortoises etc., but even these species benefit from being misted every now and then.

Reptiles, like birds, are susceptible to renal disease because the waste product of protein metabolism is predominantly the insoluble uric acid. If the reptile is not kept adequately hydrated, it will reduce the excretion of uric acid through the kidneys. This leads to deposition of uric acid inside the body, a condition known as *visceral gout*. Once deposited, the uric acid forms a tough mineralised coating to the lining of blood vessels, the kidneys, the heart and many other organs, leading to hypertension and multiple organ failure.

Maintenance energy requirements (MER)

Every species has a level of energy consumption per day which is needed to satisfy basic maintenance requirements. This is the energy used purely to maintain current status under minimal activity and is the minimum energy requirement to support that reptile or amphibian's life. In reptiles, basic maintenance requirements vary widely depending on activity level and environmental temperature, so calculations are made at that animal's optimum environmental temperature. Energy requirements will also vary according to the animal's stage of life. For example the MER will be more than doubled in active egg laying females during disease or growth.

MER is dependent on the basal metabolic rate (BMR – the energy requirement when at complete rest) and metabolic body weight as follows:

$$MER = 1.5 \times BMR$$

where $BMR = constant\ (k) \times (body\ weight)^{0.75}$

The constant, k, varies with family groups, and has been estimated at 10 for reptiles in general.

If the foods offered are so low in kilojoules that the reptile or amphibian has to eat more of it than will fit into its digestive system in 24 hours, that animal will rapidly lose condition (Figs 10.1 and 10.2).

For example, vegetables such as lettuce and celery have an energy content of 12.6 kJ/g dry matter (or in real terms 0.75 kJ/g wet food), whereas meat-based foods such as rodent prey have a much higher energy density of 19–21 kJ/g dry matter (or in real terms 6–7.5 kJ/g wet food) (Donoghue, 1998). From this we can see that in 'as fed' terms, i.e. wet food, one would need to feed eight times as much weight of vegetable matter to give the same energy dose in animal prey. This volume may well exceed the gut capacity of the reptile or amphibian.

Conversely many pet reptiles and amphibians will continue eating until their digestive tracts are full, and if all they are offered is high energy density food then they will rapidly achieve their MER, exceed it and become obese.

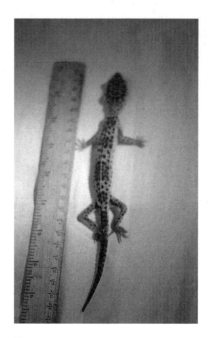

Fig. 10.1 Malnutrition in a leopard gecko.

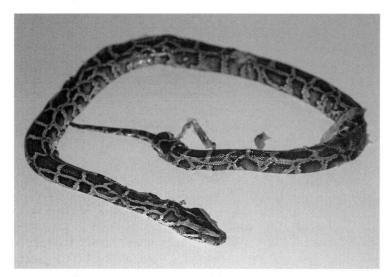

Fig. 10.2 Malnutrition and blister disease in a Burmese python.

Protein and amino acid requirements

Proteins are assembled from groups of amino acids – indeed a protein can contain up to 22 amino acids. In general terms, for humans, and it seems for reptiles and amphibians, ten amino acids are essential and need to be provided in the diet. The others may be manufactured from these ten. The essential amino acids are:

- leucine
- lysine
- methionine
- phenylalanine
- threonine
- tryptophan
- isoleucine
- valine
- arginine
- histidine.

In addition, it is known that for diets low in the amino acids methionine or arginine, an extra supplement of the amino acid glycine is required.

Proteins are therefore assessed on their ability to provide these essential amino acids, with poor proteins supplying only non-essential ones. This is quantified by the term *biological value*, a high-biological-value foodstuff containing more of the essential amino acids.

For herbivorous reptiles, levels of 25% protein content as metabolisable energy in the diet have been shown to be adequate (Donoghue, 1998). Most of this protein source in herbivores seems to come from leafy greens, but deficiencies are seen in herbivorous reptiles fed high cellulose, low protein foods such as the ubiquitous lettuce, and fruits. Chronic protein deficiencies are often presented as gradual wasting conditions, with increased susceptibility to infections.

Deficiencies in amino acids in carnivorous reptiles and amphibians is extremely rare because they eat whole prey. This gives them a 30–60% protein content as metabolisable energy. Herbivorous deficiencies specific amino acids are possible although not well documented.

In general, waste products of protein metabolism in land-based reptiles are converted into the relatively insoluble uric acid. Alligators may produce ammonia as the waste product, as may many amphibians, depending on their state of hydration, but adult frogs may excrete urea. Protein excesses, such as those produced by feeding cat or dog foods to predominantly herbivorous species, can lead to an excess production of uric acid and visceral gout, renal failure and death may result.

Fats and essential fatty acids (EFAs)

Fats provide high concentrations of energy. They also supply the reptile or amphibian with essential fatty acids, which are required for cellular integrity and as the building blocks for internal chemicals such as prostaglandins (which play a part in reproduction and inflammation). Fats also provide a carrier mechanism for the absorption of fat-soluble vitamins such as vitamins A, D, E and K.

The primary EFA for reptiles is linoleic acid, as it is for mammals, with the absolute dietary requirement of this fatty acid being 1% of the diet. If the diet becomes deficient in this essential fatty acid a rapid decline in cellular integrity occurs. This is manifested clinically by the skin becoming flaky and inelastic and prone to recurrent infections, and also to fluid loss through the skin which in turn leads to polydipsia (Wallach & Hoff, 1982).

In herbivores, less than 10% of the diet on a dry matter basis is composed of fats, the chief energy sources being carbohydrates and proteins. However, fermentation of fibre in the lower bowel produces short-chain fatty acids which can be used for energy. For carnivores, fat forms a major part of the energy source in the diet, as much as 40–70% of the calories, with protein chiefly making up the rest.

The problem of overconsumption of fats in pet reptiles which are not exercising regularly is well known and high fat foods such as dog and cat food fed to herbivores, or extremely fat rodent prey fed to snakes, are prime culprits for this. Obesity can lead to a number of problems, high amongst which is fatty degenerative change in the liver (*hepatic lipidosis*) which can lead to liver failure. This is particularly common in tortoises.

Carbohydrates

Carbohydrates are primarily used for rapid energy production. This is particularly important in herbivores which consume plant matter only, and so gain the majority of their energy source from carbohydrates and proteins. Carnivorous reptiles do not utilise carbohydrates much at all.

Fibre

Dietary fibre is extremely important for herbivorous reptiles. Indeed, the presence of fibre acts both as a bulking agent, encouraging gut motility, and as a source for fermentation by the intestinal microflora, essential for fatty acid and B vitamin production. Snakes and other carnivores do not have a dietary fibre requirement, and indeed if provided will not be utilised. Ultimately it will dilute the energy concentration of the diet necessitating feeding more frequent and larger meals.

Vitamins

These compounds are grouped together although they are widely differing in nature, but all animals have a requirement for various numbers of these. They are categorised into fat soluble (vitamin A, D, E and K) and water soluble (the B vitamin complex and vitamin C).

Fat-soluble vitamins

Vitamin A: in herbivore reptiles the most important plant precursor in terms of how much vitamin A can be produced from it is beta-carotene. Carnivorous reptile and amphibians will gain the preformed vitamin A in their prey food.

Hypovitaminosis A is a frequently seen problem in chelonians, particularly tortoises and young red-eared terrapins. If a deficiency in vitamin A occurs then mucous membranes become thickened and oral and respiratory secretions dry up. This is due to blockage of salivary and mucous glands with cellular debris – a condition known as *squamous metaplasia*. This leads to poor functioning of the ciliary mechanisms which have a role in removing foreign particles from the airways. Swelling of the periorbital membranes – a condition known as *xerophthalmia* – is also seen.

Vitamin A's role in immune system function means that a deficiency makes respiratory and digestive tract infections more common. The most frequently seen example of this is the increased susceptibility to pneumonias seen in red-eared terrapins and manifested in the lop-sided position they adopt when swimming. This is because of lung collapse or congestion which reduces buoyancy on the affected side.

Tortoises may suffer more frequently from upper respiratory tract infections when a deficiency is present. Evidence of sterile pustules and cornified plaques inside the mouth are commonly seen, with overgrowth of the beak due to hyperkeratosis.

Vitamin A also has a role in bone growth and structure, the normal function of secretory glands such as the adrenals and also in reproductive function. Finally renal damage may occur in hypovitaminosis A, with evidence of oedema in the inguinal and axillary regions secondary to failure of the renal tubular filtration system.

Because it is fat soluble, vitamin A can be stored in the body, primarily in the liver. Recommended minimum dietary levels are 200–300 IU/kg for reptiles (Wallach & Hoff, 1982).

Hypervitaminosis A rarely occurs naturally but may be induced by overdosing with vitamin A injections at 1000 times or more the daily recommended doses. If this occurs acute toxicity develops with mucus membrane and skin sloughing and frequently death within 24–48 hours. Vitamin A supplements are therefore often given orally as, due to slower absorption, this reduces the risk of this condition developing.

Vitamin D: vitamin D_3 is the most active form for calcium homeostasis, and plants are not effective as suppliers of this compound.

Cholecalciferol, the precursor of vitamin D_3, is manufactured in the reptile or amphibian's skin in a process enhanced by ultraviolet light. For this reason indoor animals produce much less of this compound unless supplied with an effective artificial ultraviolet light source.

Hypovitaminosis D_3 causes problems with calcium metabolism, and leads to rickets. This is exacerbated by low calcium high phosphorus-containing diets. A typical sufferer would be a young growing reptile, kept indoors with no ultraviolet light supplementation and fed on a low calcium diet – for example lettuce/celery/cucumber for herbivores, or meat only/day old mice/chicks for carnivorous species. The condition so produced is referred to as 'metabolic bone disease'.

An animal so affected is frequently apparently 'well-muscled', due to poorly mineralised bones which increase their thickness to maintain their strength. There is often flaring of the epiphyseal

plates at the ends of the long bones, with concomitant bowing of the limbs. Green iguanas and other herbivorous species such as terrestrial chelonians are particularly susceptible, with the lizards showing *rachitic rosettes* (Frye, 1991) due to flaring of the epiphysis in the ribs at the costochondral junction.

Chelonia develop 'lumpy shell', a deformity of the carapace in particular, where the edges roll upwards creating a 'Cornish pasty' effect, and the muscles which attach the limbs to the inside of the shell, pull the carapace downwards creating pits either side cranially and caudally (Fig. 10.3). Recommended maximum levels are 50–100 IU/kg every other day.

Hypervitaminosis D_3 occurs due to over supplementation with D_3 and calcium and leads to calcification of soft tissues, such as the medial wall of the arteries, and the kidneys, creating hypertension and organ failure. This often occurs in herbivores such as tortoises fed on tinned cat and dog food.

Vitamin E: hypovitaminosis E may occur due to a reduction in fat metabolism or absorption, such as can occur in small intestinal, pancreatic or biliary diseases, or due to a lack of dietary green plant material for herbivores. A relative deficiency will occur in species eating large amounts of polyunsaturated fats, for example marine fish such as tuna and mackerel. These use up the

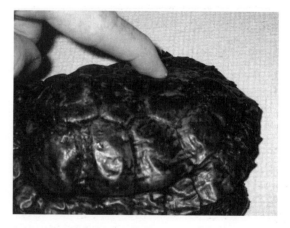

Fig. 10.3   Red-eared terrapin, *Trachemys scripta elegans*, with hypovitaminosis D_3.

body's vitamin E reserves. A condition called steatitis, wherein body fat starts to necrose, has been seen in gharials (a fish-eating crocodilian) (Frye, 1991) and terrapins.

Hypervitaminosis E is extremely rare.

Vitamin K: because of its production by gut bacteria, it is very difficult to get a true deficiency, although absorption will be reduced when fat digestion or absorption is reduced as in biliary or pancreatic disease. The consumption of warfarin and coumarin derived compounds (as found in sweet clovers) can increase the demand for clotting factors, and this may also be seen in snakes consuming prey which has been killed by these rodenticides. Disease so caused is characterised by increased internal and external haemorrhage, but vitamin K also has some function in calcium/phosphorous metabolism in bone so this may also be affected. Frye (1991) has recorded disease in crocodiles exhibiting gingival bleeding without petechiation. Recommended minimum levels for reptiles are 1 ppm (Wallach & Hoff, 1982).

Water-soluble vitamins

Vitamin B_1 (thiamine): a source of thiaminases, enzymes which destroy thiamine, is raw salt-water fish which may be fed to some snakes, crocodilians and turtles, such as garter snakes, red-eared terrapins and gharials. There are thiamine antagonists as well in blackberries, beetroot, coffee, chocolate and tea when considering herbivores. When a relative deficiency occurs, neurological signs such as opisthotonus, weakness and head tremors may be seen. In garter and water snakes, a classical inability to right itself occurs, with the snake continually flipping onto its back. In addition, fungal infections are reported as more likely after a B_1 deficiency. The recommended minimum level for reptiles is 20–35 mg/kg food offered. In addition, if sea-fish such as smelt, which are high in thiaminases, are to be fed, cooking the fish for 5 minutes at 80°C deactivates the thiaminase. In a reptile with thiamine deficiency, doses of 50–100 mg/kg body weight should be given. Because of this problem it is often advised feeding garter and water snakes on rodent prey rather

than sea-fish. They may be encouraged to eat this by wiping the rodent prey with the fish to which it is accustomed to cover the scent.

Biotin: deficiencies do occur commonly in gila monsters, beaded lizards and monitor lizards all of which enjoy raw eggs in the wild. In this state the majority of eggs are fertile, and contain little avidin (an antibiotin vitamin). However, unfertilised hen's eggs are high in avidin and so a relative biotin deficiency may occur. Deficiencies produce muscular weakness, occasionally with skin lesions. It is therefore recommended that minimal levels of raw eggs are fed to such reptiles.

Folic acid: a deficiency of folic acid is rare but can lead to severely impaired cellular division. This can lead to a number of obvious problems such as females reproductive tracts not maturing, a macrocytic anaemia due to failure of red blood cell maturation and immune system cellular dysfunction. A relative deficiency of folic acid may occur in some individuals fed a very high protein diet, as folic acid is needed to produce the waste products of protein metabolism in reptiles, uric acid. In addition there are inhibitors of folic acid in some foods such as cabbage and other brassicas, oranges, beans and peas, and the use of trimethoprim sulphonamide drugs also reduces gut bacterial folic acid production.

Vitamin B_{12}: vitamin B_{12} is produced generally by intestinal bacteria and so deficiencies are uncommon but may occur after prolonged antibiotic medication. Deficiency produces slow growth, muscular dystrophy in the legs, poor hatching rates, high mortality rates and hatching deformities in young reptiles and amphibians.

Choline: choline may be synthesised in the body, but not in enough quantities for the growing reptile. Because of interactions, the need for choline is dependent on levels of folic acid and vitamin B_{12}. Excess protein therefore, as with folic acid, increases choline requirements, as does a diet high in fats. Deficiency causes retarded growth, disrupted fat metabolism and fatty liver damage.

Vitamin C: there is no direct need for this vitamin in reptiles and amphibians as vitamin C may be produced from glucose in the outermost portions of the kidneys. However, during disease processes, particularly those which affect liver function, it may be beneficial to the recovery process to provide a dietary source of vitamin C. It is required for the formation of elastic fibres and connective tissues and is an excellent anti-oxidant similar to vitamin E. Deficiency leads to 'scurvy' where there is poor wound healing, increased bleeding due to capillary-wall fragility and bone alterations. Deficiency has been postulated as the cause of skin splitting in snakes fed rodent prey that had been starved for 24–48 hours prior to being fed (Frye, 1991). This allowed the emptying of their gastrointestinal tract, and hence reduced levels of vitamin C from the plant material therein. It has also been suggested that increasing vitamin C levels by supplementation at levels of 10–20 mg/kg intramuscularly or orally (Frye, 1991) may be useful in the treatment of chronic infections, such as 'mouth rot' in snakes.

Minerals

As with mammals there are two main groups of minerals, those classified as macro-minerals, i.e. those present in large amounts in the body, such as calcium and phosphorus, and micro-minerals, or trace elements, such as manganese, iron and cobalt, which are all necessary for normal bodily function.

Macro-minerals

Calcium: calcium has a wide range of bodily functions, the two most obvious being its role in the formation of the skeleton and mineralisation of bone matrix, and its requirement for muscular contractions. The active form of calcium in the body is the ionic double charged molecule Ca^{2+}. Low levels of this form, even though the overall body reserves of calcium are normal, leads to hyperexcitability, fitting and death, conditions seen in gravid female egg-bound green iguanas.

The ratio of calcium to phosphorus is important – as one increases the other decreases and vice versa. This is controlled by the hormones calcitonin, parathyroid hormone and the accessory hormone vitamin D_3. A ratio of 2:1 calcium to phosphorus is desirable in growing reptiles, and 1.5:1 for adults. In high egg laying periods though, to keep pace with the output of calcium into the shells, a ratio of 10:1 may be needed.

Calcium deficiency causes nutritional osteodystrophy, or metabolic bone disease, and is often accompanied by deficiency in vitamin D_3. Normal levels of vitamin D_3, however, may exacerbate this disease as they encourage further calcium resorption. Deficiency may be seen in lizards such as green iguanas and water dragons, and chelonians fed on high fruit, lettuce, celery etc. diets. Diets with excessive levels of oxalates, compounds which bind up calcium and prevent it being absorbed, such as spinach and beetroot or rhubarb leaves, can also lead to a deficiency.

Calcium deficiency may also be seen in insectivorous species, such as geckos, and bearded dragons, fed on insects without supplementation (Fig. 10.4). Insects have little or no calcium, their tough outer coat is made of a protein known as chitin. To provide adequate calcium therefore, the insect must be dusted with a calcium powder *immediately* before being fed (if not, by the time the reptile has caught the insect most of the powder has fallen off!). Alternatively, the insect is pre-fed on a calcium supplement. This is mixed in with the insect's food and fed for the 24–48 hours prior to feeding the reptile, so that the insect's gut is pre-loaded with calcium.

Extensive resorption of calcium occurs from the bones during dietary deficiencies, leaving only fibrous tissue. This is considerably weaker and so the 'bones' thicken to maintain their strength. Even so the bones are weakened, and bowing of long bones and spontaneous fractures occur in lizards, collapsing of spinal vertebrae and deformities in most reptiles and deformed, lumpy shells in chelonians. Excessive calcium in the diet (>1%) though reduces the use of proteins, fats, phosphorus, manganese, zinc, iron and iodine, and can lead to soft tissue mineralisation if in conjunction with adequate or excessive vitamin D_3 levels. Red-eared terrapins have been shown to have a

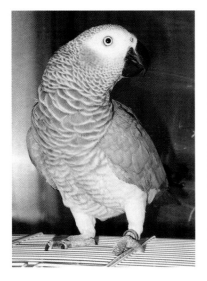

Plate 1.1 The African grey parrot is a commonly seen pet and makes one of the best talkers.

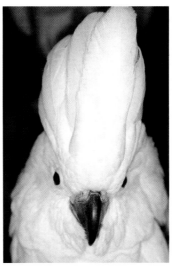

Plate 1.2 Many parrots such as this umbrella cockatoo are striking birds.

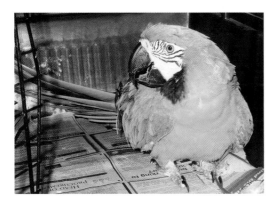

Plate 1.3 Parrots beaks make impressive crushing tools such as this blue and gold macaw, *Ara ararauna*.

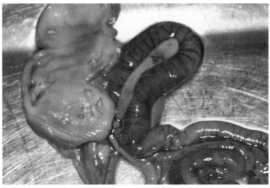

Plate 1.4 The normal lining of the ventriculus or gizzard is known as the koilin, and is often stained green with bile pigments. Note the cream coloured pancreas between the loop of descending and ascending duodenum.

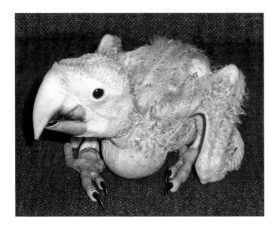

Plate 2.1 Young Psittaciformes are altricial like most avian species, and born with little or no feather covering.

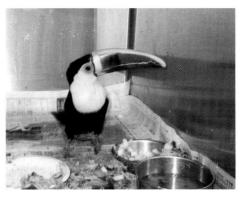

Plate 3.1 Rhamphastids, such as this red-billed toucan, have impressive beaks which need careful handling.

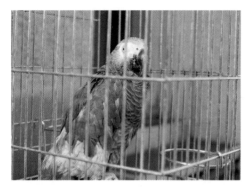

Plate 5.1 Viral diseases such as psittacine beak and feather disease in this African grey parrot may cause feather colouration changes (note multiple red feathers on the main body).

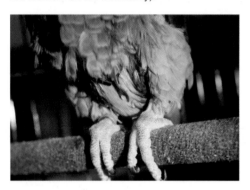

Plate 5.3 Ascites will show as ventral abdomen distension and may indicate liver disease. In this case rarely the skin has become jaundiced, a condition not commonly seen in avian species with liver failure.

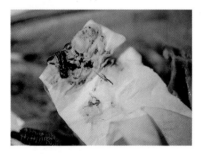

Plate 5.4 Lime green urates in raptors may indicate lead poisoning.

Plate 7.2 Ventral view of a bearded dragon, *Pogona vitticeps*, post mortem. The heart may be seen at the top of the picture, immediately below which are the dark coloured lungs, and then the red coloured liver. Below this lies the stomach and intestines. The two dark masses reflected ventrally are abdominal fat pads. Note the overall large amounts of dark melanin pigment found in the internal organs of many desert dwelling species.

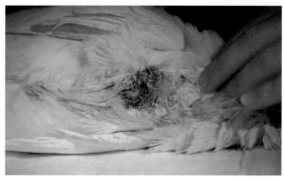

Plate 5.2 Crop burns may be caused by feeding of too hot a rearing formula.

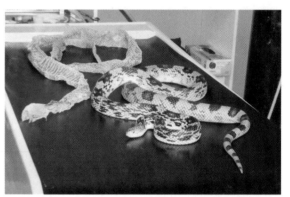

Plate 7.1 Snakes should perform a whole body slough when shedding their skin, such as that seen in this pine snake.

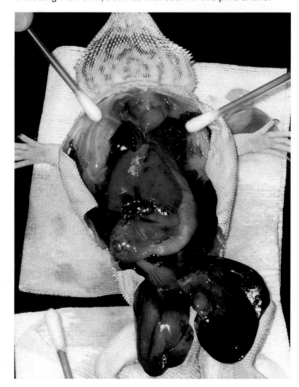

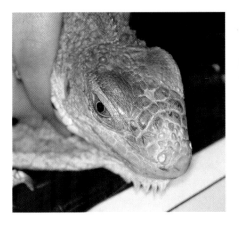

Plate 7.3 Head of green iguana showing the parietal or third eye lying at the midline on the dorsal aspect of the head.

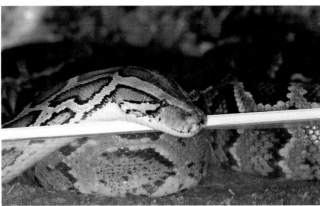

Plate 8.1 Large vivaria are needed for large species of snake such as this Burmese python, which may reach 16 feet in length. Note bark substrate of tank.

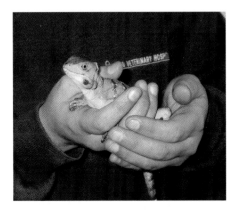

Plate 9.1 Restraint of a docile species such as this female plumed basilisk. Note facial abscess.

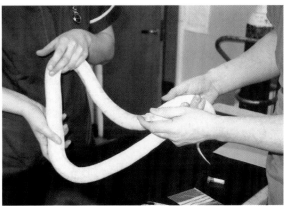

Plate 9.2 While large snakes must be handled by more than one person, even smaller species such as this corn snake are best handled by two people. Note the control of the head between thumb and forefinger.

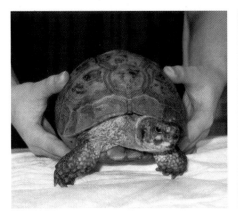

Plate 9.3 Correct position to lift a tortoise with both hands either side of the shell between the front and rear limbs.

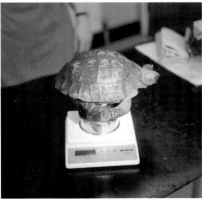

Plate 9.4 Method of short-term restraint of Chelonia by placing the animal on a pedestal so that it rests on the plastron.

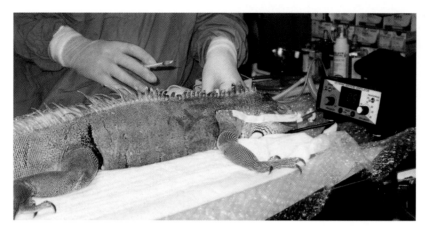

Plate 9.5 Intubation of reptiles, such as this green iguana, allows the use of intermittent positive pressure ventilation, which is being performed here by a mechanical ventilator unit (Vetronic Services).

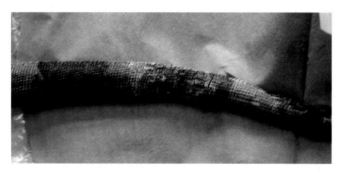

Plate 11.1 Fungal granulomatous disease in the tail of a green iguana.

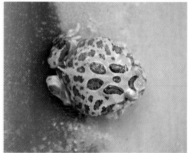

Plate 11.3 Redleg in an Argentinian horned frog.

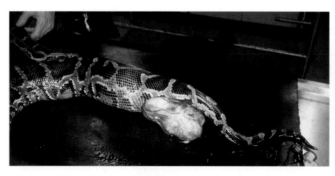

Plate 11.2 Dystocia is uncommon in snakes, but may cause prolapse of the oviduct as here.

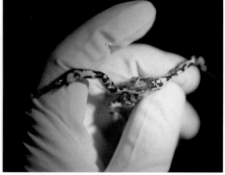

Plate 11.4 Saprolegniasis in a fire-bellied toad.

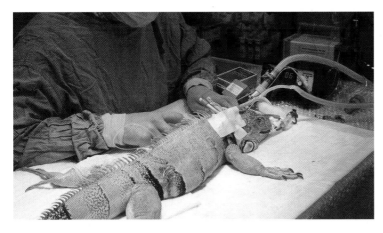

Plate 12.1 Surgical placement of a pharyngostomy tube in an anorectic green iguana.

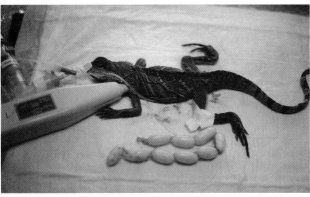

Plate 12.2 Surgical speying of a water dragon with post-ovulatory stasis.

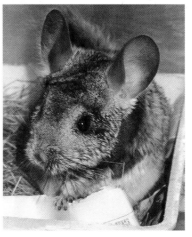

Plate 13.1 Chinchillas have fine bones and are prone to fractures, which are often compound. If these become badly infected amputation may be necessary.

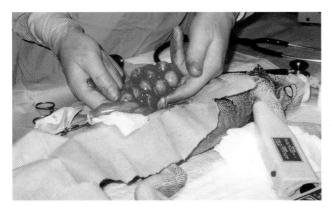

Plate 12.3 Surgical speying of a female green iguana with pre-ovulatory stasis. Note multiple yellow yolks of the ovaries.

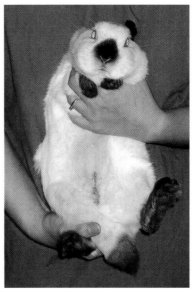

Plate 15.1 Method of holding a rabbit for examination of the ventrum.

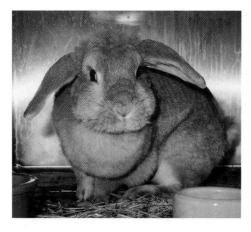

Plate 17.1 Lop breeds of rabbit are more prone to dental disease due to their foreshortened heads, which may lead to uneven molar wear.

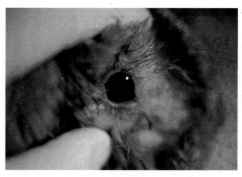

Plate 17.2 Ocular disease may be associated with rabbit snuffles but often starts in the tear duct rather than the eye. Dental problems are sometimes the cause.

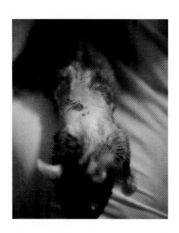

Plate 17.3 Mite infestation in mice may be intensely pruritic.

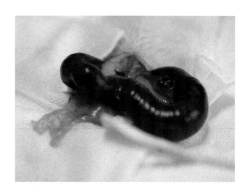

Plate 17.4 Rodents such as the rat are prone to pyometras.

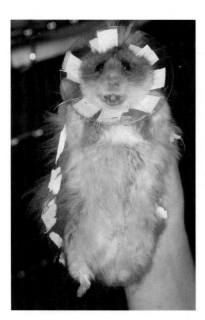

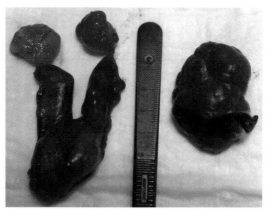

Plate 17.5 (Left) Leg amputation is not uncommon for compound fractures of hamsters after falls from the ceilings of wire cages. Note Elizabethan collar to prevent wound trauma.

Plate 17.6 (Above) Cystic ovarian disease is common in older female guinea pigs. The cystic ovaries and uterus are shown here after removal under anaesthetic.

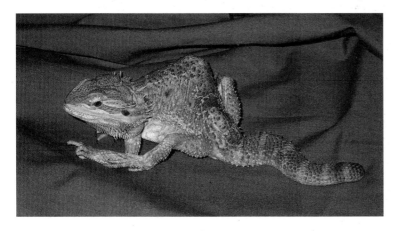

Fig. 10.4 Bearded dragon, *Pogona vitticeps*, with metabolic bone disease and resultant spinal and limb deformity.

requirement for 2% calcium on a dry matter basis (Kass *et al.*, 1982).

Phosphorus: phosphorus is widespread in plant and animal tissues, but in the former it may be bound up in unavailable form as phytates. Levels of phosphorus are controlled in the body as for calcium, the two being in equal and opposite equilibrium with each other. Therefore, if dietary phosphorus levels exceed calcium levels appreciably the parathyroid glands become stimulated to produce more parathyroid hormone and nutritional secondary hyperparathyroidism occurs. This leads to progressive bone demineralisation and renal damage due to high circulating levels of parathyroid hormone. High dietary phosphorus also reduces the amount of calcium which can be absorbed from the gut, as it complexes with the calcium present there. This can be a problem in reptiles fed pure meat with no calcium or bone supplement, and in herbivores which are predominantly fruit and lettuce consumers as these are high phosphorus low calcium foods. Green vegetables or supplementation with calcium powders may therefore be necessary. In addition, low calcium/high phosphorus levels frequently allow bladder stones to form in those species (such as chelonians, green iguanas etc.) that have a bladder.

Magnesium: most magnesium is absorbed from the small intestine, and is affected by large amounts of calcium in the diet which reduce magnesium absorption. Deficiencies rarely occur, but muscular weakness can be the result.

Potassium: as with mammals, potassium is the major intracellular positive ion. Rarely is there a dietary deficiency, but severe stress can cause hypokalaemia through increased kidney excretion because of elevated plasma proteins. This can lead to cardiac dysrhythmias, muscle spasticity and neurological dysfunction.

Sodium: sodium is the main extracellular positive ion and regulates the body's acid base balance and osmotic potential. In conjunction with potassium, it is responsible for nerve signals and impulses. Rarely does a true dietary deficiency occur, but hyponatraemia may occur due to chronic diarrhoea or renal disease. Many reptiles have salt glands found outside the kidneys responsible solely for the excretion of excess sodium whilst conserving water. The green iguana's salt glands, for example, are present inside the nostrils, and white crystalline deposits of salt may be seen here and are frequently sneezed out. It may be necessary to supplement the diet of marine species with sodium chloride if kept in fresh water situations, or if fed freshwater plants or fish.

Chlorine: this is the major extracellular negative ion and is responsible for maintaining acid–base balances in conjunction with sodium and potassium. Deficiencies are rare.

Micro-minerals (trace elements)

These elements include zinc, copper, iron, manganese, cobalt and sulphur all of which have an important part to play in cellular function. However, so far no actual deficiencies specifically related to these elements have been reported in reptiles or amphibians. The exception is iodine.

Iodine: iodine's sole function is in thyroid hormone synthesis, which affects metabolic rate. Deficiency causes goitre and fluid retention (*myxoedema*). It has knock-on effects on growth, causing stunting and neurological problems and in amphibians may prevent metamorphosis from intermediate tadpole stages to the adult form. In reptiles it is most often encountered in giant terrestrial tortoises, which will exhibit goitre swelling of the neck. It can also occur due to overfeeding with iodine-binding plants, such as cabbage, cauliflower, broccoli, kale and Brussels sprouts. Excess iodine added to the water may cause species such as the amphibian axolotl (a neotenic salamander – that is its 'adult' form has the external gills more typical of a tadpole or intermediate lifestage) to shed its external gills. Levels of 0.3 μg/kg body weight have been quoted (Donoghue & Langenburg, 1996).

Specific nutritional problems in reptiles

Below are some common presentations of nutritional problems in reptiles.

Post-hibernation anorexia (PHA)

PHA occurs in the Mediterranean species of tortoise (Hermann's, Greek or spur-thighed, marginated and Horsefield's), which hibernate during the winter months. The commonest presentation is that of an inappetant tortoise after coming out of hibernation, often with signs of systemic or respiratory tract infections (such as the 'runny nose syndrome') and often with a low body weight in

relation to length (a low Jackson's ratio). In addition the blood glucose levels are frequently below 3.2 mmol/l, which appears to be the minimum level required for appetite stimulation (Lawrence, 1987), with high levels of urea.

Dehydration is apparent in these cases, and treatment requires aggressive fluid therapy and nutritional support, using glucose-containing fluids and liquid food stomach tubing, as well as warming the tortoise to its optimum temperature (20–27°C) (Fig. 10.5).

Causes of this condition could involve any one of the following:

- Disease during or prior to hibernation
- Poor nutrition leading to poor fat reserves prior to hibernation
- Owner failure to observe recovery from hibernation for several days, so no food offered at the critical time
- A period of cold weather immediately after recovery.

It is the rising plane of blood glucose post hibernation that acts as the stimulus for appetite in these chelonians, and failure of this rise, due to malnutrition or failure to eat whilst the levels are still high, may lead to unresponsive anorexia.

To prevent PHA, therefore, it is important to attend to disease *prior* to hibernation, and, if severely affected or underweight, the tortoise should not be hibernated, but kept indoors at its

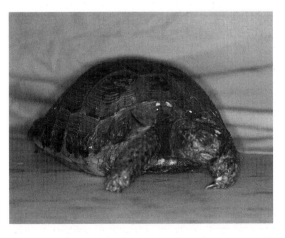

Fig. 10.5 Spur-thighed tortoise, *Testudo graeca*, with post-hibernation anorexia.

optimum temperature range and fed throughout the winter. The tortoise should also be checked regularly once in hibernation, around once or twice a week, to ensure if the tortoise does come out of hibernation early, it has food and water available immediately. Bathing the tortoise immediately after waking in warm water, cleaning the nose, eyes and mouth especially can also stimulate appetite, and no tortoise having recovered from hibernation should be allowed to rehibernate that same winter. Finally, stomach tubing with fluids and soluble carbohydrates, such as the basic sugar and protein containing liquid food Critical Care Formula produced by VetArk or vegetable baby food porridges, early on in the course of the problem can be useful.

Visceral and articular gout

Gout is a condition caused by the unique way that many reptiles deal with the waste products of protein metabolism. Most reptiles are uricotelic, that is the main excretory product of protein metabolism is uric acid. This compound is relatively insoluble in water, which has its advantages as reptiles are therefore able to reduce the water lost in excreting it. Unfortunately, if the reptile becomes dehydrated, either acutely or chronically, or consumes diets with excessive protein levels, particularly a type of protein called purines, or suffers kidney damage, then uric acid levels build up in the bloodstream. If allowed to do so, they will eventually exceed the precipitation point and form crystals inside the body.

Diet is important, as purine proteins which are found mainly in animal protein, are converted readily to uric acid on degradation in the body. Therefore, if herbivorous species, such as green iguanas, which are not used to large volumes of purines, are fed a diet rich in animal protein, such as cat or dog food, they will produce excessive amounts of uric acid and develop gout.

There are two forms of gout, *visceral* and *articular*. Articular gout can easily be diagnosed ante mortem, as it causes gross swelling and inflammation in the joints where the uric acid crystals form. Visceral gout is more difficult to diagnose ante mortem, because it occurs where uric acid crystals are deposited in the soft tissues of the body,

primary sites being the kidneys, the pericardial sac, the lungs, spleen and liver. Once deposited, it is almost impossible to move the crystals medically and permanent damage is often done.

Obesity

Obesity is a common problem in many reptiles and amphibians kept in captivity. Many species are overfed because of owners' ignorance of natural feeding intervals and of food types commonly eaten in the wild. Examples include feeding dog food to tortoises and green iguanas, both of which are totally herbivorous in the wild but both of which will eat meat if offered it. The resulting problems are as mentioned above with excess protein causing gout, excess calcium and vitamin D_3 causing soft tissue mineralisation and excess animal fat causing fatty liver syndrome (hepatic lipidosis) wherein the liver cells are filled with fat deposits impeding their function. Snakes also suffer from these conditions when fed overfat laboratory rodents, or simply fed too often. A rough idea of feeding frequencies is given in Table 10.1.

The aim should be a reptile which does not appear emaciated, but lean.

Hypoglycaemia in crocodilians

It has been reported that crocodiles kept in high density conditions, or are otherwise stressed, are prone to hypoglycaemic fits (Scott, 1992). It is interesting to note that crocodiles' blood sugar levels vary throughout the year, being lower in the winter and highest in the summer. A rising blood sugar level appears to be the stimulus to eat, as seems to be seen with Mediterranean tortoises after hibernation.

Environmental temperature and its effects on nutrition

Because reptiles and amphibians are ectothermic, that is they rely on their surroundings to maintain their body temperature, environmental temperature is important in all aspects of husbandry.

There is an optimum preferred temperature zone that will allow their enzymes and metabolic pathways to function at their optimum levels, so

Table 10.1 Feeding frequencies and food types for various reptile species.

Species	Feeding frequency and food types
Herbivores (e.g. iguanas, tortoises)	Daily grazing of food advised
Small insectivores (e.g. leopard geckos, collared lizards)	Fed 2–3 times weekly on live insect prey 'to appetite'
Small carnivores (e.g. garter snakes, corn snakes)	Fed 2–3 times weekly on rat pups, 'fuzzies' (furred baby mice) or 'pinkies' (nude baby mice) according to size
Medium carnivores (e.g. kingsnakes, ratsnakes)	Fed 1–2 times weekly, adult mice or small rats
Large carnivores (e.g. boa constrictors, Burmese pythons)	Fed once weekly or fortnightly (the larger the snake the less often) on adult rats or small rabbits

environmental temperature will influence the rate of digestion of the food offered. It may take 2–3 days for a rat consumed by a large boa constrictor to pass through its digestive system if kept within its preferred temperature zone of 25–30°C, but if kept 5–10°C cooler this will often slow down to 5–7 days, and if kept much lower than this digestion may not occur before the prey item becomes rancid inside the snake. Similarly, if kept at too high a temperature, the reptile may not be stimulated to eat at all and dehydration and heat stress may set in.

A general guide to feeding reptiles

Fresh food should always be fed to reptiles. It should also be remembered that at the increased temperatures of most vivaria, the food offered will spoil very quickly and will need to be replaced frequently.

Snakes

It is important to note that it is illegal to feed live vertebrate prey to another animal in the United Kingdom. All rodent prey fed to snakes and lizards must therefore have been humanely killed

first. In addition, live prey may damage the reptile if the latter is not hungry and does not kill the prey quickly.

To encourage anorectic snakes to eat, a number of tricks may be employed including:

- Warming the prey briefly before offering by heating it in a pot of hot water
- Breaking the prey item open to release the scent of blood
- Teasing the snake by moving the dead prey item around the cage with forceps, to mimic live prey
- Trying a variety of colours of prey – some snakes will only take dark-furred rodents
- To get a snake (such as a garter or water snake) used to eating rodent prey after only eating fish or amphibians (hog-nosed snakes), wipe the rodent to be offered with the previously taken food item to transfer scent
- Ensure that there are plenty of areas to hide; some boids and pythons like to consume their prey in a box or hide
- Leave the prey in overnight because some species prefer to hunt at night
- Choose the next smallest size of rodent, so if adult mice were previously offered try fuzzies, if juvenile rats, try adult mice, etc.

NB The term 'pinkies' refers to nude neonatal rat and mice pups, 'fuzzies' refers to week-old rat and mice pups with a thin covering of fur and 'furries' refers to juvenile rat and mice pups between 1–3 weeks of age which have a soft but longer covering of fur.

Refeeding syndrome

If anorexia in a snake or other reptile has persisted for some time it is essential to rehydrate the patient before attempting to feed. Indeed, initial feeding after this should be started off at very low levels. This is because excess calories and proteins cause a rapid uptake of glucose from the bloodstream into the cells, which takes potassium and phosphorous with it. This can lead to a life-threatening hypokalaemia and hypophosphataemia. The monitoring of blood phosphorus and potassium is therefore to be recommended when treating chronically anorectic reptiles, whether carnivorous or herbivorous.

Herbivores

If using a commercial pelleted food for iguanas or tortoises, then be sure to soak the pellets thoroughly before feeding, otherwise they swell up inside the reptile causing colic and bloat. Commercial pelleted diets are a useful adjunct to the diet of herbivorous reptiles and many companies now produce iguanid and chelonian diets which are well supplemented with minerals and vitamins and also contain moderate levels of fibre for gut motility enhancement.

The feeding of certain foods to herbivores should be prohibited. Animal proteins are one, as are certain fruit and vegetables. We have already discussed the problems of excessive volumes of largely water-containing vegetables such as lettuce, cucumber and celery, the goitrogenic properties of cabbage, kale, broccoli and cauliflower and the anti-calcium effect of oxalate-containing plants such as spinach, beetroot and rhubarb leaves. In addition, fruits such as banana can cause a sugar ferment in herbivorous reptiles causing colic, as well as adhering to the mouthparts and encouraging local infection. Avocados have an extremely high fat content and should not be fed to herbivorous reptiles due to potential secondary fatty degeneration of the liver.

Sample diet for green iguanas

Pelleted soaked commercial food may be fed at around 25% of daily intake. The rest can be based on the following: Up to half of the plant material offered can be made of calcium-rich vegetables such as kale, dandelions, chicory, watercress, cabbage, flat-leaved parsley, basil, coriander etc. The other half may be made up of other vegetable matter such as peas, beans, carrots, sweet peppers, courgettes or marrows, cauliflower florets and flowers of plants such as nasturtiums, dandelions, roses etc. To this mixture can be added small amounts of fruit such as apples, pears, tomatoes, plums, strawberries, raspberries, melon, passion fruit, papaya etc., or fibrous foods such as bran cereals, brown bread and cooked brown rice.

This combination should be thoroughly mixed so as to prevent selective feeding and to it should be added a supplement of calcium in the form of calcium lactate or gluconate, or a natural calcium source such as cuttlefish or oyster shells. In addition the use of a vitamin D_3/calcium supplement once or twice a week, particularly for growing iguanas and egg-laying females, is advised.

Sample diet for Mediterranean tortoises

The majority of the diet is to be composed of vegetable matter of a leafy nature such as dandelions, kale, watercress, flat-leaved parsley, chicory and bok-choy. To this may be added peas, beans, hay or dried grass, fresh grass (not cut), grated carrot, grated pumpkin and sweet peppers.

To this may be added small volumes of fruit such as apples, pears, melon, papaya, passion fruit, strawberries, plums, flowers such as dandelions, nasturtiums, roses and sprouted seeds such as mung beans, lentils, and chick peas.

For more tropical species, such as the red and yellow footed tortoises (*Geochelone carbonaria* and *Geochelone denticulata*), the amount of fruit and flowers may be doubled.

For grassland species, such as leopard tortoises (*Geochelone pardalis*) and Indian starred tortoises (*Geochelone elegans*), a good provision of fresh uncut grass or good quality hay is advised.

For more omnivorous species, such as box turtles (*Terrapene carolina*), up to 50% of the above fruit and vegetable diet may be replaced with adult maintenance dry dog foods (soaked), mealworms, crickets, earthworms and even baby mice (pinkies). Juveniles of this species tend to be more carnivorous than the adults.

In all of these diets it is recommended that daily supplementation with calcium lactate or gluconate be included, with a calcium/vitamin D_3 supplement added once or twice weekly depending whether the tortoise is a juvenile (higher requirement) or an adult (lower requirement).

Diets for snakes and insectivorous species have been mentioned. The latter need calcium supplementation as discussed in the section considering calcium as a macro-mineral which may either be dusted onto the insects, or pre-fed to them to load their digestive contents with the calcium.

References

Donoghue, S. (1998) Nutrition of pet amphibians and reptiles. *Seminars in Avian and Exotic Pet Medicine* **7**, 3.

Donoghue, S. and Langenburg, J. (1996) Nutrition. In *Reptile Medicine and Surgery* (Mader, D., ed), pp. 148–174. W.B. Saunders, Philadelphia.

Frye, F. (1991) A practical guide for feeding captive reptiles. In *Biomedical and Surgical Aspects of Captive Reptile Husbandry Vol 1*. Krieger Publishing Inc, Malabar, Florida.

Kass, R.E., Ullrey, D.E. and Trapp, A.L. (1982) A study of calcium requirements of the Red-eared slider turtle *(Pseudemys scripta elegans)*. *Journal of Zoo Animal Medicine*, **13**, 62.

Lawrence, K. (1987) Post hibernational anorexia in captive Mediterranean tortoises *(Testudo graeca and T. hermanii)*. *Veterinary Record* **120**, 87.

Scott, P.W. (1992) Nutritional diseases. In *Manual of Reptiles* (Beynon, P.H., Lawton, M.P.C. and Cooper, J.E., eds), pp. 138–152. BSAVA, Cheltenham.

Wallach, J.D. and Hoff, G.L. (1982) Metabolic and nutritional diseases of reptiles. In *Non-infectious Diseases of Wildlife* (Hoff, G.L. and Davis, J.W., eds), pp. 155–168. Iowa State Press, Ames.

Further reading

Barten, S.L. (1996) Lizards. In *Reptile Medicine and Surgery* (Mader, D., ed), pp. 47–60. W.B. Saunders, Philadelphia.

Boyer, J.H. (1996) *Turtles, tortoises and terrapins*. In *Reptile Medicine and Surgery* (Mader, D., ed), pp. 61–77. W.B. Saunders, Philadelphia.

Frye, F. (1995) *Reptile Clinicians Handbook*. Krieger Publishing Co, Malabar, Florida.

Zimmerman, E. (1995) *Reptiles and Amphibians: Care, Behaviour and Reproduction*. TFM Publishing Inc, Neptune City, New Jersey.

Chapter 11

Common Reptile and Amphibian Diseases

Skin disease

Dysecdysis

Dysecdysis occurs when the normal process of skin shedding (known as *ecdysis*) fails. It occurs in snakes, and to a lesser extent, lizards. The process of ecdysis involves the forming of a new skin beneath the old one. Once this is complete, a series of proteolytic enzymes and lymphatic fluid is secreted between the new skin layer and the overlying old one. This lifts the old layer and separates the two, and makes the snake appear dull and lack-lustre with the eyes noticeably blueing. This lasts for 5–7 days on average in the snake. Once complete the fluid is reabsorbed, and the snake appears to return to its normal hue. After a further 5–7 days the skin is shed, in the case of the snake, in one piece, from the head end first. It is initiated in snakes by rubbing the face on an abrasive surface to loosen the first piece of skin. When the separation fails to occur, whether in part or totally, the condition is known as dysecdysis.

The causes of dysecdysis are many and varied, but can include any condition which can cause dehydration so reducing lymphatic fluid available to separate the skin layers. If the reptile is malnourished dysecdysis may occur due to a lack of proteolytic enzymes. Alternatively old scars, a lack of an abrasive surface in the vivarium upon which to start the process or severe ectoparasitism may also cause dysecdysis (Fig. 11.1).

Scale rot

Scale rot is a colloquial term for a range of conditions affecting the reptile skin which result in severe infections.

Septicaemic cutaneous ulcerative disease (SCUD)

Septicaemic cutaneous ulcerative disease (SCUD) is a condition seen in aquatic chelonians. It is caused by the bacterium *Citrobacter freundii* which, once it has gained access to the bloodstream, produces ulcers in the skin and loosening of scales with general debilitation and, in many cases, death (Fig. 11.2).

Blister disease

This is a form of scale rot seen in snakes, particularly semi-aquatic species such as garter or water snakes. It can however occur in any species which is exposed to a persistently damp substrate. The outer layer of skin develops blisters of a clear fluid which become secondarily infected with environmental bacteria such as *Aeromonas* spp or *Pseudomonas* spp. These can progress to envelop the whole of the ventral aspect of the snake, and lead to septicaemia. Occasionally these conditions may involve a fungus such as *Aspergillus* spp.

Abscesses

Abscesses have recently been quoted as being more accurately termed *fibriscesses* (Huchzermeyer & Cooper, 2001) due to the unique nature of reptile and avian abscess formation. Instead of the liquid pus we are more familiar with in mammals, reptiles and birds form a solid, caseous, dried swelling surrounded by a thick shell of fibrous tissue. This is due to the lack of lysozymes (a form of destructive enzyme found in macrophages and other immune system cells) that help liquefy foreign matter. Instead the reptile engulfs the material in immune system

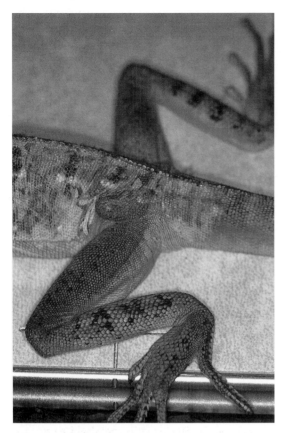

Fig. 11.1 Dysecdysis in a lizard with a subcutaneous abscess.

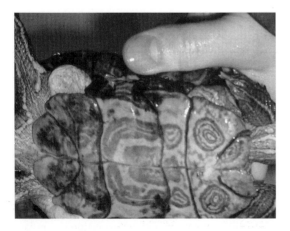

Fig. 11.2 SCUD in a red-eared terrapin, *Trachemys scripta elegans*.

cells and to contain the problem further throws up a thick connective-tissue wall around the area, forming a solid swelling (Fig. 11.1). These may form anywhere, but a common site in chelonians is the middle ear, causing a bulging of the ear drum. The pathogens involved are frequently Gram negative species, although the presence of fungi in abscesses has been well recorded.

Erythema, petechiae and ecchymoses

These three conditions may all be present at the same time or may appear individually.

Erythema is the reddening of skin tissues due to vascular congestion beneath. It can be seen in reptiles as a pink hue to the areas between scutes in the case of chelonians (Fig. 11.2) and croco-dylians, or the more generalised reddening of the skin seen in snakes. Erythema is often suggestive of a generalised medical condition such as septicaemia.

Petechiae are the pin-point haemorrhages seen in many reptiles. They can be seen in areas such as caused by the mouth, where they often suggest the incidence of an oral infection such as 'mouth rot'. They may be seen over the whole of the body suggesting the possibility of septicaemia. Other conditions include clotting deficiencies such as are caused by the consumption of rodent prey which has itself consumed a warfarin-type poison.

Ecchymoses are larger areas of haemorrhage, and may be caused by severe local infection or conditions mentioned above.

Overgrown beaks and claws

Overgrown beaks are common in chelonians, and are often due to a lack of abrasive foodstuffs or abrasive surfaces from which to eat them. The beak may become so overgrown that the reptile is unable to feed itself. Beaks may be trimmed using a slow-speed dental drill, or a battery-powered hand-held drill in much the same way as a bird's overgrown beak can be trimmed.

Overgrown claws can also be a problem in lizards and chelonians due to the lack of abrasive substrates in their environment. It should be noted however that some species have perfectly normal apparently 'long' claws. An example is the male red-eared terrapin which uses his claws as a display aid to attract and mate the female. Otherwise, trimming the claws with a standard pair of feline claw clippers is advised.

Pigment changes

An example of a physiologically normal colour change is seen in the Chameleonidae which will often blend with their surroundings and darken in colour as they become stressed. Green iguanas often become yellow brown in colour as they become stressed or unwell, and many of these species will exhibit darkening at the site of an injection. Areas of previous trauma may become whitened.

Ectoparasitic

Mites

The most commonly seen mite in snakes is *Ophionyssus natricis* which appears as red to dark-coloured pin-head mites hiding under the overlapping edges of scales. They may be seen in water dishes in which the reptile has been bathing. They can cause severe irritation, pruritus and self-trauma, as well as potentially causing anaemia and conditions such as dysecdysis. In addition, they can be responsible for transmitting *Aeromonas* spp bacteria, which may cause septicaemia. There are other mites, such as the cloacal mites of aquatic turtles of the family *Cloacarus* spp. In addition, there is of course the non-parasitic harvest mite or *Neotrombicula autumnalis* which may be brought in on straw and hay bedding material. The adult itself is not irritant but the six legged larval stage is and may cause the reptile to traumatise itself.

Ticks

Wild-caught species are common sufferers of ticks, but ticks are also seen in reptiles kept in owners' gardens, such as tortoises. In the United Kingdom the species *Ixodes ricinus* (the sheep or deer tick) and *Ixodes hexagonous* (the hedgehog tick) are seen. These attach to soft, thin-skinned areas. In tortoises these are naturally the areas around the neck inlet and in front of the hind legs. They may cause local damage and can transmit a range of viral and bacterial pathogens. These include the bacteria *Staphylococcus aureus*, the cause of tick pyaemia and *Borrelia burghdorferi*, the cause of Lyme's disease.

Blowfly myiasis

Myiasis is a particular problem for any reptile kept in insanitory conditions or those with diarrhoea. In particular, tortoises are at high risk during the summer months. Members of the blue bottle, black bottle and green bottle family are all capable of laying eggs on a tortoise. In peak conditions these can hatch into larvae or maggots within 1–2 hours. These then burrow away from the light, into the body of the tortoise causing severe trauma, infections, shock and ultimately death.

Leeches

Leeches tend not to be such a problem in the United Kingdom, but can affect aquatic species all over the world. The family Annelidae are the most dangerous, and cause large wounds which continue to bleed after the leech has detached. These may then become secondarily infected.

Traumatic and spontaneous damage

Traumatic damage can be due to attacks by predators or other reptiles, such as those induced by males fighting over a female. In some species, such as green iguanas, the male mounting the female during mating bites the shoulder area vigorously causing open wounds. In the United Kingdom it is unlawful to feed live vertebrate prey to any animal, but invertebrate live prey can be offered and these can still cause trauma to a sick or anorectic reptile. Finally, injuries from cage furniture, are commonplace. Unprotected heat sources frequently cause severe burns.

Spontaneous skin damage wherein the skin has split as the snake has swallowed prey, has been recorded in some snakes. It has been postulated that this may be due to a deficiency in vitamin C

(Frye, 1991) or even an hereditary defect in skin elasticity.

In some chelonians, scutes may be seen to lift off, often weeping clear fluid beneath them. This is frequently associated with underlying renal disease.

Iatrogenic causes of skin damage are also seen in some reptiles such as chelonians. This can occur after overadministration of vitamin A, which can cause sloughing of the epidermal layer on the head, neck and limbs, exposing the underlying dermis.

Tumours

Fibrosarcomas of the head are commonly seen in lizards and snakes. Melanomas are also seen relatively frequently in pigmented species.

Bacterial

Many bacteria have been mentioned already. Others which have been closely associated with skin disease include *Salmonella* spp. These can cause skin abscesses, septicaemia and areas of skin sloughing. Others such as *Mycobacteria* spp may be seen associated with the appearance of swellings, producing classical tuberculous lesions. The mycobacteria found are more commonly environmental ones rather than the human or cattle tuberculosis organisms.

Fungal

Many of the fungi found in the local environment are found associated with wounds. These include *Aspergillus* spp, *Penicillium* spp and dermatophytes (the cause of ringworm in mammals). Diagnosis is by histopathological demonstration and culture. Plate 11.1 shows fungal granulomatous disease on the tail of an iguana.

Viral

There are more and more cases of viral associated disease being diagnosed in reptiles each day. Herpes viruses causing grey patch disease have been found in turtles, papilloma viruses in lizards, and pox viruses in caimens (a member of the family Crocodylia).

Hereditary

Many species exhibit scale and skin abnormalities. These vary from cleft palates, to failure of scales to develop at all. In addition many colour variations have been specifically bred for.

Digestive disease

Oral ('mouth rot')

'Mouth rot' is the colloquial term for the oral infections, or *stomatitis*, commonly seen in many reptiles. It is particularly seen in snakes and chelonians, in the latter species often after hibernation and associated with anorexia.

The causes are many and varied. In the case of chelonians it has been associated with a herpes virus. In many snakes and tortoises however it is caused by secondary infections with Gram negative bacteria. The initial cause of the damage can be rubbing of the snout on vivarium glass, particularly in snakes. The use of opaque tape stuck to the outside of the glass helps the snake to 'see it', preventing this injury. Stomatitis may also be due to the overzealous force-feeding of anorectic reptiles, or simply due to other disease or stresses leading to reduced immune system function.

Vomiting and regurgitation

These two conditions are seen commonly in members of the snake family, but rarely in chelonians, crocodylians or saurians (lizards).

In snakes, regurgitation may simply occur due to rough handling, particularly soon after the snake has eaten. Snakes will also regurgitate if fed, or force-fed, food and then kept at suboptimal environmental temperatures.

Parasitic

In snakes, one of the more frequently encountered forms of stomach disease is cryptosporidiosis. It is caused by a single-celled parasite, *Cryptosporidia serpentes*, which invades the outer membrane of cells lining the stomach, most specifically the combined acid and pepsinogen secreting cells responsible for starting the digestive process. This

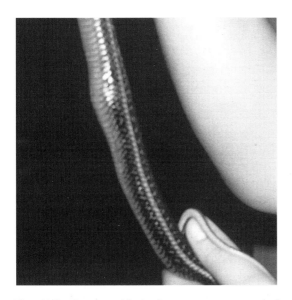

Fig. 11.3 Cryptosporidiosis is a common cause of swellings in the stomach of snakes.

bers of the python family the tapeworm *Bothridium* spp has been reported as a cause of vomiting.

Bacterial and fungal

Bacterial and fungal infections, granulomas and abscesses may also cause damage to the stomach, or pressure on it, and so lead to regurgitation or vomiting.

Tumours

Finally, stomach tumours such as gastric adenomas and adenocarcinomas have been reported. These can lead to vomiting, and often physical enlargement of the stomach may be seen externally.

Lizards and chelonians tend not to regurgitate or vomit. They have a better-developed cardiac sphincter in the stomach. However, it may still occur and is often a very grave indicator of poor health status.

Intestinal disease

Parasitic

Snakes: snakes suffer from a variety of nematode and cestode problems. Species involved include the hookworm *Kalicephalus* spp, ascarids, strongyles such as *Strongyloides* spp and tapeworms such as *Bothridium* spp in pythons and *Ophiotaenia* spp in garter and water snakes.

In addition, snakes may suffer from the parasitic condition *entamoebiasis* caused by the single celled parasite *Entamoeba invadens*. Nearly all species of snake may be affected, and its life cycle is direct, i.e. spread directly from one reptile to another. After incubating in the lining of the small intestine, each infective cyst produces eight uninucleate amoebae which invade cells lining the large intestine of the same snake. The amoebae may also penetrate into the blood stream and so end up in the liver via the hepatoportal blood stream. Here they cause a necrotising hepatitis. The symptoms of entamoebiasis include a bloody mucoid diarrhoea, distension of the snake's large intestine, central nervous system symptoms due to liver damage, often septicaemia due to bacterial blood poisoning from the damaged intestines and occasionally vomiting. Diagnosis is by finding the

results in a reduction in the ability of the snake to digest food, and the increased risk of gastritis due to opportunistic bacterial infections. With time, it also causes a thickening of the stomach lining as immune system cells move into the area to attempt to contain the problem, and new stomach-lining cells are produced. This narrows the lumen of the stomach and so reduces its elasticity, making it difficult to keep food items down.

Diagnosis of the disease is made on clinical signs and recovery of the egg sachets or oocysts shed in the faeces or recovered from a stomach wash, or via biopsy of the stomach wall. The course of the disease can vary from 4 days in severe cases to 2 years in chronic ones. Externally the snake often shows signs of a mid-body swelling, due to the thickening of the stomach wall. The parasite is passed directly from one snake's faeces or regurgitated fluids to another. The condition is difficult to treat and frequently results in the death of the snake (Fig. 11.3).

Other forms of parasitism may cause vomiting or regurgitation in snakes. These include the nematode worm *Kalicephalus* spp (the snake hookworm) which may cause extensive ulceration of the digestive system. Large numbers of roundworm ascarids may also cause vomiting. In mem-

small amoebae or cysts in the faeces (×400 magnification is required). Many herbivorous reptiles, such as green iguanas or Mediterranean tortoises, may carry this parasite without any sign of disease as the 'parasite' feeds off plant material in the herbivore's gut. In carnivores this is not possible and so the parasite damages the gut lining. This is one reason why particular care should be taken to prevent transmitting this parasite when dealing with a carnivorous reptile after handling a herbivorous one.

Chelonians: chelonians are mainly affected by species of the ascarid family such as the large roundworm *Angusticaecum* spp (10–20 cm in length!). Some may be affected by oxyurid pinworms. In most cases no symptoms are apparent. Some worm burdens may be large enough to debilitate a tortoise, particularly prior to and subsequent to hibernation, and occasionally actual intestinal obstructions due to the number of worms present have been recorded. Roundworms are passed directly from chelonian to chelonian in the faeces in the infectious egg form, and may be diagnosed by the detection of these eggs in a faecal smear.

The most important group of intestinal parasites of Chelonia, is the flagellate family. These include *Trichomonas* and *Hexamita* spp. The symptoms produced are rapid in onset and include anorexia, occasionally diarrhoea and frequently the passage of undigested food in the faeces. Additionally, there is often polydipsia, due partly to the inability of the damaged intestines to absorb water, and partly, in the case of *Hexamita parva*, due to kidney damage, as this organism migrates up the ureters from the cloaca into the kidneys. Diagnosis is made by viewing the very fast-moving organisms microscopically using a ×400 magnification, although a fresh faecal specimen is required, as when it dries, the organisms die and so do not move. Transmission is directly from the faeces of one tortoise to another. The prognosis may be extremely poor for any chelonian severely parasitised by this organism, due to its ability to cause irreparable damage to the intestinal mucosa.

Another family of single-celled, mobile parasites afflicting Chelonia is the ciliate family.

Organisms such as *Balantidium coli* and *Paramecium* spp may be seen normally in the healthy stool of a Chelonian. But they may be present in such large numbers as to cause weight loss and intestinal damage.

Lizards: worm burdens in lizards are particularly common from the Strongyloides family. Due to the direct life cycle of these parasites (that is the eggs passed in the faeces of one lizard are then immediately infective to other lizards, or even the same lizard), levels may become very high, enough to produce intestinal damage and debilitation. Diagnosis is by finding the eggs in the faeces.

The single-celled parasites of the coccidia family are also important parasites in lizards, particularly the gecko and chameleon families. Clinical signs include anorexia, weight loss, diarrhoea, dysentery and general debilitation. Diagnosis is by finding the eggs or oocysts in the faeces, and the life-cycle is direct.

Cryptosporidiosis has caused problems in some species of lizard, such as the gecko family. As in snakes it is often impossible to treat. The symptoms include weight loss, diarrhoea and anorexia.

Entamoeba invadens may also be seen in carnivorous lizards, producing colic and progressive weight loss with diarrhoea. It does not affect herbivorous lizards though.

Bacterial

In all species, but particularly snakes and chelonians, members of the family Salmonellae are commonly recovered. They are of course potentially zoonotic bacteria. Current advice is that providing the *Salmonella* spp is not causing clinical disease in the reptile, no antibiotics should be given. This is to prevent antibiotic resistance, and on a practical basis no one has satisfactorily proven that such treatment can clear a reptile permanently of the bacterium.

Salmonella spp may be carried by perfectly healthy individuals, but during other disease processes, such as parasitism, or during periods of stress, they can become opportunistic pathogens. Many septicaemic reptiles are being attacked by bacteria present within their own digestive systems that have breached the gut–blood barrier.

Other bacteria found in the normal digestive system of reptiles can act as opportunistic pathogens including many members of the *E.coli* family, *Pseudomonas* spp, *Campylobacter* spp, *Clostridia* spp, and *Aeromonas* spp.

Physical

Foreign bodies are not uncommon in chelonians and lizards, which may consume stones, sand, soil or any other substrate present. There have been a number of possible reasons put forward for this behaviour. It is true that some reptiles will consume foreign objects at the same time as their food item, due to adherence or proximity to it. However, stones may be eaten if the reptile is deficient in some mineral such as calcium in its offered diet. Another possible cause is the presence of internal parasites or indeed to help grind food which is fibrous in nature. Surgery may be required to remove some foreign bodies, although many may be passed with the aid of oral liquid paraffin and fluid therapy.

Other physical obstructions include tumours within the intestines. These are not uncommon, particularly in snakes, and may present as a swelling, or produce symptoms such as vomiting, diarrhoea, constipation or anorexia.

Liver disease

Snakes

Possible causes of liver damage in snakes (*Entamoeba invadens*) have already been mentioned above.

Other parasitic causes include some forms of the single-celled parasites of the coccidia family which gain access to the liver from the small intestine via the bile ducts.

Both a herpes virus and an adenovirus have been isolated from damaged snake livers.

Chelonia

The single-celled flagellate *Hexamita parva* has been associated with intestinal, renal and hepatic disease in Chelonia. Clinical signs have been described as lethargy, weight loss and poor growth rates.

Hepatic lipidosis, or fatty liver syndrome, is common in tortoises fed inappropriate diets, more specifically regular amounts of cat or dog food. The excessive amount of fat consumed causes deposition of fat within the liver cells themselves, enlarging the liver and, more importantly, severely affecting its function. This can lead to jaundice, anorexia and death.

Post-hibernation jaundice is often a temporary finding in tortoises immediately after hibernation. It may however persist, indicating liver damage due to any one of the above or due to hepatitis from bacteria such as *Salmonella* spp and *Aeromonas hydrophila*. In addition some forms of herpes viruses and iridoviruses have been isolated from damaged tortoise and other chelonian livers.

The liver may become calcified due to over-supplementation of the diet with calcium and vitamin D_3.

Lizards

Bacterial hepatitis due to *Salmonella* spp, *Aeromonas* spp or *Pseudomonas* spp have all been recorded. These may be associated with heavy worm burdens, many of which may migrate through or to the liver, often carrying bacteria with them.

Respiratory disease

Signs of respiratory disease

Respiratory disease in reptiles is exacerbated by the inability of many reptiles to remove fluid, mucus and debris from their airways by coughing (Fig. 11.4). This is because reptiles do not possess a true diaphragm, and have no cough reflex. Secretions pool in the dependent parts of the lungs and so make the course of the disease more chronic and difficult to treat. Signs of respiratory disease are given in Table 11.1.

Causes of respiratory disease

Parasitic

These are mainly due to the larger species of worm. However the single-celled parasite *Enta-*

moeba invadens can cause respiratory disease in snakes. The commoner parasites though include the worms known as nematodes. These are represented by:

- *Kalicephalus* spp (the hookworm of snakes). This species can migrate through the skin of the snake, or be eaten. The worm then migrates through the snake's body, often passing through the lungs as it develops, before finally ending up as the adult hookworm in the gut.
- The family Ascaridae (the roundworm family). In carnivorous reptiles, the ascarid infection is frequently acquired via an amphibian or rodent prey item which has been used as its intermediate host. The worm larvae once consumed then migrates through the liver and lungs of the reptile.

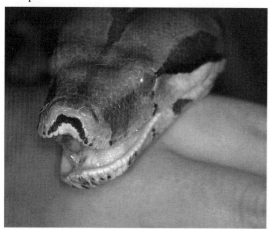

Fig. 11.4 Mouth breathing and excess oral mucus are often seen in advanced cases of respiratory disease as in this boa constrictor.

- *Rhabdias* spp (the lungworm of snakes). The snake ingests the infective eggs from the faeces of other snakes or the infective larvae may penetrate the skin of the snake as with *Kalicephalus* spp. The larvae then migrate to the lungs, where they all develop into adult female worms. The eggs are therefore produced by parthenogenesis (female giving birth to female).

Other less common parasitic causes of respiratory disease in reptiles include:

- Flukes such as *Dasymetra* spp which live in the oral cavity and respiratory tract of snakes. These parasites are also known in texts as *renifers* and are rarely pathogenic. Diagnosis is made by finding the fluke eggs in the snake's faeces.
- Pentastomes, also known as 'tongue worms'. These are the adult stage of an arachnid organism related to spiders and ticks, rather than a true worm. It uses the lungs of snakes, crocodiles or lizards as the final host, shedding eggs which are coughed up and swallowed and passed in the faeces. These then are ingested by an intermediate host such as rodents, or even humans, making this a zoonotic disease. The larvae encyst in the intermediate host. If this is then consumed by the reptile, the larvae are reactivated and migrate to the lungs where they can grow to several centimetres in length, causing severe damage. They are generally only found in wild-caught specimens, due to the lack of native prey to transmit the parasite in captivity.

Table 11.1 Signs of respiratory disease in reptiles.

Common signs of respiratory disease in reptiles	Less frequently seen signs of respiratory disease in reptiles
Mouth breathing (particularly snakes) Excess mucus at nares and mouth Lethargy Anorexia	Cyanosis Hypopyon (pus in the anterior chamber of the eye – particularly Chelonia) Subspectacular abscess in snakes (abscess beneath the eye spectacle)

Bacterial

Many bacteria have been isolated from the lungs of pneumonic reptiles. Some are primary pathogens and some are secondary invaders, following damage caused by organisms such as the above-listed parasites, or secondary to septicaemic states or oral infections such as 'mouth rot'. Examples of the bacteria seen in pneumonias include *Aeromonas* spp, *Pseudomonas* spp, *Klebsiella* spp and *Pasteurella* spp.

'Runny nose syndrome' or *rhinitis* seen in Chelonia is mainly seen in members of the tortoise family, particularly the Mediterranean species. No one pathogen has been determined as the true cause, although many bacteria, and a herpes virus have all been isolated.

Bacterial sampling

Gaining access to the bacteria causing the pneumonia may be difficult. There are two main techniques involved in sampling bacteria or parasites that cause pneumonias:

- **Lung wash**: This involves passing a sterile catheter into the trachea of the reptile. This method is usually reserved for snakes and lizards and may be done in the conscious animal due to the lack of the cough reflex. Fractious animals may require sedation. Through this catheter, sterile saline may be infused, at doses equal to 0.5–1 ml per 100 g body weight, and immediately aspirated. This sample can then be cultured to identify the pathogen. Sample collection may be enhanced by holding the reptile upside down whilst aspirating.
- **Direct sampling**: This involves taking a swab directly from the site of the problem. This may be done via laparotomy or endoscopically. In the case of Chelonia, the reptile may be anaesthetised, the shell overlying the pneumonic lesion aseptically prepared and a small hole drilled through to enable the bacteriological swab to be passed.

Viral

Paramyxovirus: paramyxovirus is becoming increasingly commonly seen in snakes in captivity.

This virus is highly infectious, being shed in respiratory secretions. It causes a haemorrhagic pneumonia and viraemia which affects other organs as well. There is no current treatment and it can be fatal. Diagnosis is based on clinical signs and serological tests on a blood sample.

Boiid inclusion virus: this has been associated with pneumonia in snakes – primarily pythons and boas. There is no treatment.

Herpes viruses: herpes viruses have been recorded in Mediterranean tortoises associated with upper respiratory tract infections which may lead to secondary pneumonias. Treatment can be attempted with the anti-viral drug acyclovir.

Cardiovascular disease

Infectious disease

There are few pathogens which specifically affect the cardiovascular system. Many of those which cause systemic illness and septicaemia are responsible for cardiac damage. In many cases the damage is due to a bacterial endocarditis which then causes micro-thrombi to seed off into the rest of the body as well as causing heart failure. Many of the Gram negative bacteria seen in reptiles, such as *Aeromonas* spp and *Pseudomonas* spp, are associated with heart disease. Diagnosis requires ultrasonography and radiology to determine heart size and internal structure. Electrocardiograms can also be used to aid diagnosis. Final proof of the organism involved depends on blood culture, which may be performed by direct cardiocentesis in a sedated or anaesthetised reptile.

Parasitic disease

There are several parasitic nematode worms which release microfilaria into the blood stream. These are microscopic young which may be transmitted from reptile to reptile by mosquitos and ticks. These parasites may cause thrombi to develop in any of the major blood vessels, causing ischaemic necrosis or cardiac damage. Other parasites, such as members of the fluke family, have also been isolated. The adult fluke is not normally the problem, but the eggs laid into the blood stream cause thrombi to form and so block capillary beds.

Nutritional disease

Hypoiodinism in chelonians has been associated with cardiac disease and goitre. The feeding of mineral-poor foods such as cucumber and lettuce or goitrogenic foods such as brassicas (e.g. cabbage, Brussels sprouts), may lead to this.

Oversupplementation with vitamin D_3 and calcium may lead to calcification of the *tunica media* of the major arteries, causing a decrease in their elasticity and so increased blood pressure. This may lead to heart failure or aneurysm formation.

Dietary deficiencies in vitamin E and/or selenium can lead to a condition known as white muscle disease, and can cause a dilated cardiomyopathy to develop. It may occur due to a dietary deficiency, or to overfeeding with high fat foods, such as snakes fed overweight rodents or fish, such as tuna and mackerel, which are high in polyunsaturates and increase the demand for vitamin E.

Urinary tract disease

Renal disease and gout

Damage to kidney function in terrestrial reptiles can lead to increasing blood levels of uric acid, the main excretory product of protein metabolism. Uric acid is not very water soluble, which means it rapidly reaches its precipitation point when crystals start to form and come out of solution. This may occur in internal organs such as the heart, kidneys and liver when it is known as visceral gout. It may also occur in the joints, when it is known as 'articular' gout, particularly of the distal limbs.

Many factors can contribute to renal damage and gout. Diet plays a role. Diets high in protein, in species designed for lower levels of protein, such as the herbivorous tortoises and green iguanas, when fed commercial cat or dog foods, cause excessive production of uric acid. In addition, these commercial mammalian diets often have too high levels of vitamin D_3 and calcium for the average herbivorous reptile. This leads to calcification of soft tissue structures, such as the *tunica media* of the arterial walls, and the kidneys themselves, leading to renal dysfunction and elevated blood uric acid levels.

Causes of renal disease

Parasitic

Flagellates, such as *Hexamita* spp, *Trichomonas* spp and *Giardia* spp have been reported in chelonians as well as in snakes and lizards, with involvement of the renal system. *Hexamita* spp are particularly damaging to the chelonian kidneys.

Kidney flukes are found in several species of kingsnake, and members of the Boiidae. They may block renal tubules and in high enough quantities cause kidney failure.

Coccidial parasites have also been seen in snakes, migrating from the digestive system by way of the cloaca, back up the ureters and into the kidneys.

Bacterial

Almost any bacteria found in the digestive system or environment of the reptile has the potential to cause renal disease if that reptile is stressed or debilitated in any way. Stresses can include incorrect environmental temperatures, incorrect feeding, malnutrition, rough and overhandling of the reptile. Bacteria commonly implicated include the *Salmonella* spp, *Aeromonas* and *Pseudomonas* spp. In some chelonians, the bacteria responsible for septicaemic cutaneous syndrome, *Citrobacter freundii*, may also cause disease. These bacteria gain access either via haematogenous spread from the gut, or via the cloaca, ascending the ureters.

Iatrogenic

Iatrogenic causes include certain nephrotoxic drugs, such as the aminoglycoside antibiotic family (e.g. gentamicin, amikacin etc.), and the diuretic frusemide. In addition, if sufficient muscle bruising occurs, such as when too firm a grasp is used when handling the patient, then myoglobin is released. This causes damage to the kidney filtration membrane.

Reproductive tract disease

Egg-binding or post-ovulatory stasis

Dystocia is common in many species of reptile, the commonest being chelonians and many of the lizard family such as green iguanas. It is often due to hypocalcaemia because of an inappropriate diet, however other causes include malformed eggs, fractured pelvic bones, cystic calculi, lack of nesting material or malnutrition of the female.

Dystocias can be difficult to diagnose in snakes, as they normally tend to be relatively quiet creatures. This difficulty is exacerbated in those species (e.g. garter snakes) which are viviparous (that is give birth to live young rather than eggs) in that any abdominal swelling is much less pronounced. Any previous history of passing eggs, and then the presence of a persistent caudally-located mass is of course highly suggestive. In addition, any evidence of a prolapse of the cloaca or distal reproductive tract also indicates dystocia (Plate 11.2).

In lizards, the patient may be obviously distended with eggs, and becomes progressively more moribund and lethargic. Many snakes can survive prolonged periods of dystocia, but lizards are not so resilient and dystocia may prove fatal within days.

Chelonia may show signs of discomfort and straining or they may show no signs at all. Radiographs are often the only way to tell if a chelonian is gravid.

Pre-ovulatory stasis

A condition recorded in both Sauria and Chelonia is pre-ovulatory stasis. This is when the ovaries produce follicles, which enlarge but do not shed into the reproductive tract. This results in two ovaries containing anywhere up to 30–40 yolks, displacing all other coelomic organs. Over time the affected reptile becomes anorectic and lethargic and often succumbs to secondary diseases and malnourishment. The cause of the condition is not fully understood.

Musculoskeletal disease

Metabolic bone disease

The disease is common in young growing lizards and chelonians that are being fed on a calcium deficient diet, often in conjunction with a vitamin D_3 deficiency due to a lack of ultraviolet light. (See also pages 152 and 154.)

The disease presents in lizards as an individual which is often weak and lethargic. The limbs are markedly swollen due to thickening of the bones. A lack of mineralisation causes the now primarily fibrous bone structure to weaken. The bones compensate for this by increasing their width. In addition, pathological fractures are common. Also softening of the jaws is common, and this can cause foreshortening of the mandible, due to the pull of the tongue and neck muscles.

In chelonians the disease is often seen as a softening and pyramiding of the shell. The plastron and carapace are weakened due to the hypomineralisation which allows the muscles to deform their structure. This is particularly obvious over the internal attachments of the fore- and hind limbs where depressions are seen. In some chelonians, for example, the softened shell allows the corners of the carapace to roll upwards.

Fractures

These may be pathological, as is seen in nutritional deficiencies of calcium, often combined with a lack of ultraviolet lighting. Alternatively they may be traumatic in origin.

Autotomy (tail shedding)

Autotomy, or spontaneous shedding, with subsequent regrowth of the tail is seen in some saurian species such as the gecko and iguanid families.

These lizards have fracture planes in their tails allowing a clean break, with minimal bleeding, to occur should a predator attack or a handler be overzealous in restraint attempts. The tail will subsequently regrow, but when it does so the lost coccygeal vertebrae are replaced with a rod of cartilage, and the scale pattern is frequently much more haphazard.

In iguanids, once the individual matures, autotomy is often lost. This can occur over the age of 2.5–3 years in the green iguana for example.

Neurological disease

Nutritional

Hypocalcaemic collapse

This is commonly seen in gravid lizards, such as green iguanas, when the blood calcium levels drop too low. The female becomes flaccidly paralysed, and unresponsive. Occasionally fine muscle tremors will be seen.

Hypovitaminosis B₁

This has been mentioned on page 153. It is seen in primarily fish eating reptiles such as garter snakes. The thiaminases present in salt-water fish break down the vitamin B_1 present in the food leading to a functional deficit. The presenting signs include opisthotonus and a lack of a righting reflex.

Biotin deficiency

This is seen in species fed mainly on unfertilised hen's eggs that contain large amounts of the antibiotin vitamin, avidin. This produces a relative deficiency in biotin which leads to muscle tremor and general weakness. Monitor lizards are commonly affected.

Hypoglycaemia

This is a condition seen in crocodiles. It is unknown why it occurs, but muscle tremor and weakness are seen.

Environmental

This can occur due to freezing injuries. These are seen in chelonians overwintering outside in the United Kingdom. Frost damage causes blindness, vestibular disease and death. There is no treatment.

Parasitic

Acanthamoebic meningoencephalitis is a condition seen primarily in snakes due to the gut parasites of the acanthamoeba family. Fits and opisthotonic seizures are seen. Treatment is generally unsuccessful.

Viral

Paramyxovirus

These have been reported in many species of snake. The virus causes haemorrhagic pneumonias but will also cause neurological signs such as the loss of righting reflexes. There is no current treatment.

Inclusion body disease of boiids

This is another viral condition seen primarily in boas and pythons. In pythons the disease is severe with infectious stomatitis, pneumonia and neurological signs such as loss of the righting reflex, disorientation and blindness often followed rapidly by death. In boas, the disease is fatal in young individuals. In older patients, the disease produces more chronic neurological signs with anorexia, vomiting and pneumonias. Neurological signs are milder, with a loss of ability to chew and swallow prey, and a loss of the striking reflex. There is no treatment for this disease.

Overview of reptile biochemistry

Blood for biochemical parameters is best collected in a heparinised container. This also applies for haematological parameter measurements as potassium EDTA-coated tubes often cause lysis of reptilian red blood cells, particularly in chelonians.

Liver parameters

There are no liver-specific enzymes in reptiles. The use of the enzyme aspartamine transaminase (AST) has been widely noted. Levels in excess of 150–200 IU/l are suggestive of problems, but as there is much species variation and this enzyme is found in the skeletal muscle as well it is only a guide.

Renal parameters

Uric acid is useful for uricotelic species such as most terrestrial chelonians, lizards and snakes. Levels over 450 µmol/l suggest renal problems, but care should be taken in carnivorous species such as snakes to ensure that they have not recently consumed a meal as this will falsely elevate uric acid levels. Uric acid levels will only be pathologically elevated if greater than 75% of the renal mass ceases to function, so this is not a sensitive test. Urea is much less useful, although it has been used in Chelonia immediately after hibernation to assess dehydration. Creatinine appears to be of no use in reptiles.

Glucose

Levels below 3 mmol/l are seen in the hypoglycaemic syndrome of crocodiles. Fits, incoordination and weakness are a common sign in malnourished reptiles, which will also show low blood glucose levels.

Calcium and phosphorus

Calcium levels vary between 2–5 mmol/l in most reptiles. Levels below 2 mmol/l can be seen in gravid female lizards with egg-binding, and young growing reptiles with metabolic bone disease. Calcium levels will increase up to four-fold in females producing eggs. Phosphorus levels vary from 0.3 mmol/l to 1.8 mmol/l. Calcium to phosphorus ratios of less than 1:1 have been used to indicate early renal disease.

Total proteins

Total protein levels are used to indicate general nutritional status and liver function. Dry chemistry techniques such as those commonly used in practice blood analysers are not accurate for albumin and globulin levels. Total protein values of 30–80 g/l have been quoted as normal.

Diseases of amphibians

Bacterial

Redleg

Redleg is a common disease seen in amphibians caused by the bacteria *Aeromonas* spp. It causes ulcerating red wounds, which give it its name (Plate 11.3). The bacteria also causes a septicaemic syndrome with the amphibian becoming bloated and rapidly going into renal and hepatic failure. Poor environmental conditions are often blamed.

Mycobacteria

Mycobacterial infections are caused by environmental species such as *Mycobacterium marinum*, which are extremely resistant species and cause classical tuberculous lesions mainly on the limbs or internal organs. The affected amphibian loses weight rapidly becoming emaciated. There is no effective treatment.

Fungal

Saprolegniasis

This is a common environmental fungal disease seen in all aquatic species. It is seen classically as strands of white, cottonwool-like material adhering to the skin surface (Plate 11.4). The condition is worsened in warmer waters.

Phycomycosis

This is due to common moulds such as *Mucor* spp. These are often darkly pigmented. These moulds will often affect amphibian eggs.

Viral

Herpes virus

A well-known viral condition of the North American leopard frog is casued by the herpes virus that induces a form of renal adenocarcinoma, known as Lucke's renal tumour. The tumour grows during the warmer months, with the virus being shed in the spring to infect other frogs. Renal failure occurs with chronic weight loss and death. There is no treatment for this condition.

Parasitic

Nematodes

The commonest nematode seen in anurans is the lungworm *Rhabdias* spp, the same family group of parasite as is seen in reptiles. In large numbers this parasite may cause pnuemonia. The parasite has a direct life cycle.

Other nematodes of the Strongyloides family may parasitise the gut and coelomic cavity, with large burdens resulting in poor growth and intestinal blockages.

Protozoa

Entamoeba ranurum: can cause damage to the large intestine of anurans, as well as causing liver infections and abscesses. These may lead to weight loss, diarrhoea with blood, anorexia and dehydration. This protozoa has also been associated with kidney damage in some species of toad and ascites and oedema of the limbs may be seen.

Oodimium pillularis: is a motile protozoan which affects many aquatic animals including amphibians. It damages the skin, and in tadpole stages damages the gills leading to anoxia. It is able to swim through the water from amphibian to amphibian and can therefore spread rapidly.

Metabolic bone disease

This is common, particularly in frogs and toads (anurans). There is often softening of the lower jaw which bulges laterally, weakness and paralysis of the limbs, with spontaneous fractures.

References

Frye, F. (1991) *Biomedical and Surgical Aspects of Captive Reptile Husbandry Volume 1.* Kreiger Publishing, Malabar, Florida.

Huchzermeyer, F.W. and Cooper, J.E. (2001) Fibriscess, not abscess, resulting from localised inflammatory response to infection in reptiles and birds. *Veterinary Record* **147**:515–516.

Further reading

Bone, R.D. (1992) Gastrointestinal system. In *Manual of Reptiles* (Beynon, P.H., Lawton, M.P.C. and Cooper, J.E., eds), pp. 101–116. BSAVA, Cheltenham.

Cranfield, M.R. and Grazyk, T.K. (1996) Cryptosporidiosis. In *Reptile Medicine and Surgery* (Mader, D.R., ed), pp. 359–363. W.B. Saunders, Philadelphia.

Lane, F.J. and Mader, D.R. (1996) Parasitology. In *Reptile Medicine and Surgery* (Mader, D.R., ed), pp. 185–203. W.B. Saunders, Philadelphia.

Wright, K.M. (1996) Amphibian husbandry and medicine. In *Reptile Medicine and Surgery* (Mader, D.R., ed), pp. 436–459. W.B. Saunders, Philadelphia.

Chapter 12

An Overview of Reptile and Amphibian Therapeutics

FLUID THERAPY

Maintenance requirements

Every reptile or amphibian has a fluid maintenance requirement, that is, fluid intake to replace everyday fluid losses. These losses, as for cats and dogs, occur in several ways, such as urine output, insensible losses through respiration, panting (often referred to as gular fluttering, as with birds) and salivation.

In most reptiles very little water is lost through the skin as sweat as reptiles have little or no skin sweat glands. Amphibians, however, will lose fluid readily across their semi-permeable skin membranes, and so need to remain close to a water source for nearly all of their lives.

Some reptiles will lose water through gular fluttering, examples are members of the Crocodylia as well as many desert-dwelling lizards.

Reptiles in particular are extremely good at conserving water. Most species are uricotelic, excreting uric acid instead of urea as their main form of urinary protein waste product. Uric acid requires very little water to be excreted with it, unlike urea in mammals, and so maintenance requirements are very much lower for these reptiles than for cats, dogs and other mammals. Other reptiles, mainly the aquatic and semi-aquatic species, excrete protein waste products as ammonia and urea. In the case of totally aquatic amphibians, species such as caecilians, ammonia is excreted, whereas the more terrestrial amphibians, such as toads, excrete urea, and one or two may produce uric acid.

Maintenance requirements can therefore vary widely. A desert-dwelling, uricotelic species may be able to cope with some water deprivation, while an ammontelic species, such as an aquatic turtle or amphibian, is used to large, regular fluid intakes and outputs and therefore has a higher maintenance requirement.

However, if a uricotelic reptile is deprived of water for prolonged periods of time, uric acid waste will not be excreted. This leads to a build-up of uric acid in the bloodstream. Once levels exceed 1500 μmol/l of uric acid, precipitation of uric acid crystals occurs inside the body, a condition known as 'visceral gout'. Once uric acid crystals are deposited in and around vital organs, such as the kidneys and heart, they cannot be removed and permanent damage has been done.

The volume of water consumed daily, then, varies from species to species. So do the sources of water. Herbivorous reptiles such as the Mediterranean tortoises get the majority of their daily fluid requirement from their diet. However, other herbivorous species, such as the green iguana, are used to living in tropical rainforest conditions where the relative humidity is 100%. Place this reptile into an arid vivarium and it will, with time, lose fluid progressively through its skin if it is not also provided with daily misting of its tank. Many reptiles will not drink from water bowls, only taking water from droplets on leaves in the wild. An example of this are many of the chameleon family as well as the previously mentioned green iguana.

To add to this, whenever ectothermic species such as reptiles are kept, it is important to take into account the environmental temperature requirements of that species. If the reptile is not kept within its preferred optimum temperature zone (POTZ), then it cannot achieve its preferred body temperature (PBT) and its internal physiological processes will not operate at their optimal rates, leading to inefficient water usage and consumption. A list of optimum temperature requirements can be found on page in Table 8.1.

The effect of disease on fluid requirements

Fluid loss may be rapid, due to water loss alone, such as occurs with acute diarrhoea, thermal burns or vomiting. In this case, the remaining extracellular fluid (ECF) becomes reduced, but is still of the same composition (*isotonic*). Alternatively, fluid loss may be due to long-term anorexia, producing a reduction in electrolytes and creating a *hypotonic* ECF. Finally, water deprivation or oral trauma preventing drinking will lead to increases in the tonicity of the ECF, and create a *hypertonic* dehydration.

With any disease, the need for fluids increases, even if no obvious fluid loss has occurred. This is due to a number of reasons. It may involve renal changes, such as increases in the glomerular filtration rate or reduction in water reabsorption by the collecting ducts so causing increased urine output. Or there may be reduced absorption of water from the small or large intestine.

Respiratory disease is a not uncommon finding in reptiles, especially tortoises and septicaemic snakes. In these animals chronic levels of lung infection can occur, with increased respiratory secretions being the result. Fluid loss via this route can be appreciable.

Another less obvious route is fluid and electrolyte loss through skin disease. Reptiles often suffer from serious burns from unprotected basking lamps and faulty heaters. Not only will there be serious fluid and electrolyte loss via full-thickness skin burns but these reptiles will succumb to secondary skin infections from environmental bacteria such as *Pseudomonas* spp. These produce lesions which resemble chemical or thermal burns, and leave large areas of weeping exudative skin for further fluid loss.

Finally we have to consider the need for fluid therapy during other forms of medical therapy, such as antibiotic treatment. Many of the more commonly seen bacterial infections in reptiles are caused by Gram negative bacteria, therefore the aminoglycoside family of antibiotics (gentamicin,

tobramycin, amikacin etc.) has been widely used for treatment. This family of antibiotics has several serious side-effects, particularly in the dehydrated patient. The most serious of these is renal damage if for any reason the drug accumulates in the kidney. This can happen if there is reduced renal perfusion because of dehydration. Levels of the drug then reach toxic concentrations very quickly. The renal damage so caused can be easily enough to kill even a healthy reptile.

Post-surgical fluid requirements

Surgical procedures are more and more frequently being performed on reptiles and amphibians in both routine and emergency situations. Causes of fluid loss include the possibility of intrasurgical haemorrhaging. This will call for vascular support with an aqueous electrolyte solution or, in more serious blood losses (greater than 10% blood volume), colloidal fluids or even blood transfusions.

Even if surgery is relatively bloodless there are inevitable losses via the respiratory route. This is due to the drying nature of the gases used to deliver the anaesthetics commonly used in reptile and amphibian surgery. As many of these species are small in size they have a large lung surface area in relation to volume and hence a greater loss of fluid per unit time/per breath than larger animals. To exacerbate the situation, many patients are not able to drink immediately after surgery, and so the period without water or food intake may stretch to a few hours – enough time for any reptile or amphibian to start to dehydrate. Finally, some forms of surgery will lead to inappetance for a period, as for some forms of head trauma – such as the repair of tortoises that have gone ten rounds with the family lawnmower!

Electrolyte replacement

Other diseases, such diarrhoea, will cause fluid loss and metabolic acidosis due to the prolonged loss of bicarbonate. This is not uncommon in reptiles, and is often due to parasitism, such as amoebiasis, in snakes. There may also be chronic losses of potassium, in cases of chronic diarrhoea, due to the reduced absorption of this electrolyte by the large intestine.

Snakes will vomit after a meal if stressed, and may suffer from diseases of the stomach such as *cryptosporidiosis*, causing loss of fluid and hydrogen ions, and a resultant metabolic alkalosis. Other reptiles such as tortoises will rarely vomit, so the likelihood of fluid loss via this route is less common.

Fluids used in reptilian practice

Lactated Ringer's/Hartmann's

As with cats and dogs, lactated Ringer's solution is useful as a general purpose rehydration and maintenance fluid. It is particularly useful for reptiles and amphibians suffering from metabolic acidosis, such as those described above with chronic gastrointestinal problems, but can also be used for fluid therapy after routine surgical procedures.

Glucose/saline combinations

Glucose/saline combinations are useful for reptiles and amphibians, as they may have been through periods of anorexia prior to treatment, and therefore may well be borderline hypoglycaemic.

There is some evidence that in reptiles, and probably amphibians, the isotonicity of the extracellular fluids is lower than that of mammals. Studies on non-marine reptiles suggest that isotonicity for the majority is 0.8% rather than the 0.9% saline assumed for mammals. Because of this, a number of fluid combinations utilising the above two types of crystalloid support have been derived as follows:

- One third each of 5% glucose with 0.9% saline, lactated Ringer's solution and sterile water
- Nine parts 5% glucose with 0.9% saline to 1 part sterile water.

Many texts still advise that straightforward, undiluted lactated Ringer's solution or 4% glucose with 0.18% saline may be used, and glucose/saline solutions are particularly useful for amphibia, where the use of potassium-containing fluids should be avoided initially.

It is important that whatever fluid is administered it be warmed to the reptile or amphibian's preferred body temperature (approximately 30–35°C) before being given.

Protein amino acid/B vitamin supplements

Protein and vitamin supplements are useful for nutritional support. Products such as Duphalyte® (Fort Dodge) may be used at the rate of 1 ml/kg/day. They are used to replace nutrients in cases where the patient is malnourished or has been suffering from protein-losing enteropathy, such as may occur with heavy parasitism, or a protein-losing nephropathy, as in renal failure. It is also a useful supplement for patients with hepatic disease or severe exudative skin diseases, such as heater burns, in which blood proteins will be reduced.

Colloidal fluids

Colloidal fluids have been used in reptilian practice when intravenous administration has been possible. This limits their usefulness, as some reptiles are just too small to gain full vascular access, although there is some evidence that they may be used via the intraosseous route. They are used when a serious loss of blood occurs, in order to support central blood pressure. This may be a temporary measure whilst a blood donor is selected, or, if none is available, the only means of attempting to support such a patient.

Blood transfusions

Blood transfusions are indicated when the packed cell volume (PCV) has dropped below 0.05 l/l, and they may be given via intravenous or intraosseous routes. Cross-matching of blood groups does not appear to be necessary for one-off transfusions, but the same species should be used each time, i.e. green iguana to green iguana, boa constrictor to boa constrictor. In an emergency, it is possible to transfuse a member of a family group with another from the same group, i.e. iguanid to iguanid and boiid to boiid. Up to 2% body weight as blood may be taken from healthy species (Klingenberg, 1996), preferably into a pre-heparinised syringe before immediately transfusing into the recipient.

Oral fluids and electrolytes

Oral fluid administration may also be used in reptile and amphibian practice for those patients experiencing mild dehydration, and for home administration. Many products are available for cats and dogs, and may be used for reptiles. However, as with the crystalloid fluids, it is advisable to dilute these oral electrolytes by approximately 10%, otherwise their concentration will be greater than the reptile's extracellular fluid (ECF) and so water will move from the body into the gastrointestinal tract rather than the other way around. The inclusion of a probiotic with the electrolytes may aid recovery by normalising gut flora and digestion.

Calculation of fluid requirements

Fluid requirements may be calculated as for cats and dogs. It is worth noting that a lot of the fluid intake is normally consumed in food e.g. in the form of fresh vegetation for herbivorous species. This is difficult to take into consideration, and therefore it is safer to assume that the debilitated reptile will not be eating significant enough amounts for this to matter in the calculation. In any case, levels of fluid replacement rates have received relatively little research. Consequently for the vast number of reptiles and amphibians a calculated guess has to be made!

Frye (1991) recommends that levels of 20–25 ml/kg/day be used for hydration purposes in both reptiles and amphibians, and current literature suggests that rates across several species vary from 10–50 ml/kg/day.

The factor that limits the volume of fluids that can be administered is that, although intravenous and intraosseous routes may also be used, most fluids are given intracoelomically to the debilitated reptile. Reptiles and amphibians do not possess true diaphragms, therefore the thorax and abdomen are all interconnected in a coelom. When fluids are placed in this cavity, it is equivalent to giving intraperitoneal fluids to a mammal, but as there is no diaphragm these fluids can cause pressure to build up on the lungs. Excessive fluids may severely compromise respiration.

Excessive fluids given intravenously or intraosseously may also overload the circulation and cause pulmonary oedema. It can result in cardiac and renal overperfusion and solute wash-out, with potassium in particular being excreted with the increased diuresis causing a hypokalaemic crisis to develop. This may manifest itself initially as an anorectic reptile, but will progress to cardiac arrhythmias, coma and death.

As with cats and dogs, one can assume that 1% dehydration equates with a need to supply 10 ml/kg fluid replacement in addition to the maintenance requirements. It is also possible to make some qualitative assessment of the level of dehydration from the elasticity of the skin. Although reptile skin is not as elastic as mammalian, it should be freely mobile and recoil, albeit slowly, after tenting. Other factors to assess are the brightness of the corneas in species with mobile eyelids. In those without mobile eyelids (e.g. snakes) the collapse of the spectacle (the clear fused eyelids) is suggestive of dehydration. Other assessments of thirst and urate output can be made over 24 hours.

It is possible to estimate the degree of dehydration of a reptile patient as follows:

- 3% dehydrated – increased thirst, slight lethargy, decreased urates
- 7% dehydrated – increased thirst, anorexia, dullness, tenting of the skin with slow return to normal, dull corneas, loss of turgor of spectacles in snakes
- 10% dehydrated – dull to comatose, skin remains tented after pinching, desiccating mucous membranes, sunken eyeballs, no urate/urine output.

The alternative is to compare packed cell volumes and total protein levels to assess dehydration (Table 12.1), again with 1% increase in PCV suggesting 10 ml/kg fluid replacements are needed (this assumes no anaemia in the patient).

Table 12.1 Examples of normal packed cell volumes (PCV) and total blood proteins in selected species of reptile.

Species	PCV l/l	Total protein g/l
Green iguana (*Iguana iguana*)	0.25–0.38	28–69
Tortoise (*Testudo* spp.)	0.19–0.4	32–50
Ratsnake (*Elaphe* spp.)	0.2–0.3	30–60
Boa constrictor (*Boa constrictor constrictor*)	0.2–0.32	46–60

It is important not to exceed 25–30 ml/kg/day as a maximum for reasons mentioned above, whatever the level of dehydration of the patient. So rehydration of severely debilitated reptiles may take days to weeks. As with avian patients, therefore, making good the fluid deficit may need to be split over several days.

Equipment for fluid administration

Catheters

The most useful catheters for small reptiles and amphibians are the series of butterfly catheters available, often adapted from human paediatric medicine. These are extremely useful for the small and fragile vessels in these patients, as they have a short length of tubing attached to the needle. If the syringe or drip set is connected to this piece of flexible tubing, rather than directly to the catheter, there is less chance of the catheter becoming dislodged if the reptile moves. Also, the piece of clear tubing on the catheter allows you to see when venous access has been achieved, as blood will flow back into this area without the need to draw back thus collapsing the fragile veins.

To make effective use of a butterfly catheter, it is advisable to flush it with heparinised saline prior to use to prevent clotting. 25–27 gauge sizes are recommended. They may also be used to give intracoelomic fluids to reptiles, as the conscious patient may continue to move (particularly a problem in snakes) without dislodging the needle.

For larger patients, such as adult iguanas, monitor lizards and Crocodylia, 21–25 gauge over-the-needle Teflon®-coated catheters used for cats and dogs can be used.

Hypodermic or spinal needles

Hypodermic needles are useful for the administration of intraosseous, intracoelomic or subcutaneous fluids.

Intraosseous fluids may be the only method of central venous support in very small patients or patients in which vascular collapse is occurring. The proximal femur, tibia or humerus may be used. Entry can be gained using spinal needles. These have a central stylet to prevent clogging of the lumen of the needle with bone fragments after insertion. 23–25 gauge spinal needles are usually sufficient.

Straightforward hypodermic needles may also be used for the same purpose, although the risks of blockage are higher. Hypodermic needles may also be used, of course, for the administration of intracoelomic and subcutaneous fluids. Generally 23–25 gauge hypodermic needles are sufficient for the task.

Pharyngostomy or oesophageal tubes

Pharyngostomy tubes are often used in reptiles in order to provide nutritional support in as stress-free manner as is possible. They are also useful as a route for some fluid administration, as only liquid formulas will pass through these narrow (3.5–6.5 french) tubes. It should be noted though that in severely dehydrated individuals there is a real possibility that gut pathology may exist, so this route may need to be supplemented by others. This route therefore has limited use in facilitating fluid replacement, and is used mainly for nutritional support and rehydrating and replenishing the gut microflora.

Syringe drivers

For continuous fluid administration, such as is required for intravenous and intraosseous fluid administration, syringe drivers are being used more and more. The units themselves vary from the inexpensive, semi-disposable, battery-operated units available to the veterinary profession, right through to the more expensive digital units requiring mains electricity. As an investment for the practice they are well worthwhile, as they may be used for cat and small dog fluid administration as well. Their advantage is that small volumes, such as a fraction of a ml may be administered accurately per hour. An error of 1–2 ml in some of the smaller species dealt with over an hour could be equivalent to overperfusion of 50–100%! In addition it is almost impossible to keep gravity fed drip sets running at these low rates without blocking every few minutes.

Intravenous drip tubing

Particular fine drip tubing is available for attachment to syringes and syringe-driver units. It is useful if these are luer locking as this enhances safety and prevents disconnection when the patient moves.

Routes of fluid administration in reptile

As with cats and dogs the same medical principles broadly apply with five main routes of administration available as follows:

- Oral
- Subcutaneous
- Intracoelomic
- Intravenous
- Intraosseous.

Table 12.2 gives the advantages and disadvantages of each of the five routes.

Oral

Snakes

The oral route is not very good for seriously debilitated animals, but useful for those with pharyngostomy feeding tubes in place, or if the owner or handler is experienced in stomach tubing. This makes it useful for mild cases of dehydration where owners wish to home treat their pet. A stomach tube is passed by restraining the snake's head gently but firmly and then inserting a plastic or wooden tongue depressor to open the mouth. A lubricated feeding tube is then passed through the labial notch (the area at the most rostral aspect of the mouth without teeth) and to a depth of one third of the snake's length.

Lizards

Gavage (stomach) tubes or avian straight crop tubes or straightforward feeding tubes can be used to administer fluids directly into the oesophagus or stomach. The reptile needs to be firmly restrained to keep the head and oesophagus in a straight line. The mouth is opened with a plastic or wooden tongue depressor and the tube inserted to a depth of one third to one half the torso length of the reptile. This method is often stressful for the reptile. The alternative is to syringe fluids into the mouth, but this risks inhalation in a debilitated reptile. A pharyngostomy tube may be placed for nutritional support, and so may be used for fluid therapy.

Chelonians

The oral route can be used as for lizards and snakes. A pharyngostomy tube may be implanted as described below, and levels of 10 ml/kg at any one time can be administered. Alternatively, a stomach tube may be inserted each time it is needed. The feeding tube is first measured from the tip of the extended nose to the line where the pectoral and abdominal ventral scutes connect. It can then be lubricated and passed after extending the head and gently prising the mouth open with a wooden or plastic speculum (Fig. 12.1).

Placement of pharyngostomy tubes

Pharyngostomy tubes may be placed in any species of reptile, but are particularly useful in chelonians, such as the leopard tortoise (*Geochelone pardalis*) which can retract its head deep

Table 12.2 Advantages and disadvantages of various fluid therapies for reptiles and amphibians.

	Advantages	Disadvantages
Oral	• Minimal stress with experienced handler • Physiological route for fluid intake • Less risk of tissue trauma • Home therapy possible • Rapid administration	• Stressful with inexperienced handler • No use in cases of digestive tract disease • May damage stomach if the stomach tube is inserted too roughly • Rehydration rates are slow • Risk of inhalational pneumonia • Limited volumes may be administered at any one time
Subcutaneous	• Large volumes may be given at one time • Rapid administration possible, minimising stress • Uptake may be better than oral route in cases of digestive tract disease • Minimal risk of internal organ damage during administration	• May be uncomfortable for patient • Risk of muscle and subcutaneous tissue trauma • Rates of rehydration poor if severely dehydrated and peripheral vessels are collapsed • Only isotonic or hypotonic fluids may be administered • Darkening of the skin at injection site in many lizards such as chameleons and iguanas
Intracoelomic	• Large volumes may be administered at one time, increasing dosing intervals • Uptake is faster than subcutaneous route in dehydrated patients • Generally relatively painless route of administration	• Large volumes may cause pressure on the lungs (no diaphragm) • Rehydration rates may still be slow in severely hypovolaemic patients • Only isotonic or hypotonic fluids may be given • Increased risk of organ damage
Intravenous	• Rapid rehydration in even severely dehydrated patients is possible • Colloidal fluids and blood transfusions possible • Use of intravenous catheters and syringe drivers makes accurate, continuous, reduced-stress dosing possible	• Size of reptile may prevent venous access • Species of reptile (e.g. snakes) may make venous access difficult without minor surgery • Veins are more fragile than mammalian vessels • Increased skill levels and equipment requirements
Intraosseous	• Rapid rehydration possible even with collapsed peripheral vasculature • Accurate dosing and continuous perfusion possible • Use of colloidal fluids and blood transfusions possible • Useful in smaller species and species where venous access is difficult	• Not useful in presence of infection (osteomyelitis) or skeletal nutritional disease (metabolic bone disease) • Sedation, local or general anaesthesia is required • Tolerance may be poor in some species

inside its shell, making repeated stomach tubing impossible. It also significantly reduces the stress and trauma of repeatedly passing a stomach tube in long-term anorectic reptile patients.

The steps for placement are as follows:

(1) Sedation or anaesthesia is required, and good analgesia post implantation.

(2) Surgically prepare the site with 0.25–0.5% povidone-iodine, being particularly scrupulous as reptile skin is notoriously dirty. In chelonians, the implantation site is the ventral aspect of the lateral neck, 3–4 cm caudal to the angle of the jaw. In snakes and lizards it is the ventrolateral aspect of the throat region, 5–10 cm caudal to the angle of the jaw.

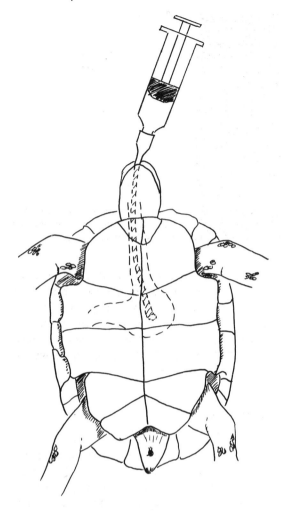

Fig. 12.1   Placement and depth of insertion of a stomach tube in a chelonian.

(3) A pair of curved haemostats is placed in through the mouth and pushed laterally and ventrally, tenting the skin above them.
(4) A sharp incision is made with a scalpel blade, over the point of the haemostats, through the skin and the underlying muscle.
(5) The tubing, preferably as large a diameter as will comfortably fit down the oesophagus (Foley catheters are useful in tortoises), is grasped with the haemostats as they protrude out through the incision, and then pulled into the pharynx and pushed down into the oesophagus.

NB The tube should be measured prior to implantation so the depth of insertion is known. It is measured in tortoises from the site of the tube incision to the mid-portion of the plastron, halfway through the abdominal scutes (page 116). A further length should then be allowed, in order to attach the end of the feeding tube to the dorsal aspect of the carapace.

(6) Once in place, two pieces of zinc oxide tape may be attached to the tube close to the skin surface. Through this, sutures may be placed, attaching this to the skin itself. The tube may then be attached to the midline cranial carapace in tortoises, or taped to the side of the neck for snakes and reptiles, and a bung inserted (Fig. 12.2, Plate 12.1). Care of the tube is as for nasogastric tubes in cats and dogs. For example, plain water should be flushed through the tube prior to administering food to ensure correct placement. This should also be done after feeding to flush food debris out of the tube.

Subcutaneous

Snakes

The lateral aspect of the dorsum of the snake, in the caudal third of its body, is the ideal site for subcutaneous fluid administration. This is a good technique for use for routine post-operative administration of fluids to patients undergoing minor surgical procedures such as skin mass removals. If positioned correctly, there is a lymph sinus running lateral to the epaxial muscles on either side, just subcutaneously, which can be used for moderately large volumes. It may however still be necessary to use several sites.

Lizards

The lateral thoracic area is easily used for smaller volumes of fluids at any one site. There is a risk of the reptile developing a darkened, pigmented area over the injection site, particularly in the chameleon family.

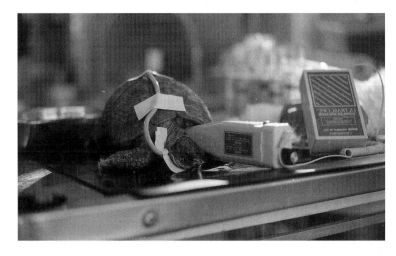

Fig. 12.2 A pharyngostomy tube in place in an anorectic spur-thighed tortoise (*Testudo graeca*).

Chelonians

The subcutaneous route is easily used for postoperative fluids and mild dehydration in this species. Fluids may be given in the area just cranial to the hind limbs, or in the skin folds just lateral to the neck. Relatively large volumes may be given via this route.

Intracoelomic

Snakes

The intracoelomic route is useful for more seriously dehydrated reptiles, as there is a greater vasculature at this site for absorption. The needle or butterfly catheter is inserted two rows of lateral scales dorsal to the ventral scutes in the caudal third of the snake, but cranial to the vent. The needle is inserted so that it just penetrates the body wall, the plunger of the syringe is pulled back to ensure no organ puncture has occurred and the fluids administered. If correctly inserted there will be no resistance to the injection.

Lizards

Because of the positioning necessary for administration, the intracoelomic route may be a stressful method of fluid administration. As for small mammals, the lizard should be placed in dorsal recumbency with its head downwards to encourage the gut contents to fall cranially and away

from the injection site. The needle, preferably 25 gauge or smaller, is advanced slowly to just pop through the abdominal wall in the lower right ventral quadrant. The syringe plunger should be pulled back to ensure that no organ has been penetrated, and the fluids can be administered without any resistance.

Chelonians

The intracoelomic route can be used in tortoises up to a maximum of 20–25 ml/kg/day only, otherwise, due to the confines of the rigid shell, the fluids will place too much pressure on the lung fields. The area cranial to the hind limbs is used, i.e. the same site as for subcutaneous routes, but the chief difference is depth. The concern with this route is that the bladder lies in this area, and if full may be punctured. The other route is the cranial access site. This is located lateral to the neck and medial to the front limb and is more epicoelomic than truly intracoelomic. The needle is kept close and parallel to the plastron and a $^3/_4$-in needle may be inserted to the level of the hub.

Intravenous

Snakes

There are no major vessels for intravenous use in snakes which are easily accessible. If an intravenous route is to be used one of the following is required.

Ventral tail vein: this is more of a plexus of veins, and may be accessed from the ventrum. The needle is inserted midline, one third of the tail length from the vent, and advanced until it touches the coccygeal vertebrae at a 90-degree angle. The needle is then retracted slightly whilst drawing back on the syringe until blood flows into the hub. Fluids may then be given slowly.

Palatine vein: this is present on the roof of the mouth, as its name suggests, and is paired. Cannulation may be performed with a 25–27 gauge butterfly catheter although the snake usually has to be sedated or anaesthetised to gain access.

Jugular vein: these also can only be accessed in an anesthetised or sedated snake. To gain access, a full-thickness skin cut-down procedure may be performed 5–7.5 cm caudal to the angle of the jaw, two rows of scales dorsal to the ventral scutes. The jugular vein can then be seen medial to the ribs. An over-the-needle catheter is best for this, and should then be sutured in place, therefore a catheter with plastic wings is advised.

Intracardiac: this site can be used in emergencies. The heart may be catheterised under sedation or anaesthesia only. On turning the snake onto its back, the heart may be seen to beat against the ventral scale, approximately one quarter of its length from the snout. A 25–27 gauge over-the-needle catheter may be inserted between the scales, ventrally, in a caudocranial manner at 30 degrees to the body wall into the single ventricle. A bolus may be administered, or it may be taped, glued or sutured in place for 24–48 hours.

Lizards

The intravenous route can be difficult in small lizards, and frequently requires sedation or anaesthesia. Several veins may be tried.

Cephalic vein: this is approached in the anaesthetised lizard by performing a cut-down procedure on the cranial aspect of the middle of the

antebrachium, perpendicular to the long axis of the radius and ulna. The vessel may then be catheterised using an over-the-needle catheter, which is then sutured in place. This technique is really only useful for lizards over 0.25 kg in weight.

Jugular vein: this vessel may be accessed via a cut-down technique in the anaesthetised or sedated lizard. An incision is made in a craniocaudal direction from 2.5 cm caudal to the angle of the jaw. An over-the-needle catheter may then be sutured in place.

Ventral tail vein: this is more of a plexus of veins. It is accessed from the ventral aspect of the tail and can be performed in the conscious lizard. It is frequently only suitable for one-off bolus injections, and special care should be taken with species which exhibit autotomy (spontaneous tail shedding) such as day geckos and green iguanas. The needle is inserted at 90 degrees to the angle of the tail and advanced until it touches the coccygeal vertebrae. It is then withdrawn slightly while drawing back on the syringe. When blood flows into the syringe, the infusion may begin (Fig. 12.3).

Chelonians

There are two main intravenous routes, the dorsal tail vein and the jugular veins.

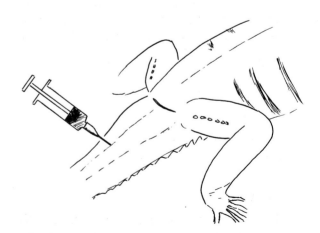

Fig. 12.3 Green iguana in dorsal recumbancy for ventral tail vein fluid administration or blood sampling.

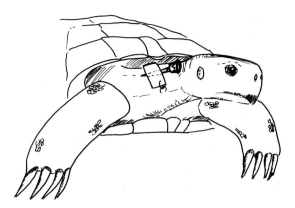

Fig. 12.4 Placement of a jugular catheter in a chelonian.

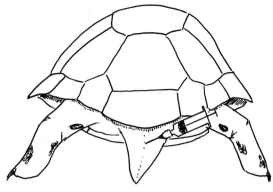

Fig. 12.5 Access to dorsal tail vein in chelonian for fluid administration or blood sampling.

Jugular vein: these may be accessed for catheter placement in the sedated or anaesthetised tortoise. The neck is extended and the head tilted away from the operator to push the neck towards him or her. The jugular vein runs from the dorsal aspect of the eardrum along the more dorsal aspect of the neck (Fig. 12.4). An over-the-needle catheter may be placed directly, or, in thicker-skinned animals, a cut-down technique employed.

Dorsal tail vein: this is more of a plexus of veins. Therefore it is often not possible to give large volumes of fluids, and certainly not possible to place a catheter. Access is midline, on the dorsal aspect of the tail. The needle is inserted at a 90-degree angle until it hits the coccygeal vertebrae. The needle is then pulled back, drawing back on the syringe at the same time, until blood flows into the hub (Fig. 12.5).

Intraosseous

Snakes

The intraosseous route is not possible in the snake.

Lizards

The intraosseous is a good route for the smaller species of lizards, where venous access is restricted or difficult. There are a few access points to choose from. Hypodermic or spinal needles of 23–25 gauge sizes may be used.

Proximal femur: this may be accessed from the fossa created between the greater trochanter and the hip joint. This route may be difficult due to the 90-degree angle the femur often forms with the pelvis.

Distal femur: this is relatively easy to access from the stifle joint. It does restrict the movement of the stifle, but it is easier to bandage the catheter in to this site and access to the medullary cavity of the femur is certainly easier via this route. Sedation or anaesthesia is required. See below for the placement technique.

Proximal tibia: this again is possible in the larger species. Anaesthesia and sedation is needed, and the spinal needle or hypodermic needle may be screwed into the tibial crest region in a proximodistal manner.

Placement of distal femoral intraosseous catheters in lizards

The technique for placement of a distal femoral intraosseous catheter in a lizard is explained in detail below.

(1) Sedation or anaesthesia (local or general) is needed, and in all cases it is advised that good analgesia is administered.

(2) Surgically scrub the area overlying the craniolateral aspect of the stifle joint using povidone-iodine. It is important that placement of the catheter or needle is performed as aseptically as possible.

(3) Take a 20–23 gauge spinal or hypodermic needle and insert it in through the ridge just proximal to the stifle joint, screwing it into the bone in the direction of the long axis of the femur proximally.

(4) Flush the needle with heparinised saline (the advantage of a spinal needle is that it has a central stylet which helps prevent it from becoming plugged with bone fragments).

(5) Tape the needle securely in place and apply an antibiotic cream around the site. It may be worthwhile radiographing the area to ensure correct intramedullary placement of the needle.

(6) Once the needle or catheter has been correctly placed, attach the intravenous tubing and bandage it securely in place by wrapping bandage material around the leg of the patient.

(7) Finally, it may be necessary to immobilise the limb by bandaging it to a splint to prevent dislodgement of the catheter, which should now be attached to a syringe driver.

Chelonians

Two main intraosseous sites can be used.

Plastrocarapacial junction/pillar: this is the pillar of shell which connects the plastron to the carapace. It is approached from the caudal aspect, just cranial to one of the hind limbs. The spinal or hypodermic needle (21–23 gauge) is screwed into the shell attempting to keep the angle of insertion parallel with the outer wall of the shell, so entering the shell bone marrow cavity (Fig. 12.6). In larger older species, the shell may be too tough to allow penetration.

Proximal tibia: this may be approached as for lizards. The area is thoroughly scrubbed with 0.25–0.5% povidone-iodine and the hypodermic or spinal needle is screwed into the tibial crest in the direction of the long axis of the tibia distally.

Routes of fluid administration in amphibians

Cutaneous

The cutaneous route is unique to amphibians and makes use of their semi-permeable skin. It can be used only with mildly dehydrated amphibians, and should only involve the use of dechlorinated, plain water. It should be warmed to the amphibian's preferred body temperature and be well oxygenated before immersing the patient. Absorption will occur across the skin membranes.

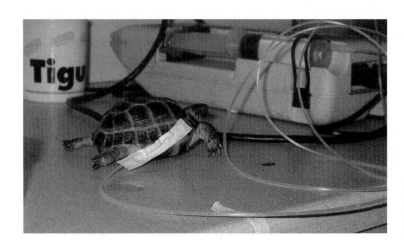

Fig. 12.6 Intraosseous fluid administration via the plastrocarapacial pillars. Note syringe driver in background.

Oral

This route can be used for hypotonic fluid therapy via a small feeding tube inserted orally. The danger is that trauma can easily occur during restraint and opening of the amphibian's mouth during this procedure. In addition the process is moderately stressful.

Intracoelomic

This is accessed in the right lower ventral quadrant of the 'abdomen'. The amphibian should be placed in dorsal recumbency and with its head down to allow coelom contents to fall away from the injection site.

Intravenous

In the larger anurans and some salamanders, the midline ventral abdominal vein may be used for bolus fluids or blood transfusions. The vessel, as its name suggests, lies midline just below the skin surface and runs from the pubis area of the pelvis to the xiphoid of the sternum. A 25–27 gauge insulin needle may be used to gain access, although the vessel is very fragile and care should be taken not to rupture it.

Treatment of reptilian diseases

As this text is aimed at the veterinary nurse or technician it is not intended to give exhaustive lists of treatments or drug dosages, rather to give an idea of the treatments possible and the techniques useful to aid recovery. For drug dosages the reader is referred to one of the many excellent texts listed in the additional reading list at the end of this chapter.

Metabolic scaling of drug dosages

It should be mentioned that, due to the lack of research, many drugs have not been evaluated in reptiles and amphibians.

Drug doses may (with care) be extrapolated from known doses in other species. However, to do this, the differences in basal metabolic rate (BMR) or metabolism should be taken into consideration (see Chapter 10, on reptile and amphibian nutrition). Reptiles have a much lower metabolic rate than mammals, and this is reflected by the fact that they excrete drugs at slower rates. The environmental temperature at which the reptile or amphibian is kept, due to their ectothermic nature, will also greatly affect their metabolic rate and hence excretion of any drug administered. Therefore, dosages and dose rates are often much lower in reptiles than in mammals.

A formula has been derived to 'metabolically scale' the dosage of a drug in a tested species, such as a dog, to an untried one, such as a snake. For those keen to read more on this subject the reader is referred to the BSAVA Manual of Reptiles (1992 edition).

Reptile dermatological disease therapy

Table 12.3 highlights some of the treatments and therapies commonly used for the management of reptilian dermatological diseases.

Reptile digestive tract disease therapy

Table 12.4 highlights some of the treatments and therapies commonly used for the management of reptilian digestive tract diseases.

Reptile respiratory and cardiovascular disease therapy

Table 12.5 highlights some of the treatments and therapies commonly used for the management of reptilian respiratory and cardiovascular diseases.

Reptile reproductive tract disease therapy

Table 12.6 highlights some of the treatments and therapies commonly used for the management of reptilian reproductive tract diseases.

Table 12.3 Treatment of skin diseases.

Diagnosis	Treatment
Ectoparasites	
Mites	Ivermectin 0.2 mg/kg injection on 2–3 occasions at 10–14 day intervals. Can spray environmental mixture of 0.5 ml ivermectin + 1 litre water with 1–2 ml propylene glycol to aid mixing to remove remaining mites. Fipronil has also been used topically, sprayed onto a cloth and wiped over the reptile
Ticks	Manual removal, topical ivermectin/fipronil. Treat for secondary bacterial infection
Blowflies	Manual removal, often under sedation, antibiosis and treatment of initiating cause
Leeches	Manual removal after applying lignocaine to leech
Bacterial, fungal and viral skin diseases	Mycobacterial infections require surgical excision. For topical fungal infections use enilconazole washes, but difficult to treat if systemic. Some herpes virus infections may be treated with acyclovir topically as ointment or orally once daily at 80 mg/kg (Stein, 1996)
Dysecdysis	(1) Rehydrate patient (2) Treat underlying cause (3) Luke-warm water shallow bathing, allow access to abrasive surfaces for snakes, e.g. wet towels. (4) Retained spectacles in snakes may be removed carefully with viscous tear drops and moistened cotton buds.
Scale rot	(1) Isolate bacteria/fungi involved and obtain sensitivity. (2) Blisters treated topically dilute povidone iodine, silver sulfadiazine cream/enilconazole washes. (3) Parenteral antibiosis (4) Prevention geared to reducing substrate moisture and increase hygiene.
Abscesses	Surgical therapy due to fibrous nature. Requires debridement and topical antiseptic with systemic antibiosis based on culture and sensitivity.

Table 12.4 Treatment of digestive system diseases.

Diagnosis	Treatment
Mouth rot	Antibiosis based on culture and sensitivity. Necrotic tissue should be debrided under sedation/anaesthesia. Topical compounds containing silver sulfadiazine and framycetin are useful. Intralesion injections of antibiotic and vitamin C advised (Frye, 1991). For Chelonian herpesvirus, use topical iodine washes and acyclovir ointment.
Stomach diseases	*Tumours:* surgical option. *Nematodes:* ivermectin 0.2 mg/kg once, or fenbendazole 100 mg/kg orally once, or oxfendazole 60 mg/kg once. Note: dose may require repeating. *Cryptosporidiosis:* unrewarding, but metronidazole may be used (may be toxic in indigo and king snakes) or use spiramycin and paromycin. Raising environmental temperature to 80°F may help.
Intestinal diseases	*Nematodes:* see stomach diseases. **NEVER USE IVERMECTIN IN CHELONIA AS IT IS LETHAL** *Entamoebiasis:* metronidazole 160 mg/kg orally once daily for 3 days (beware toxicity in indigo and king snakes). *Coccidiosis:* sulfadimidine, orally, 50 mg/kg once daily for 3 days *Flagellates:* (Chelonia particularly) metronidazole 260 mg/kg orally once.
Liver diseases	*Entamoebiasis:* see intestinal diseases. *Hepatic lipidosis:* supportive nutritional and fluid therapy. Use of anabolic steroids and thyroxine in Chelonia may be helpful.

Table 12.5 Treatment of respiratory and cardiovascular system diseases.

Diagnosis	Treatment
Parasitic respiratory disease	***Nematodes:*** Ivermectin may be used at 0.2 mg/kg **EXCEPT IN CHELONIA**. Alternatively, fenbendazole and oxfendazole may be used (see intestinal disease treatment, Table 12.4). ***Pentastomes:*** Manual removal or levamisole at 5 mg/kg may help.
Bacterial respiratory disease	Based on culture and sensitivity results. Lung washes may be used to collect samples for this, and to flush out infection if antibiosis is used in the lung wash.
Cardiovascular disease	***Heart failure:*** may use furosemide, but care should be taken as nephrotoxic in the long-term. ***Filariasis:*** Ivermectin 0.2 mg/kg. Raising environmental temperature may help to kill adult worms. ***Goitre:*** Iodine supplement at 2–4 mg/kg orally once weekly (Stein, 1996).

Table 12.6 Treatment for reproductive system diseases.

Diagnosis	Treatment
Dystocia (post-ovulatory stasis, Fig. 12.7)	Provide nesting material and quiet location. Supplement with calcium gluconate 100 mg/kg intramuscularly if you believe hypocalcaemic paralysis has occurred. Oxytocin at 5–35 IU/kg once. Fluid therapy to correct dehydration. Percutaneous/per cloacal aspiration of egg contents via needle and syringe (see Table 6.6) to collapse egg. Surgical caesarian (Fig. 12.8, Plate 12.2) may be required as a last resort.
Pre-ovulatory stasis	Surgical spey advised – seen in Sauria and Chelonia, with supportive therapy initially (Plate 12.3).

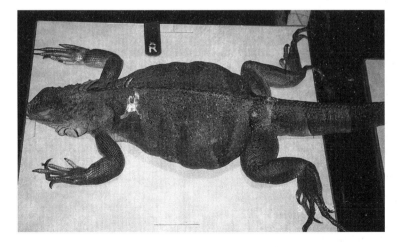

Fig. 12.7 Heavily pregnant female green iguana with post-ovulatory stasis.

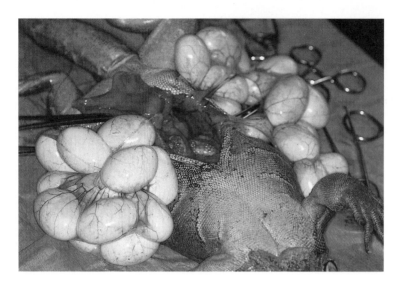

Fig. 12.8 Surgical removal of eggs from same iguana.

Table 12.7 Treatment of musculo-skeletal diseases.

Diagnosis	Treatment
Metabolic bone disease	Correction of dietary deficiency and possible UV light deficiency. In cases of hypocalcaemic paralysis 100 mg/kg calcium gluconate intramuscularly is advised.
Fractures	In cases of metabolic bone disease it is better to correct diet and splint fractures than repair surgically. *Lizards:* for one fore limb fracture bandage limb to body wall (see Fig. 12.9). For bilateral humeral fractures use a coaption splint. For one hindlimb fracture bandage limb to tail base. For digital fractures ball bandage as for avian patients. *Chelonia:* possible to bandage limb into shell. This is useful in cases of metabolic bone disease. Spinal fractures should be splinted as neural control may be regained. All species may require external coaption or internal surgical fixation to mend fractures.
Tail loss	For young iguanids and geckos treat stump as an open wound and dress with topical silver sulfadiazine cream or iodine antiseptic (dilute). For agamids or species not showing autonomy (tail re-growth) and older iguanids which lose this ability, suture the stump surgically.

Reptile musculoskeletal system disease therapy

Table 12.7 highlights some of the treatments and therapies commonly used for the management of reptilian musculoskeletal system diseases.

Reptile neurological system disease therapy

Table 12.8 highlights some of the treatments and therapies commonly used for the management of reptilian neurological system diseases.

Treatment of amphibian diseases

Table 12.9 highlights some of the treatments and therapies commonly used for the management of amphibian diseases.

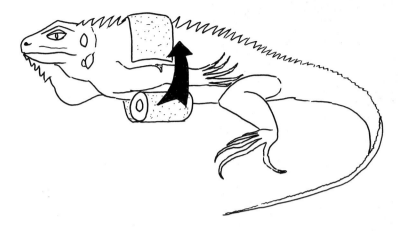

Fig. 12.9 Bandaging a fore limb to the body wall as a conservative method of treating a humeral fracture in a lizard.

Table 12.8 Treatment of nervous system diseases.

Diagnosis	Treatment
Hypocalcaemic tetany	Over the short-term use calcium gluconate 100 mg/kg intramuscularly. Over the long-term, administer dietary calcium, vitamin D3 and UV light supplementation.
Hypovitaminosis B1	Over the short-term, thiamine injections 25 mg/kg once daily. Over the long-term cook food to destroy thiaminases, or change to a non-thiaminase containing diet, or supplement with thiamine at 35 mg/kg of food given.
Biotin deficiency	Over the short-term give a vitamin B complex by injection. Over the long-term, supplement the diet with vitamin B complex powder or stop feeding unfertilised hens eggs.
Hypoglycaemia	Oral administration of 3 g/kg glucose solution (Stein, 1996)

Table 12.9 Treatment of diseases of amphibia.

Diagnosis	Treatment
Redleg	Based on sensitivity results. Enrofloxacin at 5 mg/kg orally daily. Tetracyclines, e.g. oxytetracycline, at 50 mg/kg
Saprolegnia	Dilute topical malachite green (a fish preparation).
Phycomycosis	Dilute topical malachite green (not always successful).
Parasitic nematodes	Fenbendazole orally 50 mg/kg once, or ivermectin 0.2 mg/kg orally once.
Protozoal diseases	*Entamoeba ranarum* in anurans may be treated with metronidazole at 100 mg/kg orally once. *Note*: may be toxic.
Metabolic bone disease	Dietary supplementation with calcium and vitamin D3. Flaked fish foods also contain these two nutrients.

References

Frye, F.L. (1991) Infectious diseases. In *Biomedical and Surgical Aspects of Captive Reptile Husbandry*, *2nd edn*, Vol 1. Kreiger Publishing, Malabar, Florida.

Klingenberg, R.J. (1996) Therapeutics. In *Reptile Medicine and Surgery* (Mader, D.R., ed). W.B. Saunders, Philadelphia.

Stein, G. (1996) Reptile and amphibian formulary. In *Reptile Medicine and Surgery* (Mader, D.R., ed), pp. 465–472. W.B. Saunders, Philadelphia.

Cranfield, M.R. and Grazyk, T.K. (1996) Cryptosporidiosis. In *Reptile Medicine and Surgery* (Mader, D.R., ed), pp. 359–363. W.B. Saunders, Philadelphia.

Pokra, M.A., Sedgewick, C.J. and Kaufman, G.E. (1992) Therapeutics. In *Manual of Reptiles* (Beynon, P.H., Lawton, M.P.C. and Cooper, J.E., eds). BSAVA, Cheltenham.

Wright, K.M. (1996) Amphibian husbandry and medicine. In *Reptile Medicine and Surgery* (Mader, D.R., ed), pp. 436–459. W.B. Saunders, Philadelphia.

Further reading

Bone, R.D. (1992) Gastrointestinal system. In *Manual of Reptiles* (Beynon, P.H., Lawton, M.P.C. and Cooper, J.E., eds), pp. 101–116. BSAVA, Cheltenham.

Small Mammals

Chapter 13

Basic Small Mammal Anatomy and Physiology

Classification of small mammals

The commonly seen species of small mammals in veterinary practice are classified in Table 13.1.

RABBIT

Biological average values for the domestic rabbit

Table 13.2 below gives the basic biological parameters for domestic rabbits.

Musculoskeletal system

The skeletal system of rabbits is extremely light. As a percentage of body weight the rabbit's skeleton is 7–8% whereas the domestic cat's skeleton is 12–13%. This makes rabbits prone to fractures, especially of the spine and the hind limbs. This is because of a combination of the powerful musculature of their hind legs and their habit of kicking out.

Skull

The mandible is narrower than the maxilla, and the temperomandibular joint has a wide surface area allowing lateral movement of the mandible in relation to the maxilla.

Axial skeleton

The cervical vertebrae are box-like and small and give great mobility. The thoracic vertebrae possess attachments to the twelve paired ribs which are flattened in comparison to cats ribs. The pelvis is narrow and positioned vertically. The ilial wings meet the ischium and pubis at the acetabulum, where an accessory bone unique to rabbits, called the *os acetabuli*, lies. The pubis forms the floor of the pelvis and borders the obturator foramen which is oval in rabbits as compared to the cat where it is round.

Appendicular skeleton

The scapula is slender and distally has a markedly hooked suprahamate process projecting caudally from the hamate process. The scapula articulates with the humerus which in turn articulates with the radius and ulna. In rabbits, the ulna fuses to the radius in older animals and the two bones are deeply bowed. The radius and ulna articulate with the carpal bones which in turn articulate with the metacarpals and the five digits.

The hind limbs are similar to a cat's excepting the femur is flatter ventrodorsally and the tibia and fibula are fused in the rabbit. The tibia articulates distally with the tarsal bones where there is a prominent calcaneous bone. The tarsals articulate with the metatarsals which articulate with the four hind limb digits.

The hind limbs are well muscled and powerful. Lagomorph muscle is a pale colour, unlike the domestic cat's which is a deeper red.

Respiratory anatomy

Upper respiratory tract

The paired nostrils can be closed tightly shut in lagomorphs. Rabbits, like horses are nasal breathers, with the nasopharynx permanently

Table 13.1 Classification of commonly seen small mammals.

Order		Rodentia				Carnivora
Suborder	**Lagomorpha**	**Myomorpha**		**Hystricomorpha**	**Sciuromorpha**	**Fissepedia**
Family	Leporidae	Muridae	Cricetidae	Caviidae	Sciuridae	Mustelidae
Species	Domestic rabbit (*Oryctolagus cuniculi*)	Rat (*Rattus norvegicus*) Mouse (*Mus musculus*)	Gerbil (*Meriones unguiculatus*) Syrian hamster (*Mesocricetus auratus*) Russian hamster (*Phodopus sungorus*) Chinese hamster (*Cricetulus cricetus*)	Guinea pig (*Cavia porcellus*) Chinchilla (*Chinchilla laniger*) Degu (*Octodon degus*)	Siberian chipmunk (*Tamias sibericus*)	Domestic ferret (*Mustela putorius furo*)

Table 13.2 Biological parameters for the domestic rabbit.

Biological parameter	Average range
Body weight (kg)	1.5 (Netherland dwarf) to 10 (New Zealand whites and Belgian hares)
Rectal body temperature (°C)	38.5–40
Respiratory rate at rest (breaths/min)	30–60
Heart rate at rest (beats/min)	130 (New Zealand whites) to 325 (Netherland dwarf)
Gestation length (days)	29–35 (average 31)
Litter size	4–10
Age at sexual maturity (months) –	
Male	5–8
Female	4–7
Life span (years)	6–10

locked around the epiglottis, hence upper respiratory disease or evidence of mouth breathing are poor prognostic signs. The nasolacrimal ducts open onto the rostral floor of the nasal passage. The epiglottis is not visible easily from the oral cavity making direct intubation difficult. It is narrow and elongated and leads into the larynx which has limited vocal fold development. The larynx leads into the trachea which has incomplete C-shaped cartilage rings for support.

Lower respiratory tract

The trachea bifurcates into two primary bronchi. There are two lungs, which are relatively small in proportion to the overall rabbit's body size.

This means that even minor lung disease may cause serious problems. The majority of the inspiratory effort comes from the movement of the diaphragm and abdominal musculature rather than the intercostal muscles and ribcage movement. Each lung has three lobes, with the cranial ones being the smallest.

Respiratory physiology

Much of the impetus for inspiration derives from the muscular contraction and flattening of the diaphragm. In rabbits the lungs are the 'shock organ' (for cats and dogs it is the gut). The lung parenchyma possesses a cellular population that is well supplied with anaphylactic mediating chemicals. These are strong enough to cause fluid extravasation and blood pooling as well as spasms within the walls of the main pulmonary arterial supply, leading to rapid right-sided heart failure. This is of particular importance when performing chest surgery and anaesthetising a rabbit.

Digestive system

Oral cavity

The dental formula is

I 2/1 C 0/0 Pm 3/2 M 3/3

The roots of all of the teeth are open, allowing continual growth throughout the rabbit's life. The molar enamel is folded providing an uneven occlusal surface with the ipsilateral jaw which allows some interlocking of the teeth. Wear is kept even by the lateral movement of the mandible allowing independent left and right arcades to engage in mastication. The incisors differentiate the order Lagomorpha from Rodentia, as the rabbit and hare have two smaller incisors, or 'peg teeth', behind the upper two forming an angled wedge, whereas rodents have only two upper incisors. The larger incisors only have enamel on the labial surface, whereas the smaller maxillary peg teeth have enamel on the labial and lingual sides. This allows the wedge-shaped bite plane of the incisors wherein the lower incisors close immediately behind the upper large incisors and fit into a groove made by the peg teeth. The permanent incisors are present at birth, although the peg teeth are replaced by permanent peg teeth at around the second week of life. The deciduous premolars present at birth are replaced and joined by permanent molars by the fourth week of life. There are no canines, instead there is a gap, or *diastema*, between the incisors and premolars (Fig. 13.1).

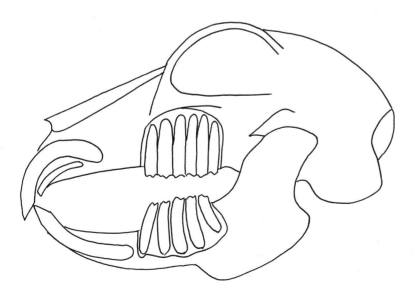

Fig. 13.1 Lateral diagram of a normal rabbit skull showing the relation of tooth roots to the orbit and jaw bones. Note peg-teeth incisors behind main incisors in maxilla.

Stomach

The stomach is a large, simple structure, with a strong cardiac sphincter. This makes vomiting in the rabbit virtually impossible. There is a main body, or fundus, and a pyloric section with a well-formed pyloric sphincter. The lining of the stomach wall contains acid-secreting and separate pepsinogen-secreting cells. The pH of the rabbit's stomach contents is surprisingly higher than a cat or dog's at 1.5–1.8. In addition, a healthy rabbit's stomach never truly empties, so an empty stomach on radiography is an abnormal finding.

Small intestine

The total length of the small intestine in the average rabbit may be some 2–3 feet!

Caecum and large intestinal anatomy

At the junction of the ileum and caecum lies the *sacculus rotundus*. This is a swelling of the gut, infiltrated with lymphoid tissue and a common site for foreign body impactions. The caecum is a large, sacculated and spiral-shaped organ, finishing in a blind-ended, thickened, finger-like projection known as the vermiform appendix which also contains lymphoid tissue. The bulk of the caecum is thin walled and possesses a semi-fluid digestive content.

The start of the large intestine is the *ampulla coli* which sits near to the sacculus rotundus and caecum. It is a smooth-walled portion of the gut with some lymphoid infiltration of its walls, unlike the rest of the large intestine. It is also distinguished by having bands of fibrous tissue (known as *taeniae*) which create sacculations (also known as *haustra*). At the end of the proximal colon the taeniae and haustra cease, and the gut is then known as the *fusus coli*, its walls becoming thickened and smooth because of the presence of large members of nerve ganglia. These nerve cells act as pacemakers for contraction waves in the large bowel. The distal descending colon then continues through the pelvis to empty through the rectum and anus. There are a couple of anal glands just inside the anus, one on either side, emptying their secretions onto the faecal pellets.

Large intestinal physiology

Two types of faecal pellet are produced by the rabbit. One is a true faecal pellet, comprising waste material in a dry and light brown spherical form. The other is a much darker, mucus-covered pellet known as a *caecotroph*. The caecotroph is eaten directly from the anus, as soon as it is produced, which in the wild is during the middle of the day when the rabbit is often underground. In captivity they are often produced overnight, but may be produced at any time. The caecotroph contains plant material from which all of the nutrients have yet to be extracted.

The large bowel can produce two types of pellet due to the unique contraction waves in the large intestine and caecum. Food accumulates in the multiple haustra of the proximal colon, and reverse peristaltic waves flush fine particulate matter back into the caecum. Here bacterial and microbial fermentation occurs, breaking down the tough cellulose and hemicellulose walls of the plant material. The larger fibre particles, which would not be digested adequately in the caecum, are selected out by the proximal colon and pass out of the gut as the caecotroph pellet. This will be re-eaten directly from the rabbit's anus, and so undergo a second digestion process. The caecotrophs are mucus covered to protect their microbial contents from the acidic stomach contents, allowing further microbial breakdown of the fibre. The smaller fibre particles which were flushed back into the caecum, once broken down as far as possible, will then be passed out of the caecum, back into the colon, and excreted as the true, dry faecal pellet.

Liver

The rabbit liver has four lobes. There is a gall bladder, which has an opening separate from the pancreatic duct into the proximal duodenum. The main bile pigment is biliverdin, rather than the more usual bilirubin seen in cats and dogs.

Pancreas

The pancreas is a diffuse organ, suspended in the loop of the duodenum. There is one single pancreatic duct, separate from the bile duct, emptying into the proximal duodenum.

Urinary anatomy

Kidney

The kidneys are similar in shape to the cat's kidneys. The right kidney is slightly more cranial than the left, and they are often separated from the ventral lumbar spine by large fat deposits. A single ureter arises from each kidney and traverses across the abdominal cavity to empty into the urinary bladder.

Bladder

The bladder lining is composed of transitional cell epithelium. The urethra in the male rabbit exits through the pelvis and out through the penis. In females the urethra opens onto the floor of the vagina.

Renal physiology

Like most herbivores, rabbits' urine is alkaline in nature, with a pH varying between 6.5–8, but it will become acidic if the rabbit has been anorectic for 24 hours or more. The urine will contain varying amounts of calcium carbonate due to the rabbit's unique method of calcium metabolism. The rabbit has no ability to alter how much calcium is absorbed from the gut. This means any excess calcium must be excreted by the kidneys into the urine, where, owing to its alkaline nature, crystals of calcium carbonate form. This can be seen as a tan-coloured silt. Other pigments may also be seen in rabbits' urine. These are known as *porphyrins*. These are plant pigments, and make the urine appear anywhere from a dark yellow to a deep wine red in colour. This may mimic haematuria, so to diagnose blood in the urine, it is often necessary to examine it microscopically.

Cardiovascular system

Heart

The rabbit heart is relatively small in relation to body size. The right atrioventricular valve has only two cusps instead of three, unlike cats and dogs. The pulmonary artery also has a large amount of smooth muscle in its wall which can contract vigorously during anaphylactic shock, causing immediate right-sided cardiac overload and failure.

Blood vessels for sampling

Vascular access in rabbits include the lateral ear vein which, as its name suggests, runs along the lateral margin of either ear. It may be entered using a 25 or 27 gauge needle or catheter and used for slow intravenous injections and blood sampling. Application of local anaesthetic cream to the area 2–3 minutes prior to venipuncture is recommended to avoid the rabbit jumping at the critical moment and to encourage vasodilation.

The central ear artery runs along the midline of the outer aspect of each pinna. It is a large vessel, and is generally avoided for blood sampling due to fear of causing thrombus formation, which would cut off the blood supply to the ear tip, leading to avascular necrosis. It may however be used with care in an emergency using a 25–27 gauge needle, and applying pressure to the vessel once sampled.

Cephalic vein

The cephalic vein runs in a similar position to that seen in cats and dogs. It may be split into two in some individuals, but may be used for intravenous fluids and sampling (Fig. 13.2).

Saphenous vein

The saphenous vein runs across the lateral aspect of the hock, as in cats and dogs, and may also be used for venipuncture.

Jugular vein

The jugular veins are prominent in the rabbit but they form the major part of the drainage of blood from the orbit of the eye. Therefore if a haematoma and thrombus forms and blocks the lumen of a jugular vein, severe orbital oedema may occur, with possible damaging effects.

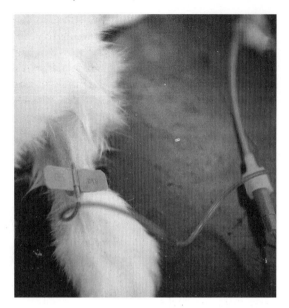

Fig. 13.2 Cephalic vein access in a rabbit using a pre-heparinised butterfly catheter.

Eye plexus

The eye also has a large venous plexus at the medial canthus, draining the orbit. This is an important structure to avoid when enucleating the eye.

Lymphatic system

Spleen

The spleen is a flattened structure, oblong in nature and attached to the greater curvature of the stomach, and is thus found predominantly on the left side.

Thymus

The thymus is a large structure in the cranial thoracic compartment even in the adult rabbit. It has the same functions as for any other mammal, in that it provides the body with the T-cell population of lymphocytes.

Lymph nodes

The root of the mesentery supporting the digestive tract is well supplied with lymph nodes, as is the hilar area of the lungs where the two main bronchi diverge to supply each lung. In addition there are superficial lymph nodes in the popliteal, prescapular and submandibular areas, although these are much smaller deposits than are found in dogs and cats.

Reproductive anatomy

Male

The paired testes can move from an inguinal position within the thin-skinned scrotal sacs, to an intrabdominal position through the open inguinal canal. The scrotal sacs are sparsely haired and lie either side of the anogenital area.

The accessory sex glands which are found in the buck attached to the urethra in the caudal abdomen are a dorsal and a smaller ventral prostate, a bilobed vesicular gland, a bilobed coagulating gland and a bilobed bulbourethral gland. There is no evidence of an os penis. The prepuce has numerous small preputial glands in the dermis and there are a couple of inguinal glands situated either side of the penis which secrete a brown-coloured sebum clearly seen adjacent to the anus.

Female

The ovaries are small, elongated, bean-shaped structures, supported by the ovarian ligament and lying caudal to each respective kidney. The ovarian artery often splits into two parts after leaving the aorta, and it, along with the rest of the reproductive tract, is frequently encased in large amounts of fat, as the doe's reproductive tract is a fat deposition site.

The uterus is duplex – there is no common uterine body. Instead there are two separate uteri with separate cervices emptying into the vagina. The vagina is large and thin walled, with the urethra opening onto its floor cranial to the pelvis. The vulva therefore is a common opening for the reproductive and urinary systems unlike many rodents. It lies just cranial to the anus, and is flanked on either side by the inguinal glands, as with the buck.

The doe has on average four pairs of mammary glands extending from the inguinal region up to the axillary areas.

Reproductive physiology

Male

The buck rabbit has the same sexual hormones as in cats and dogs, but they are on a seasonal time clock triggered by the lengthening daylight of the spring. This is mediated through the pineal gland in the brain. This has neural links from the retinas, and controls the hormone melatonin. It in turn controls the pituitary release of follicle stimulating and luteinising hormones which then act upon the testes.

Female

Does are induced ovulators. Waves of follicles swell and regress during the course of the season, starting to increase in activity in early spring. If not mated, these follicles will often dominate the cycle for 12–16 days at a time. There is no real anoestrus phase in does, instead a slight waning in activity for 1–2 days occurs before a return to heat. During peak sexual activity the vulva is often deeply congested and almost purple in colour and considerably enlarged.

Once mated, the male's semen may form a copulatory plug, which is a gelatinous accumulation of sperm which drops out of the doe's vagina 4–6 hours post mating. Gestation lasts from 29–35 days, with the foetus forming a haemochorial placenta (where the outer chorion layer of the foetal placental membrane burrows into the lining of the uterus so that it directly attaches to the blood in the intrauterine vessels) at about day 13. This is a common time for abortions to occur. A pregnant doe will often remove fur from her ventrum to line the nest in the latter few days prior to parturition.

Dystocia is uncommon. The doe only nurses the kittens once a day for 20 minutes or so, often in the early morning. It is therefore not uncommon for owners to think that the doe is neglecting her young, as she will often spend the rest of the time eating and away from the litter.

Pseudopregnancy or phantom pregnancy is not uncommon and often occurs after an unsuccessful mating or mounting activity by another buck or doe. A corpus luteum forms and this lasts for 15–17 days during which time the doe may produce milk, and build a nest. At this time the doe is susceptible to mastitis.

Neonatology

The young kits or kittens are *altricial* in nature, i.e. they are totally dependent on the mother for nutrition and survival for the first few weeks of life. They are born blind, deaf and furless. Fur growth appears around days 5–6, the eyes open at 8–10 days and the ears at 11–12. Weaning occurs around 6 weeks of age, with the young taking solid food from 2–3 weeks.

Sexing

The young may be sexed from 4–5 weeks of age. Gentle pressure is placed either side of the reproductive/anal area to protrude the vulva or penis. The vulva of the young doe is rounded and has a central slit in midline and projects cranially. The penis of the young buck is more conical and pointed, with no central slit and tends to project caudally when protruded. Once the buck is older, the testes descend into the scrotum.

Skin

Lop breeds, particularly does, have extra skin folds called 'dewlaps' around the ventral neck region. In addition, such extra folds of skin may be found around the anogenital area, leading to increased risk of urine and faecal soiling.

Rabbits do not have the keratinised foot pads that are found in cats and dogs. Instead they have thick fur covering the areas of the toes and metatarsals which are pressed flat to the ground.

In addition to the para-anal scent glands mentioned above, there are a series of discrete submandibular chin glands. These are used to mark territory and also, in the case of does, to mark their young to distinguish them from others.

The rabbit has no skin sweat glands except a few along the margins of the lips. This means that they are very prone to heat stress at temperatures greater than 28°C.

The presence of many vibrissae or sensitive hairs around the lips and chin are important, as rabbits cannot see anything immediately below their mouths, and so rely on touch to manipulate food towards the mouth.

Eyes

Rabbits have prominent eyes, which allow a near 360° field of vision. There is a prominent third eyelid which moves from the medial canthus of the eye, and possesses a large amount of reactive lymphoid tissue within its structure and a Harderian tear gland at its base. This is often enlarged in the buck during the breeding season and possesses two lobes in both the sexes. There are two blind spots, just in front of the rabbit below the mouth and immediately behind the head. The former means that the rabbit detects its food at close range by smell and by touch with the sensitive whiskers known as vibrissae which fringe the lips.

Haematology

The most notable difference between rabbit and feline or canine haematology is the staining of the rabbit neutrophil, which makes it resemble the cat or dog eosinophil, which is why it is often known as the *pseudoeosinophil*. Many rabbits have more lymphocytes than pseudoeosinophils, resembling other mammals such as cattle, rather than cats and dogs, where the neutrophil is the commonest white blood cell.

In other respects the red and white blood cells of the rabbit resemble those of the domestic cat and dog.

RAT AND MOUSE

Biological average values for the rat and mouse

The normal biological values for the rat and mouse are given in Table 13.3 below.

Musculoskeletal system

Skull

The skull of both species is elongated. The eyes are laterally situated and there is a long snout and a shallow cranium. The maxilla is narrower than the mandible, the reverse of the rabbit. The temperomandibular joint is elongated craniocaudally allowing the mandible to move rostrally and caudally in relation to the maxilla. This allows the incisors to be engaged for gnawing whilst the molars are disengaged. Alternatively, the molars may be engaged for mastication prior

Table 13.3 Biological parameters of rats and mice.

Biological parameter		Average range rat	Average range mouse
Weight (g)		400–1000	25–50
Rectal body temperature (°C)		37.6–38.6	37–38
Respiration rate at rest (breaths/min)		60–140	100–280
Heart rate at rest (beats/min)		250–450	500–600
Gestation length (days)		20–22	19–21
Litter size		6–16	8–12
Age sexual maturity (weeks)	Male	8	6
	Female	10	7
Oestrus interval (days)		4–5	4–5
Life span (years)		3–4	2–3

to swallowing, whilst the incisors are disengaged. The two procedures cannot occur at the same time. The rostral symphysis, joining each half of the mandible, is also articulated allowing movement of each hemimandible independently of the other.

Axial skeleton

The pelvis of the female mouse is joined at the pubis and ischial areas midline by fibrous tissue. This allows separation of the pelvis during parturition in the mouse. There are no fibrous areas to the pelvis of the female rat and consequently no pelvic separation occurs.

Appendicular skeleton

Each species has shortened limbs. The scapula articulates at its coracoid process with the clavicles as well as the humerus. There are four metacarpal bones in the rat, with four digits. Occasionally the vestigial remnant of digit 1 is present.

The hind limbs have a strongly laterally-bowed fibula in both species. The tibia articulates with five metatarsal bones at the hock joint. Consequently there are five digits in the hind limb of these species. Rats and mice are plantigrade in their stance, i.e. they walk with the whole of the metatarsal bone area flat to the ground.

Male rats may still have open growth plates in many of their long bones well into the second year of their lives, whereas mice close their growth plates in the first 3–4 months of life.

Respiratory system

The nares of both species are prominent and surrounded by an area of hairless skin which do contain some sweat glands.

There is a vomeronasal organ in the floor of the nasal passages, accessed via two small stoma in the roof of the mouth just caudal to the maxillary incisors. This organ is responsible for detecting pheromones secreted by other individuals.

The right lung of the rat is divided into three distinct lobes, whereas the left lung is undivided. The chest cavity itself is smaller in proportion to the abdominal cavity than is the case in cats and dogs, leading to little respiratory reserve capacity, making damage to the lungs more of a problem in rats and mice.

Digestive system

Oral cavity

The lips of mice and particularly rats are deeply divided exposing the upper incisors, with large areas of loose folds of skin forming the cheeks.

Both species have pigmented yellow orange enamel coating the labial aspect of the incisors. The maxillary incisors are naturally one third to one quarter of the length of the mandibular incisors. There is a chisel shape to their occlusal surfaces due to the absence of enamel on the lingual aspect of the incisors making them wear quicker on this side. The mandibular incisors are also mobile and loosely rooted in the lower jaw. Their dental formula is:

I 1/1 C 0/0 Pm 0/0 M 3/3

There is no evidence of any deciduous or 'milk' teeth being present in either species. The molars grow extremely slowly and therefore appear not to develop the problems seen in rabbits and chinchillas.

Both species have a diastema as with rabbits, i.e. a gap between incisors and molars. In the case of rats, this gap is particularly noticeable, and large enough to allow them to draw their cheeks into the gap to effectively close off the back of the mouth. This enables them to gnaw, without consuming the material they are nibbling.

The tongue is relatively mobile and its surface is covered with small, backward-pointing papillae.

Stomach

The stomach of the mouse and rat is elongated and narrow. In the rat in particular the stomach is divided into two regions. The most cranial is known as the proventricular region and is covered by a thin, whitened lining of aglandular mucosa. The oesophagus enters the stomach half way along the length of its lesser curvature. The caudal area of the stomach is covered by a redder, thicker, glandular mucosa known as the pyloric region.

Small intestine

The small intestine comprises the largest portion of the gastrointestinal tract. The bile duct enters the first part of the duodenum direct from the liver in the rat, which has no gall bladder. The mouse does have a gall bladder which empties into the first part of the duodenum.

Large intestine

The ileum enters the large intestine at the junction of the caecum and the large intestine on the left side of the abdomen. The caecum is a medium sized organ in the mouse and rat, reflecting their omnivorous nature, and forms a blind-ended pouch which is flexed back on itself.

Liver

The liver is divided in both species into four lobes. There is a gall bladder present in the mouse but not the rat. The liver sits cranial to the stomach. Biliverdin is the prominent bile pigment in rats and mice.

Pancreas

The pancreas lies along the proximal aspect of the duodenal loop. In both species it empties through a series of ducts into the bile duct. Its function appears to be the same as in the cat and dog, producing both insulin and glucagon for glucose homeostasis and the digestive enzymes amylase, lipase and trypsinogen.

Urinary system

Kidney

The kidneys are of a typical mammalian structure, with a cortex and medulla. There are left and right kidneys, both bean shaped. The right kidney sits in a depression in the right lobe of the liver, the left kidney is slightly more caudal. Each empties through its ureter, which enters the bladder at the trigone area.

Bladder

The bladder is lined with transitional epithelium and empties through the urethra. In the female mouse and rat, the urethra empties through a separate urinary papilla rather than onto the floor of the vagina as it does with higher mammals. The female mouse and rat therefore has three orifices caudoventrally: the anus most caudally; the reproductive tract entrance next cranially; and the urinary papilla the most cranial of the three.

Cardiovascular system

Heart

The heart of the mouse and rat is four chambered, as in other mammals. As with rabbits, the chest compartment is relatively small in comparison to the abdomen, and the heart therefore appears relatively large in relation to the rest of the chest. The heart occupies the fourth to sixth rib spaces.

Blood vessels for sampling

Useful vessels from which to sample blood are the lateral tail veins. These are best accessed after first warming the tail, or lightly sedating the mouse or rat to allow dilation of the vessels. A 25–27 gauge needle or butterfly catheter is required. Some mild pressure at the tail base allows further dilation.

In the rat, the femoral vein may also be used for sampling. This is found on the medial aspect of the thigh, close to its junction with the inguinal area, just caudal to the femur itself. This vessel is best used only under sedation or anaesthetic due to the difficulty of accessing it in the conscious rat.

For small capillary samples, a microcapillary tube may be gently pushed into the medial canthus of the eye socket in the sedated or anaesthetised rat or mouse. This collects blood from the orbital sinus which sits here.

Lymphatic system

Spleen

The spleen of male mice is often twice the size of that in females. In both species it is a strap-like organ sitting along the greater curvature of the stomach.

Thymus

The thymus is an obvious organ in the cranial chest, and may be split into several smaller islands of tissue. It is frequently present in the adult rat or mouse.

Lymph nodes

The lymph nodes follow similar patterns to those seen in the rabbit. The mesenteric lymph nodes can become very prominent in certain bacterial infections.

Reproductive anatomy

Male

The male rat and male mouse reproductive systems are nearly identical in design.

The testes are large and can move between the abdomen and the scrotal sacs although their movement is somewhat inhibited by a large fat body attached to the tail of each testicle extending through the open inguinal canal. Each testis descends into the scrotum around the fifth week of age in the rat and the third to fourth week in the mouse.

The vasa deferentia are joined by the opening of the small ampullary glands which open into a swelling of the vas deferens known as the ampulla just before they join the urethra. Other accessory sex glands, the vesicular glands, the coagulating glands (which are joined together) and the two parts of the prostate (the ventral and dorsal lobes), open into the urethra itself. As the urethra exits the pelvic canal, a paired bulbourethral gland empties into its lumen.

These accessory glands produce nutrients and supporting fluids for the spermatozoa. In addition,

the coagulating glands are responsible for allowing a plug of sperm to form in the female's vagina immediately after mating. The penis has an os penis in both species. There is a preputial gland in the small prepuce, which is used for territorial marking. Male mice and rats have no nipples.

Female

The rat uterus has two separate uterine horns which come together at two separate cervices. From the outside these appear to merge to form a common uterine body, and so it is referred to as *bicornuate* in nature. The vagina itself has no lumen in the immature rat. Instead, at puberty, the solid mass of tissue forms its own lumen, breaking through to the surface at the time of the first ovulation.

The mouse uterus is almost exactly the same except that the two separate uterine horns do fuse just before the cervix, making it truly bicornuate and so there is just the one cervical opening into the vagina. The vagina is also non-patent in the immature state. At the first heat, the vaginal lumen is created.

Mammary tissue is extensive in both female rats and mice. In mice there are normally five pairs of mammary glands, three in the axillary region, with mammary tissue extending dorsally nearly to midline! The other two pairs of glands are in the inguinal region with mammary tissue extending around the anus and tail base. In rats there are more commonly six pairs of mammary glands. Three are located in the axillary region, again with some tissue moving onto the lateral chest wall. The other three glands are inguinally located.

Reproductive physiology

The female rat is non-seasonally polyoestrus. The commonest time for heat to occur is during the night. The first cycling activity occurs around 8 weeks of age in the female rat, with the cycle lasting 4–5 days in total. Ovulation is spontaneous and occurs towards the end of the 12-hour-long heat. There is a reduction in reproductive activity in the female rat over 18 months of age.

During mating, the semen deposited in the female rat's vagina forms a copulatory plug which sits in the cranial vagina, blocking both cervices. This dries and falls out within a few hours of mating, but seems to play an important role in the success of mating. It is often eaten rapidly after being passed.

Gestation length is around 21 days. The placentation of the rat and mouse is discoidal, i.e. the area of attachment is disc-like with the chorion of the placenta in contact with the blood stream of the dam's uterus. There may be a bloody mucous discharge from the vagina around 14 days, which is normal. This stops within 2–3 days. Mammary development occurs at around days 12–14 and at that stage the foetuses may be palpated.

Parturition is rarely complicated. There is no separation of the pelvis in the female rat, although the female mouse's pelvis does separate at the ischial and pubic sutures. Parturition occurs in the afternoon, and is followed by a post-partum oestrus.

Pseudopregnancy is seen in both rats and mice. During this time the female may nest build, there may be some mammary development and no signs of a heat for up to 2 weeks.

There are a couple of important physiological reproductive phenomena in mice and rats. One of these is the *Whitten effect*. This is when a group of anoestrus females will all come into heat spontaneously some 72 hours after being exposed to the pheromones of a male. This has beneficial effects when it comes to successful rapid breeding. The other is the *Bruce effect*. This is when a female in the early stages of gestation will reabsorb the embryos and come back into heat when presented with a new male. By preferentially allowing successful mating with a new male, this is thought to have a beneficial effect on genetic diversity.

Neonatology

Rat and mouse pups are altricial. They are born blind, deaf and hairless. The ear canals open around day 4–5 and the eyes at around 2 weeks of age. The first few hairs are also seen in the first week of life. The pups are born without teeth, the incisors becoming visible at 1–2 weeks of age with the molars developing later.

The female rat and mouse are prone to cannibalism if disturbed with their young in the first few weeks after parturition. It is therefore important to leave the female rat and mouse alone during this period, only disturbing them to replenish food and clear the worst of any cage soiling.

Sexing

Sexing may be done from 4–6 weeks of age. In males the urinary papilla is slightly larger than the female and further away from the anus. It may be possible in the sexually mature female to see the small reproductive tract entrance as a transverse slit in between the anus and urinary papilla. Also, in male mice and rats, no nipples are visible. In mature males, if the rat or mouse is gently suspended in a vertical position with the head uppermost, the testes will often descend into the scrotal sacs, and are then obvious.

Skin

Rats and mice, like rabbits, possess no generalised sweat glands and so are prone to heat stress at temperatures above 26–28°C. There are some sweat glands present on the soles of the feet as well as the nares.

There is a layer of brown fat between the shoulder blades dorsally, its function is not clearly known, but it decreases with age and may play a role in thermoregulation.

The tails of rats and mice are relatively hairless. As rats age there is an increasing number of coarse skin scales present on the tail surface making blood sampling difficult. Rats should not be grasped by the tip of the tail, as the skin may slough in this region.

White fur will often yellow in rats as they age, and most rats will show evidence of a yellow hue to the skin on the back with time.

The vibrissae around the lips and nose are important for detecting vibrations and determining where food is due to their inability, as with rabbits, to see food immediately below their mouths.

Eyes

Rats and mice have a prominent set of small eyes located laterally. The albino breeds lack pigment in their irises or retinas and so their eyes appear pink red. Many rats under stress will produce excess tears. These excess tears will stain the periocular area and run over the face, down the nasolacrimal ducts and so be transferred onto the fur of the body as they groom. They contain a porphyrin pigment which is a red-brown colour on contact with air, and so these tear stains resemble dried blood. The condition is known as *chromodacryorrhea*. These tears will also fluoresce under ultraviolet light. It is not a disease in itself, but may suggest an underlying problem causing stress.

Haematology

The haematological parameters are similar to those seen in the cat or dog, except that the lymphocyte, as opposed to the neutrophil, is the most common white blood cell.

GERBIL AND HAMSTER

Biological average values for the gerbil and hamster

Table 13.4 below gives the average normal values for the basic biological values for gerbils and hamsters.

Musculoskeletal system

Skull

The skull of the gerbil is not dissimilar to that of the rat or mouse, in the hamster the skull is shortened, particularly in the Russian and Chinese hamster subspecies.

Axial skeleton

The axial skeleton is much the same as for rats and mice, except the hamster has much fewer coccygeal vertebrae (only seven or so).

Table 13.4   Biological parameters of the gerbil and hamster.

Biological parameter	Russian Hamster	Syrian Hamster	Gerbil
Weight (g)	30–60	90–150 (male larger)	50–60 (male larger)
Rectal body temperature (°C)	36–38	36.2–37.5	37.5–39
Respiration rate at rest (breaths/min)	60–80	40–70	80–150
Heart rate at rest (beats/min)	300–460	250–400	250–400
Gestation (days)	Average 16 (Chinese hamster 21)	15–18	24–26 (up to 42 – delayed implantation)
Litter size	4–8	4–12	2–6
Age at sexual maturity (weeks):			
Male	5–6	6–8	8–9
Female	6–8 (Chinese hamster 14)	8–12	9–10
Oestrus interval (days)	3–4	4	4–6
Lifespan (months)	18–24	24–36	36–60

Appendicular skeleton

The gerbil has a longer femur and tibial length, giving them the longer hind limbs equipped for jumping. Their normal stance is bipedal, standing erect on their hind limbs. The hamster is a much shorter-legged creature, stockier in build and walks predominantly on all fours.

The forelimbs have four digits and the hind limbs have five in both species.

Respiratory system

As with rats and mice, the chest cavity is small in relation to the abdomen, but the situation is not so pronounced as that seen in rats.

Digestive system

Oral cavity

The incisors in both species are continuously erupting (open rooted) and both species have orange pigmentation of the enamel surfaces. The dental formula is:

I 1/1 C 0/0 Pm 0/0 M 3/3.

Hamsters are born with the incisors fully erupted, and use them to grasp the nipples of the female (a potentially painful situation!) enabling them to suck effectively.

The molars are also open rooted and so grow continually, but at a very slow rate. In addition, there appears to be no evidence of deciduous teeth, similarly to the rabbit, rat and mouse. Both species possess a diastema. The mandible is generally wider than the maxilla.

The cheek pouches of the hamster are its most distinguishing feature. These are not present at birth, but rather develop during the second week of life from a solid cord of cells which disintegrate, creating the cavities. The entrances to the cheek pouches open into the diastema. Each cheek pouch extends caudal to the respective ear, and so has a huge storage capacity. They are lined by stratified squamous epithelium, and have a reduced local immune system and lymphatic func-tion. This can be a problem if the cheek pouch becomes infected.

Stomach

The stomach of the hamster has two separate areas. The oesophagus enters the proximal portion. This portion is non-glandular and has a bacterial population that allows limited microbial breakdown of food. It is sharply divided by a deep groove from the distal area of the stomach, which *is* glandular, with a redder lining composed of the acid and pepsinogen secreting cells that start the process of enzymatic digestion.

The gerbil has two areas to the stomach but they are less clearly demarcated, and the proximal portion does not support a significant microbial population.

Small intestine

The hamster's small intestine is extremely long, being three to four times its own body length! The gerbil has a similar layout to the mouse.

Large intestine

In the hamster the caecum is a sacculated and enlarged organ sitting in the ventral left por-tion of the abdomen at the ileocaecal junction. It has fine divisions within it which may function to increase its surface area and aid fibre fermen-tation. The gerbil has a similar layout to the mouse.

Liver

The liver in both species is highly divided into four lobes. In both hamsters and gerbils a gall bladder is present. A bile duct empties into the duodenum accompanied by the pancreatic duct.

Pancreas

The pancreas is found adjacent to the descending duodenum. It has a similar structure and function to that seen in the rat and mouse.

Urinary system

Kidney

The kidneys are similar to the rat and mouse kidney. The gerbil is very good at concentrating its urine, being a desert dwelling species, and to do this it has very long loops of Henle which contain a countercurrent multiplying system. In the hamster, the renal papilla is particularly long and protrudes from each kidney into its ureter.

Bladder

The bladder of gerbils and hamsters is essentially the same as that seen in the rat and mouse.

Cardiovascular system

Heart

The heart is similar in form to the rat and mouse heart. The hamster is prone to thrombus formation around the atrioventricular valves, although why this occurs is not fully known.

Blood vessels for sampling

The hamster has very few accessible external vessels for blood sampling. This is principally due to its much reduced tail length, which provides the main vascular access in the rat and mouse. The gerbil's tail breaks off easily, making its use for blood sampling very restricted. Vessels used therefore include the jugular veins and the femoral veins both of which require the hamster or gerbil to be sedated or anaesthetised. Capillary samples may be taken from the orbital sinus as described in the rat and mouse.

Lymphatic system

Spleen

The structure and position of the spleen is much the same for both species as that seen in the rat.

Thymus

The thymus is again a prominent organ in the cranial chest and often persists in the adult. It provides the T-cell lymphocyte population as in other mammals.

Lymph nodes

The presence of lymphatic tissue is the same as that seen in the mouse and rat.

Reproductive anatomy

Male

The male hamster has a smaller fat body attached to the testicle than has the rat. The testes are freely moveable between the abdominal cavity and the scrotal sacs. A small os penis is present in the penile structure.

The male gerbil is similar to the male rat and mouse. The main difference is the slightly smaller size of the testes in relation to the overall body size and the presence of a pigmented scrotum.

Female

The hamster uterus is bicornuate. It has two separate cervices opening into a common vagina, although the uterine horns appear to join externally to produce a common uterine body. The vagina is, as with the rat, not patent at birth. It opens after the tenth day of life, rather than at puberty as in the rat.

The gerbil reproductive tract is similar to that of the mouse. The main difference is that, whilst there is only one cervical opening into the vagina, the division between the left and right uterine lumens persists to within a few millimetres of this single cervical orifice.

The female hamster has 6–7 pairs of mammary glands stretching in a continuous band from the axillary region to the inguinal and perianal region.

The female gerbil has four pairs of mammary glands. Two pairs are found in the axillary region and two pairs in the inguinal region.

Reproductive physiology

The female hamster is seasonally polyoestrus with cycling and fertility dropping off during the winter period. The reproductive cycle is short, lasting 4 days. The female hamster develops a creamy white vaginal discharge around the first day following oestrus. This may be mistaken for a pathological discharge as it has an odour. Ovulation is spontaneous and generally occurs overnight. Phantom pregnancy does occur in the hamster, postponing oestrus for 7–13 days. Gestation itself lasts for 15–18 days in the Syrian hamster, an average of 21 days in the Chinese hamster and an average of 16 days for the Russian hamster. Successful mating is followed by the presence of a copulatory plug of coagulated semen 24 hours post mating. Pregnancy can be confirmed by failure to produce the copious white discharge 5 days after mating, and an increase in weight at around day 10. There is no evidence of pelvic separation at parturition as is seen in the mouse. There is reduced fertility in the female hamster after one year of life.

Gerbils form a monogamous pair, i.e. they pair for life. The female gerbil is seasonally polyoestrus and a spontaneous ovulator. The oestrus cycle lasts for 4–6 days. Oestrus lasts for 24 hours, and may occur within 14–20 hours of parturition. Gestation lasts an average of 26 days, but may take up to 42 days if mating has occurred at the post partum heat. This is because when the female is still feeding the young, the fertilised ova will not implant, so prolonging the interval from mating to parturition.

Neonatology

The young hamster is altricial. The pale pink colour of the skin is replaced by some darker pigmentation after the first 2–3 days, with the eyes opening at 2 weeks of age. Weaning occurs around 3–4 weeks of age, with the female hamster becoming sexually mature at 6–8 weeks (up to 14 weeks for the Chinese hamster) and the male at 8–9 weeks.

The young gerbil is also altricial, born blind, deaf and furless. The skin is a pale pink at birth but darkens by the end of the first week with the appearance of the first few hairs. The teeth erupt in the first few days of life. The eyes open at 2 weeks of age and the ears around days 4–5. Weaning occurs at 3–4 weeks of age. The female gerbil becomes sexually mature at 9–10 weeks of age when the vaginal opening becomes patent. The male gerbil becomes sexually mature at 8–9 weeks of age, the testes descending into the scrotal sac at 5 weeks.

It is particularly inadvisable to disturb the female hamster with her young as cannibalism may then occur. However, a common protective action of the female is to place the young into her cheek pouches to move them and this may make it look as if she is 'eating' the young. Gerbils are less prone to abandoning or abusing their young if disturbed.

Sexing

This may be done from 4 weeks of age. In the immature gerbil and hamster the differences are determined by anogenital distances as with the rat and mouse. In the sexually mature hamster, the male has a pointed outline to his rear, owing to the descended testes, whereas the female has a more rounded appearance. In both gerbils and hamsters though it is relatively easy to determine the sex once mature if the individual is supported in a vertical position with the head uppermost. In this position the testes will descend into the scrotal sacs where they are clearly visible!

Skin

Hamster and gerbil skin has no sweat glands, like that of rats and mice. Gerbils, however, can tolerate wider temperature ranges, up to 29–30°C, although if the humidity levels increase above 50% they will rapidly suffer from heat exhaustion.

In hamsters, there is a pair of oval, raised, flank scent glands situated either side just cranial to the thigh region on the body wall. In the mature adult, particularly the male, they may become darkly pigmented. The secretions of these glands may matt the sparsely covered fur, increasing their prominence.

In gerbils, there is a large ventral sebaceous scent gland in the region of the umbilical scar. This is devoid of fur, secretes a yellow sebaceous fluid and is more prominent in males. This is a predilection site for the development of adenocarcinoma in adults. The tail of gerbils is fully furred, but has a series of fracture planes allowing a degloving injury if a gerbil is grasped by the tail. The soft tissue structure never regrows, and the denuded vertebrae will drop off leaving a stump.

Haematology

The lifespan of the gerbil red blood cell is short, lasting only 10 days. This is why so many gerbil red cells show the degenerative blue speckling colour when stained with Romanowsky stains. Gerbil blood is often lipaemic and this has been blamed on their high fat, predominantly sunflower seed diet. In addition the blood parameters vary depending on the sex. The male gerbil has a higher packed cell volume, white blood cell and lymphocyte count than the female. Hamster haematology is similar to that seen in mice.

GUINEA PIG, CHINCHILLA AND DEGU

Biological averages for the guinea pig and chinchilla

The average normal values for guinea pigs and chinchillas are given in Table 13.5 below.

Musculoskeletal system

Guinea pig

Skull

The skull is rodent shaped, with an elongated nose, low forehead and widely spaced eyes. There are moderately large tympanic bullae which house the middle ear, and are clearly visible on radiographs.

Axial skeleton

The vertebral structure is the same as that seen in the rat and mouse excepting the number of coccygeal vertebrae is much reduced at 4–6, and they are less mobile. There are 13 ribs, the last two are more cartilaginous than mineralised. Guinea pigs also have clavicles.

The pelvis of the female is joined at the pubis and ischium by a fibrocartilagenous suture line allowing separation of the pelvis prior to and during parturition. If the female guinea pig has not had a litter by the time she has reached one year of age, this suture line mineralises and prevents future separation. Female guinea pigs not mated before one year, should therefore not be mated for the rest of their life, as dystocia problems are common.

Appendicular skeleton

The fore- and hind limbs are relatively long in comparison to the rat and mouse, but the same

Table 13.5 Biological parameters of guinea pigs and chinchillas.

Biological parameter		Guinea pig	Chinchilla
Weight (g)		600–1200	400–550
Rectal body temperature (°C)		37.2–39.5	37.8–39.2
Respiration rate at rest (breaths/min)		60–140	50–60
Heart rate at rest (beats/min)		100–180	120–160
Gestation length (days)		59–72 (average 63)	111
Litter size		1–6 (average 3)	1–5 (average 2)
Age at sexual maturity (months	Male	2–3	6–7
	Female	1.5–2	8–9
Oestrus interval (days)		16	30–50
Lifespan (years)		3–8	6–10

bone formulas exist. The main difference is that the guinea pig has four digits on each forelimb and only three digits on each hind limb.

Chinchilla

Skull

The bones of the skull are more domed than the quinea pig, although still distinctly rodent-like (Fig. 13.3). Like guinea pigs the chinchilla has very large tympanic bullae which are clearly visible as coiled, snail-shell-like features on radiographs.

Axial skeleton

The vertebral structure is similar to that seen in the rat and mouse. Chinchillas are fine-boned and prone to fractures (Plate 13.1).

Appendicular skeleton

The fore- and hind limbs are proportionately the longest of the mammals so far considered. The hind limbs in particular have very long femurs and tibias. The chinchilla has the usual four digits on each forelimb (Plate 13.1), but, unlike the guinea pig, has four digits on each hind limb as well.

Respiratory system

The lung structure of the guinea pig is similar to that seen in the rat and mouse. The left lung is divided into three lobes, and the right into four. Chinchillas follow a similar pattern.

Digestive system

Oral cavity

The dental formula of both chinchillas and guinea pigs is:

1 1/1 C 0/0 Pm 1/1 M 3/3.

In both species all of the teeth, both incisors and premolars and molars (often collectively referred to as 'cheek teeth' as in rabbits) are open rooted and therefore continuously growing. This can lead to malocclusion problems, particularly in chinchillas, if an inappropriately non-fibrous diet is fed. The incisors of the chinchilla are orange yellow pigmented on their enamel surfaces, but those of the guinea pig are often white. In both cases a diastema is present.

Both species also have a *palatal ostium* creating an entrance through the soft palate allowing communication of the oropharynx with the pharynx. It exists because the soft palate is actually connected with the base of the muscular tongue.

Stomach

The whole stomach of the guinea pig is covered with a glandular epithelium containing acid- and

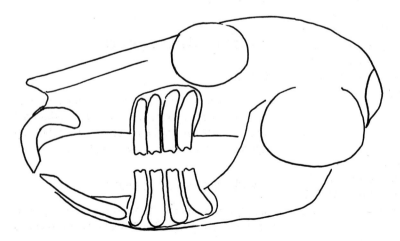

Fig. 13.3 Lateral diagram of the skull of a normal chinchilla showing the relation of tooth roots to the orbit and jaw bones. Note how close the roots of the third and fourth cheek teeth are to the inner aspect of the eye, hence root elongation often causes watering of the eyes.

pepsinogen-secreting cells and is usually full of food material. It has a strong cardiac sphincter, making vomiting a rare and grave occurrence. The stomach of the chinchilla is much the same.

Small intestine

The small intestine of both species is relatively long and pink in colour, measuring anywhere up to 50–60 cm in the chinchilla and over 120 cm in the adult guinea pig!

Large intestine

The large intestine starts at the ileocaecal junction on the left side of the abdomen where the ileum enters the caecum. The caecum is a large, sacculated organ, measuring 20 cm in length, and in the guinea pig it contains 60–70% of all the gut contents. It is attached to the dorsal abdomen, and has a series of three smooth muscle bands running along its length known as *taeniae coli*. These produce the sacculations of the caecum known as *haustrae*. In the chinchilla, the caecum is smaller, containing only 20–25% of gut contents, but it is more folded. The caecum itself forms a blind-ending sac at one end, and empties into the colon near to the ileocaecal junction.

The colon is twice as long as the small intestine in both species and is dark brown. In the chinchilla, the proximal section of the colon possesses taeniae and haustra, whereas in the guinea pig the whole of the colon is smooth surfaced. The latter half of the colon in both species can be distinguished by the presence of faecal pellets in its lumen. The guinea pig has a complicated series of coils to the large intestine, which form a spiral of bowel on the right cranial ventral aspect of the abdomen. The chinchilla's colon is much more simply arranged, and not as long.

Liver

The liver of the guinea pig has six lobes. There is also an obvious gall bladder, unlike the rat. The gall bladder empties through one bile duct into the small intestine. The chinchilla's liver has a similar format.

Pancreas

The pancreas has two limbs in the guinea pig and lies alongside the stomach and proximal duodenum. It empties via one duct into the mid-descending duodenum and performs the same functions as in other mammals.

Urinary system

Kidney

As with the hamster, the guinea pig has a relatively long renal papilla. Both kidneys in the guinea pig are surrounded by large amounts of fat, making them difficult to see at laparotomy. The chinchilla's kidneys are not so covered in fat deposits.

Lower urinary tract

The urine of the guinea pig is often yellow and cloudy in nature. Like all herbivore urine, it is alkaline under normal conditions, and may contain calcium carbonate or calcium oxalate crystals normally. In the female guinea pig the urethra empties just caudal to the vagina, but without a urinary papilla, giving the false impression of a common urogenital opening.

In the female chinchilla, cloudy alkaline urine is common. The urethra of the bladder however opens through a separate orifice from the vagina. The urinary papilla is a large structure in the female chinchilla and may easily be confused with the male penis.

Cardiovascular system

Heart

In both species, the thoracic cavity appears relatively small in comparison with the abdominal cavity, and therefore the heart appears relatively large in comparison with the lung field.

Blood vessels for sampling

The jugular veins are the vessels commonly used for blood sampling. Small doses of intravenous medications may be administered through the ear veins that are clearly visible on the non-furred ears, or via the cephalic or saphenous veins which occupy the same positions as in other species.

Lymphatic system

Spleen

The spleen of the guinea pig is a wide structure attached to the greater curvature of the stomach on the left side of the cranial abdomen.

The spleen of the chinchilla is a smaller strap-like organ attached again to the greater curvature of the stomach on the left side.

Thymus

In guinea pigs, the thymus is prominent in the cranial thorax in the immature stage, but there are often only remnants left in the adult. A similar situation exists in the chinchilla.

Lymph nodes

The guinea pig is prone to *Streptococcus zooepidemicus* infections of the cervical lymph nodes which run in a chain along the ventral aspect of the neck. Both species have prominent mesenteric lymphoid deposits.

Reproductive anatomy

Male

Guinea pig

The male guinea pig is often referred to as a boar. His testes are prominent, and occupy the scrotal sacs either side of the anus. Each testis has a large fat body projecting through the open inguinal canal into the abdomen. The vas deferens opens, with the accessory sex glands (the vesicular glands, the coagulating glands and the ventral and dorsal prostate lobes), into the proximal urethra. The vesicular glands are the most prominent, curving cranially into the abdomen for 10 cm or more. The paired bulbourethral glands lie dorsal to the urethra just before it passes into the penis,

which is Z-shaped, moving cranioventrally from the caudal brim of the pelvis and then caudoventrally so to point caudally at rest. The penis is a large structure by rodent standards and possesses a glans structure distally. There is an os penis which sits dorsal to the urethra when the penis is erect and pointing cranially. Ventral to the distal urethra are two invaginated spurs, which, when the penis is erect, project from the end of the glans as two slender spurs 4–5 mm in length. Their function is not fully known but they may aid in locking into similar grooves in the female reproductive system. The whole penis is contained in a prepuce, which possesses sebaceous glands, and is partly formed from a fold of perineal skin.

Chinchilla

There is no true scrotum. The tail of the epididymis sits lateral to the anus, whilst the testis occupies an inguinal position. A fat body projects from each testis into the abdominal cavity. The vas deferens opens into the urethra caudal to the bladder neck along with the accessory sex glands. These include the ventral and dorsal paired lobes of the prostate as well as the paired, frond-like vesicular glands. The urethra then passes caudally through the pelvis, becoming ensheathed in the ischiocavernosus muscles that control the movement of the penis and pelvic floor. The bulbourethral glands lie dorsal to the urethra in this area. The urethra then passes out of the pelvis and into the penis, which is tubular and blunt ended and points caudally when relaxed. The penis forms a Z-like flexure, similar to the guinea pig, and contains an os penis in its most caudal portion.

Male chinchillas are often prone to fur rings. This is when a band of fine fur becomes wound around the penis inside the prepuce. This may constrict and so cause ischaemic damage to the penis.

Female

Guinea pig

The female guinea pig is often referred to as a sow. Her uterus is bicornuate. It has two uterine horns, a short uterine body and a single cervix. The ovaries are closely associated with the respective kidneys. The periuterine tissues and cornuate ligaments are sites for the same fat deposition that is seen in the female rabbit. The vagina opens just cranial to the urethral opening. A small clitoris sits just ventral to the urethral opening, and the two are enclosed in skin folds to create a Y-shaped slit. The entrance to the vagina is sealed by epithelial tissues at all times other than at oestrus and immediately prior to parturition.

The female guinea pig has two mammary glands in the inguinal region (the male has two vestigial glands as well).

Chinchilla

The female chinchilla has a uterus like the rabbit. There are two uterine horns but no common uterine body. Instead two separate cervices open into the vagina. The entrance to the vagina is sealed at all times except during oestrus and just prior to parturition. The urethra opens through a separate urinary papilla.

Reproductive physiology

Guinea pig

The female guinea pig is non-seasonally polyoestrus. The cycle lasts for around 16 days, oestrus lasting for 6–12 hours, and ovulation is spontaneous. Immediately after mating (1–2 hours) a copulatory plug may be found in the cage. It is possible that this is necessary to prevent leakage of sperm back out of the reproductive tract, but it could also prevent another male from successfully mating the female. Gestation lasts on average 63 days, although it may take up to 67 days for small litters and 59 days for large ones. The average litter contains three young. Pregnancy may be detected by gentle palpation from 3 weeks. The entrance to the vagina is closed at all times other than immediately before parturition, and for 2–3 days around oestrus. There is a post partum heat within 10 hours of parturition at which the female may be successfully remated.

In the last 2 days of gestation hormones, such as relaxin and progesterone, allow the pelvic ligaments to separate the pubis and ischium by up to 2 cm, allowing the passage of the relatively large young. This only occurs if the female is under one year of age or has had her first litter under one year. Nulliparous females over one year of age have a fused pelvis and dystocias are therefore common. Many female guinea pigs will breed through to two years of age.

The guinea pig placenta is *haemochorial*. That is the membranes of the placenta (chorion) are in contact with the blood of the mother. This allows for large amounts of immune system exchange between mother and foetus during gestation.

Chinchilla

The chinchilla is seasonally polyoestrus. The reproductive season stretches from November to May, and the cycle lasts on average 40 days. The entrance to the vagina opens at oestrus, which lasts for 12–24 hours, and stays patent for 3–4 days. At this stage the perineum may darken in colour, and clear mucus may be seen from the vaginal opening. It also opens 2–3 days prior to parturition, and remains open for the commonly seen post-partum oestrus.

Chinchillas are spontaneous ovulators. A copulatory plug is frequently found the day after a successful mating. Gestation lasts on average 111 days, with typically two kits being born. Pregnancy may be diagnosed by palpation from day 60. Female chinchillas may continue to breed up to ten years of age.

The chinchilla placenta is haemochorial.

Neonatology

Both guinea pigs and chinchillas are *precocial*, that is they are born fully furred, with eyes and ears open, and often start to eat small amounts of solid food from day one. Weaning generally occurs at 6 weeks in guinea pigs and 6–8 weeks in chinchillas. Sexual maturity occurs from 2–3 months in the guinea pig to 6–8 months in the chinchilla.

Sexing

Guinea pig

Sexing of male and female guinea pigs is relatively simple and may be performed from the first few weeks of life. The female anogenital area is oval in nature. The anus is closest to the tail base, and cranial to this is a Y-shaped slit housing the small clitoris and the entrance to the urinary and genital tracts. In the male, the distance between the anus and urogenital system is larger, and gentle pressure either side of the prepuce will allow protrusion of an obvious penis.

Chinchilla

The female chinchilla has a large urinary papilla making identification difficult. The identification is made on the distance between the anus and the urinary papilla. The female's urinary papilla is close to the anus, and if examined closely it may be possible to observe the transverse slit which marks the sealed (when not in heat) entrance to the reproductive tract lying between the anus and urinary papilla. The male's prepuce, which resembles the female's urinary papilla, is much larger and more cranial, and the penis may be protruded in compliant individuals.

Females are often larger than males in the chinchilla, the reverse of many other rodents.

Skin

The guinea pig has a prominent sebaceous gland on its back, cranial to the tail base. This secretes a yellow waxy material which frequently matts the fur in this area. There are additional glands emptying into the anal sacs in the folds of skin which enclose the anus and genitalia. These can produce a creamy white, strong-smelling discharge in the boar. Guinea pig fur is often relatively coarse in nature, varying with the breed type.

Conversely, the coat of the chinchilla is renowned for its soft silky nature. It responds badly to moisture, hence the need to provide chinchillas with dust baths for cleaning. In addition, the chinchilla may experience a feature known as 'fur slip'. This is when a section of fur will drop out due to fright or stress. The alopecic area left may take several weeks to regrow its fur.

In both species the ears are prominently furless, with the chinchilla in particular having the largest pinnae.

The guinea pig has a prominent subcutaneous fat pad over the scruff region of the neck, which makes large injections at this site painful.

The chinchilla has very small claws on each digit. In comparison, the guinea pig has prominent claws on every digit. Both have defined leathery pads to the ends of each digit.

Eyes

The eyes of the guinea pig are relatively small in comparison to the size of their heads. There is a prominent third eyelid tear gland which may prolapse. The chinchilla on the other hand has large prominent eyes, and a vertical, slit-like pupil which allows the chinchilla virtually to close off all light reaching the retina. This is to protect it in its wild habitat high in the Andes of South America, which is exposed to bright sunshine.

Haematology

In both species, the morphology of the red and white cells is similar to that seen in other rodents. There are predominantly more lymphocytes than neutrophils in the white cell count. In the guinea pig, however, an intracellular inclusion known as the Kurloff body may be seen in the circulating monocytes which are therefore, known as 'Kurloff cells'. These are rare in the juvenile and male guinea pigs, but common in the female particularly during gestation, and they may play a role in the physiological immunity relationship between mother and foetus. Their origin is not clear but they are thought to come from the thymus or spleen.

CHIPMUNK

Biological average values for the chipmunk

The normal values for the basic biological parameters of the chipmunk are given in Table 13.6.

Table 13.6 Biological parameters of the chipmunk.

Biological parameter		Chipmunk
Weight (g)		55–150
Rectal body temperature (°C)		37.8–39.6 (when not hibernating)
Respiration rate at rest (breaths/min)		60–90
Heart rate at rest (beats/min)		150–280
Gestation (days)		28–35
Litter size		2–10 (average 4)
Age at sexual maturity (months)	Male	8–9
	Female	9–12
Oestrus interval (days)		Average 14
Lifespan (years)		8–12 (may be shorter in captivity)

Musculoskeletal system

The musculoskeletal system has many similarities to the rat as outlined above.

Skull

The skull is typically rodent in its long and flattened form.

Axial skeleton

The spinal vertebral layout is the same as the rat.

Appendicular skeleton

Each forelimb has four and each hind limb five digits. Their gait is a jumping sinuous movement, which makes them excellent climbers, with fore- and hind limbs a similar length. Their bodies are more elongated than those of rats or mice, and their long, prehensile tail is used for balance and support. Their bone structure is light-weight and more bird-like than the heavier structure of the rat.

Respiratory system

The lungs are divided into three lobes on the left side and four on the right. Their thoracic cavity is larger in relation to the abdomen than is the case in many other rodents.

Digestive system

Oral cavity

The incisors are open rooted, or continuously growing, and malocclusions are not uncommon. The dental formula is:

I 1/1 C 0/0 Pm 0/0 M 3/3.

They have a diastema. The mouth is narrow, the tongue fleshy and fixed firmly at the base, although the rostral tip is mobile. There are small cheek pouches communicating with the diastema of the oral cavity and extending back to the ear base. These are frequently sites for abscess formation if sharp seeds, such as unhusked oats, are fed.

Stomach

The stomach is of a simple glandular design. There is a strong cardiac sphincter which normally prevents regurgitation.

Small intestine

The small intestine is relatively long. The duodenum receives a duct from the gall bladder just after the pyloric sphincter, and one further on from the pancreas.

Large intestine

The initial part of the large intestine at the ileo-caecal junction has a small, blind-ending caecum with some sacculations, or haustrae.

Liver

The liver has four main lobes, and possesses a gall bladder and bile duct, which joins the descending duodenum.

Pancreas

The pancreas is found along the descending duodenum and the edge of the stomach. It empties through one duct which empties into the proximal descending duodenum.

Urinary system

Kidney

The kidneys are a typical bean shape. Fat deposits are often found in this area during the late summer and early autumn. Each kidney has the usual ureter passing caudally to the urinary bladder.

Bladder

The bladder is of the usual design seen in mammals. Chipmunk urine is usually alkaline in nature and may contain calcium crystals. However, due to their more omnivorous nature (they eat meat such as insects, eggs etc.), they may also produce acidic urine.

Cardiovascular system

Heart

The heart is similar to that seen in the rat and mouse.

Blood vessels for sampling

The jugular veins make the best vessels for blood sampling. The ventral tail vein may be used but care should be exercised here and the chipmunk sedated, as the tail skin can deglove and slough relatively easily.

Lymphatic system

Spleen

The spleen is a small, strap-like organ on the greater curvature of the stomach to the left side of the cranial abdomen.

Thymus

The thymus is a prominent organ in the juvenile, and persists in the cranial thorax of the adult.

Reproductive anatomy

Male

The testes sit in a caudally placed scrotum, but only during the reproductive season. During the quiescent period the testes are retracted into the abdomen. The scrotum and testes thus enlarge during the breeding season from January to September.

Female

The female chipmunk has four pairs of mammary glands, two inguinal and two thoracic. Otherwise, the reproductive tract follows a pattern similar to that of the rat.

Reproductive physiology

The chipmunk is seasonally polyoestrus, cycling between March and September. Chipmunks are spontaneous ovulators, with an oestrus cycle length of around 14 days. There is no evidence of a post-partum oestrus, and gestation length averages 31–32 days. Mammary development becomes prominent 24–48 hours prior to parturition.

Reproductive success drops dramatically after 6–7 years of age in the female.

Neonatology

Chipmunk young are altricial and so are born blind, deaf and hairless. Fur starts to appear around 7–10 days of age, and the eyes open at 4 weeks. The age at weaning is 5–7 weeks. Sexual maturity is reached at 8 months in the male and 10 months in the female.

Sexing

The male chipmunk has a clearly visible penis which points caudally. During the breeding season the scrotum is noticeably enlarged. The female has a urogenital papilla, but the distance from anus to papilla is less than the distance from anus to prepuce in the male.

Skin

Chipmunks have soft fur covering the whole of their bodies. Sebaceous glands exist around the anus in both sexes. They have five digits on their forepaws and four on the hind, which possess small pads and claws. The ears are small and furred.

FERRETS

Biological averages for the domestic ferret

Table 13.7 gives the basic normal biological values for the domestic ferret.

Musculoskeletal system

Skull

The skull is more rodent-like, in that it is pointed and flattened dorsoventrally. The eyes are for-ward facing, giving binocular vision for prey detection.

Axial skeleton

The vertebral formula for the ferret is similar to most mammals and comprises the usual seven cervical vertebrae, with the extended 15 thoracic, 5 lumbar, 3 sacral and, on average, 18 coccygeal vertebrae.

Appendicular skeleton

The form is basically similar to that seen in the cat. The forelimbs and hind limbs each have five digits.

Respiratory system

Ferret lungs are split into two lobes on the left side and four on the right. The entrance to the thoracic cavity is very small and is bounded by the first ribs. Any space-occupying lesion, therefore, such as thymic lymphoma, will cause dyspnoea and dysphagia.

Digestive system

Oral cavity

The ferret has a set of deciduous teeth, which appear at 3–4 weeks of age. These are replaced by permanent teeth at 7–11 weeks of age. The dental formula of the adult is:

Table 13.7 Biological parameters of the domestic ferret.

Biological parameter		Domestic ferret
Weight (kg)		0.5–1 females; 1–2 males
Rectal body temperature (°C)		37.8–40
Respiration rate at rest (breaths/min)		40–80
Heart rate at rest (beats/min)		180–250
Gestation length (days)		41–42
Litter size		2–14 (average 8)
Age at sexual maturity (months)	Male	4–6
	Female	4–8 (spring following birth)
Lifespan (years)		5–10

I 3/3 C 1/1 Pm 3/3 M 1/2.

The deciduous formula for the ferret is:

I 1/0 C 1/1 Pm 3/3.

The most prominent teeth are the canines, which are responsible for holding onto the prey. The molars and premolars are shearing teeth, as is typical of the carnivore family, rather than the flat grinding surface of herbivorous mammals. The tongue is fleshy and mobile.

Stomach

The stomach is of a simple form, lined with glandular epithelium containing both acid- and pepsinogen-secreting cells. It has a weak cardiac sphincter allowing easy vomition, and a pronounced pyloric sphincter. The stomach can dilate markedly when full.

Small intestine

The descending duodenum begins at the pylorus of the stomach and passes across to the right side of the abdomen. It is entered into, after the first 5 cm or so, by the common bile and pancreatic duct.

Large intestine

The large intestine is not easily differentiated from the small intestine, as it is the same width and colour, although the mesenteric lymph node marks the junction between the two. There is no caecum in the ferret or any member of the family Mustelidae. The terminal portion of the rectum has emptying into it the two anal glands which, when emptied, can give off the very unpleasant odour associated with a frightened ferret! The removal of these glands is considered an unnecessary mutilation by the Royal College of Veterinary Surgeons in the UK and so should not be done unless there is a medical reason for so doing.

Liver

The liver is deeply divided into six lobes. The right lobe has the usual renal fossa to accommo-date the right kidney. A gall bladder is present, and empties via a common duct with the pancreas.

Pancreas

The pancreas is a prominent organ, with two main lobes, one along the descending duodenum and the other along the pyloric axis. A single duct merges with the bile duct to provide a common entrance to the duodenum.

Urinary system

Kidney

The kidneys are the traditional kidney-bean shape. The right kidney sits more cranially, in a fossa in the right lobe of the liver. The left kidney is more caudal and freely suspended.

Bladder

The bladder is much the same structure as that seen in the cat or dog. The urethra passes through the penis in the male ferret, which contains a J-shaped os penis. This makes urinary catheterisation of the male difficult.

Ferret urine is naturally acidic in nature, due to its carnivorous diet. It tends to be relatively concentrated and free of turbidity.

Cardiovascular system

Heart

The heart occupies rib spaces 6–8. Its tip is connected to the sternum by a ligament which frequently contains fat, making the heart appear elevated off the sternal floor on radiographs.

Blood vessels for sampling

Blood vessels for sampling include the jugular veins, the cephalic and saphenous veins. These are found in the same places as for the cat. The ferret also has an unusual series of arteries branching from the main aortic trunk. In cats and dogs, two separate carotid arteries arise from the aortic trunk. In the ferret, a single vessel (the brachiocephalic or innominate artery 1) leaves the aortic arch. *This* then divides into the left and right carotid arteries, as well as into the right subclavian artery at the thoracic inlet. This prevents restriction of blood flow to the head which could occur due to the narrow chest inlet.

Lymphatic system

Spleen

The spleen varies greatly in size between individuals, and is attached to the greater curvature of the stomach on the left side. Its ventral tip may extend across the floor of the abdomen and back up to meet the right kidney.

Thymus

The thymus is a prominent organ in the cranial thorax of the young ferret. It dwindles to a few islands of tissue in the adult.

Lymph nodes

The lymph nodes are of a similar arrangement to the cat. The most notable lymph node is the mesenteric node, which can be used to differentiate between small and large intestine.

Reproductive anatomy

Male

The male ferret is known as a hob. The testes are situated in a perineally located scrotum. They enlarge in the breeding season (March to September). There is no movement of the testes from scrotal sac to abdomen.

A single accessory sex gland exists in the male ferret. This is the prostate, which lies at the neck of the bladder and opens into the lumen of the urethra. The urethra passes caudally through the pelvis before bending ventrally and cranially to exit at the ventrally located prepuce. The os penis is J-shaped.

Female

The female ferret is known as a jill. The ovaries are found close to the caudal poles of the respective kidneys. The uterus is bicornuate and similar to that seen in the cat, with two long uterine horns and a short uterine body. There is a single cervix opening into the vagina. The urethra opens into the floor of the vagina so there is a common urogenital opening at the vulva, cranial to the anus.

Reproductive physiology

The female ferret is seasonally polyoestrus and an induced ovulator. Ovulation occurs 1–2 days after mating. The breeding season runs from March through to September. Oestrus is demonstrated by the obviously swollen vulva, which returns to normal 2–3 weeks after a successful mating.

Gestation lasts on average 42 days. The placenta is zonary, similar to that seen in the cat and dog.

The most important point about the female ferret's reproductive cycle is that if she is not mated, or brought out of heat in some way, the persistent exposure to oestrogen can cause a fatal bone marrow suppression in one season. Female ferrets should therefore be mated by entire or vasectomised males, treated with progesterone hormone therapy to halt the oestrus or speyed to prevent heat altogether.

Neonatology

The young ferret is known as a kit. They are born altricial, blind, furless and deaf. The average litter size is eight kits. The fur starts to appear around the second day post partum, and is pronounced by 2 weeks. The eyes open around 3 weeks and the ears around 10 days. The kit is born with a prominent fat pad on the dorsum of the neck providing some energy reserves during the early stages of life. The female ferret is sexually mature from 4–8 months and the male from 4–6 months, usually in the spring following birth.

Sexing

The male ferret has an obvious prepuce on the ventral abdomen similar to that seen in the domestic dog. In addition, the male has a caudally located scrotum with obvious testes. The female has a vulval orifice just ventral to the anus.

Skin

The claws present on all four feet are not retractable. The odour of a ferret is primarily from the normal sebaceous glands present within the skin, giving them the characteristic musky smell. These glands are particularly well concentrated around the mouth, chin and perineum. The odour of the male ferret is particularly strong, due to the action of testosterone on these glands and the tendency to spray and empty the anal glands to mark territory. Neutering reduces this latter problem.

Haematology

One noticeable aspect of the ferret blood count is the consistently high packed cell volume, often in the 58–63% range in healthy adults. The white cell count on the other hand tends routinely to be lower than that seen in cats and dogs. The neutrophil is generally the predominant white cell seen.

Further reading

Harkness, J.E. and Wagner, J.E. (2000) *Biology and Medicine of Rabbits and Rodents, 5th edn*. Lea & Febiger, Philadelphia.

Hillyer, E.V. and Quesenberry, K.E. (1997) *Ferrets, Rabbits and Rodents*. W.B. Saunders, Philadelphia.

Meredith, A. and Redrobe, S. (2001) *Manual of Exotic Pets, 4th edn*. BSAVA, Cheltenham.

Okerman, L. (1994) *Diseases of Domestic Rabbits*. Blackwell Science, Oxford.

Richardson, V.C.G. (1992) *Diseases of Domestic Guinea Pigs*. Blackwell Science, Oxford.

Chapter 14

Small Mammal Housing, Husbandry and Rearing

DOMESTIC RABBIT

Breeds

There are many different breeds of rabbit, varying from the miniature breeds such as the Netherland dwarf, weighing in at 0.5–0.75 kg, through to the New Zealand whites and the Belgian hares at 8–10 kg. Other commonly seen breeds include the lop-eared crosses, the angoran breeds, the Rex and the traditional Dutch rabbits.

Cage requirements

Size and construction

The traditional hutch is a common feature of rabbit husbandry. The provision of a wooden enclosure which is sufficiently large to provide sleeping quarters, a feeding area and a toilet area is common. In general, a rough guide to a minimum width of a rabbit hutch is three times the length of the rabbit to be housed when it is stretched out at rest. The depth should be one rabbit length, and the height equal to that of the rabbit standing on hind legs. Anything smaller and the rabbit must be provided with an outside run, or allowed out of the hutch for regular exercise periods every day. Apart from being cruel, cooping a rabbit up in too small a hutch will lead to muscular and skeletal atrophy, and increase the risk of spontaneous spine and limb fractures when the rabbit overexerts itself. However many commercially available hutches are in fact too small for the adult rabbit, being the correct size only for the small juvenile or dwarf.

Wooden hutches are the standard and are satisfactory in many cases. Their disadvantage is that they will tend to rot with the absorption of urine and rain unless properly protected. Care should be taken with wood preservatives to ensure an animal friendly preservative is chosen (do not use creosote!). The roof may be further protected with the felt material used to roof garden sheds, and should slope to the rear of the hutch to avoid rain dripping into the front, or pooling on the roof. The hutches should also be raised off the floor on legs to avoid the bottom rotting from the damp ground surface. A ramp should therefore be supplied if the rabbits are to be allowed in and out of the hutch of their own accord. Wooden hutches are also much more easily destroyed by gnawing.

In commercial fur and meat producing situations, rabbits are kept in wire mesh hutches suspended above a solid floor. The wire mesh 'hutch' has one major advantage in that it prevents soiling of the fur by urine and faeces. However it can cause abrasions of the hocks in older overweight rabbits, and is not advised for housing pet rabbits.

Substrates

Substrates used for cage floor covering include straw, hay, shavings and newspaper. Many rabbits will preferentially select hay and straw for bedding over shavings and paper. One of the advantages of the former is that they allow urine to drop through the fibre framework and away from the rabbit, so reducing the likelihood of urine scolding in older and arthritic rabbits.

Positioning

Care should be taken to avoid overheating of the hutch, as rabbits cannot sweat and temperatures above 26–28°C will rapidly cause hyperthermia and death. Hutches should therefore be positioned out of direct sunlight, particularly in the summer months. Rabbits will shiver when cold, although they can tolerate colder temperatures better than hot. Care should still be taken to ensure the hutch is not overly drafty or exposed during the winter months. Bringing it into a shed or garage is often advisable in the worst weather.

Food and water bowls

Feeding bowls should be a ceramic or metal. The former are preferred, as they are heavier and harder to knock over. Plastic feed bowls should be avoided as they are easily chewed. Water feeders are better offered with ball valve drip dispensers. They allow less contamination of the water with food, urine and faeces than an open bowl. Care should be taken with these feeders, though, as some rabbits reared with water bowls will not drink from them. In addition, the ball valve often leaks and this will lead to excessively damp substrate and mould growth. Drip feeders will also suffer from bacterial build-up and need careful cleaning once or twice a week, or even daily if a large number of rabbits are housed.

Outdoor runs

It is advisable to provide outside runs attached to the hutch in the summer months. This allows the rabbit access to unfiltered sunshine, which is important for vitamin D_3 synthesis as well as for stimulating normal annual rhythms of behaviour. Fresh grass is also the food item rabbits are supremely adapted to eat. The fibre content in particular is vital for wear of the teeth and stimulation of normal gut motility. Grass should not be cut first and then offered though, as this rapidly ferments and can produce colic.

Care should be taken when securing outside runs to make them both rabbit proof *and* predator proof. For this reason it may be necessary to bury the wire sides to any run a foot or so beneath the ground surface as does in particular will burrow regularly. To prevent foxes and cats gaining access to the run, a meshed roof should be provided. Finally, all outdoor rabbits should be vaccinated against myxomatosis, the viral condition spread by fleas and mosquitos from wild rabbits, and preferably against viral haemorrhagic disease as well.

House rabbit

Many rabbits are now kept as house rabbits, with sleeping quarters and a litter tray. Rabbits can be toilet trained relatively easily. The first steps in this are to keep the rabbit in a small area with a sleeping area, the litter tray and a feeding area. Once the litter tray has been associated with urination in particular, the rabbit may then be allowed more freedom to roam.

Hazards in the home include electrical cabling, which should be hidden beneath carpets or protected inside heavy duty cable trunking, which is available from hardware stores. House plants are another problem. Many of the exotic tropical house plants are poisonous. Examples include African violet, *Dieffenbachia*, cheese plant and spider plant.

Social grouping

Rabbits are in general a social species, preferring to live in a group rather than singly. Problems arise though with keeping a number of entire males together, as bullying and sexual harassment will occur. Neutering is therefore advised where more than one male is to be kept, and may be performed in bucks from 4–5 months of age. Mixed sex groups will work well if the does are spayed. This may be safely done from 5–6 months of age, and is advised even in solitary does due to the high risk of developing a malignant uterine cancer, known as a uterine *adenocarcinoma*, in middle age.

Some owners advocate the grouping of guinea pigs with rabbits. This is to be discouraged for two important reasons. One is that the rabbit has very powerful hind legs and the guinea pig a long and fragile spine. One well placed kick from the rabbit can consequently do a great deal of damage. The other reason is that rabbits are frequently asymptomatic carriers of the bacteria *Bordetella bronchiseptica* in their airways. This bacteria can cause a severe pneumonia in guinea pigs. Other domestic pets are not advised to be mixed with rabbits, as both the cat and dog are potential predators!

Behaviour

Rabbits are a prey species and therefore communicate in a very different manner from the more commonly understood cats and dogs. Indeed, it may seem that rabbits are very poor at communicating their feelings to their owners, when in fact they may be communicating, but in a much more subtle manner.

Affection is shown by mutual grooming of a companion, or owner, with licking of the hands in the latter case common. Other signs of relaxation include coming to the owner to be fed treats, following an owner around the house and, in many rabbits, making a buzzing noise from the larynx. This may be mistaken for a disease problem by inexperienced owners as it can be quite loud!

Aggression is shown by scratching, boxing with the front legs and biting. Aggression may be initiated because of a hormonal state, such as does coming into season or bucks fighting for territory in the early spring, or it may be fear or pain driven. Aggression may also become a learnt behaviour if an act of aggression results in a desired effect, such as immediate backing off or replacing of a rabbit that has just been picked up by an owner.

Fear is shown initially by the regular thumping of the hind legs. This is a warning signal. As the object of fear approaches, the rabbit will then either freeze and remain motionless, or suddenly bolt towards an exit.

Chewing of almost everything in the rabbit's environment is a perfectly normal behaviour and no amount of training will alter this fact. Owners of house rabbits should be warned of this, and take appropriate action to prevent chewing of electric cables and other hazardous items of household furnishing.

Fostering

Rabbit kittens are difficult to hand rear. Many females will not foster a strange doe's kittens, but does kept together and lactating at the same time will often allow suckle each other's young. This is the best scenario if another known lactating doe is available. If not, as is often the case, hand rearing may be attempted.

A rearing formula has been derived (Okerman, 1994): 25 ml of whole cow's milk to 75 ml of condensed milk and 6 g of lyophilised skimmed milk powder. To this may be added a vitamin supplement. The kitten is fed twice a day only, from 2–10 ml depending on its age. This should continue until the kitten is 2 weeks old when more and more good quality hay and pellets should be introduced, aiming to wean the kitten at 3 weeks. The anogenital area should be stimulated with a piece of damp cotton wool after every feed to stimulate urination and defaecation for the first 2 weeks.

RAT AND MOUSE

Varieties

Rat

The common albino laboratory rat is widely domesticated. Other common varieties include the hooded rat and Rex groups. These are all variations on the *Rattus norvegicus* species, and the fancy rat numbers are ever increasing.

Mouse

As with rats, there are many different varieties of domesticated mouse. These vary from albinos through to the Rex, whole body colour types etc.

Cage requirements

Construction and temperature

These are similar for both rats and mice. The traditional solid, plastic-bottomed and wire mesh upper cages are to be advised. These allow good air circulation at the level of the rat or mouse. The fish-tank style of housing is much less ventilated and allows the build-up of ammonia from urine-soaked bedding. Ammonia is a heavy gas and sits just above substrate level, i.e. at rat or mouse nose level, and is thus inhaled often in high concentrations in this style of housing. Ammonia is highly irritant to the sensitive mucous membranes of the airways and will inflame and damage them, allowing secondary bacterial infection. This leads to the all too common problems of pneumonia seen in these species.

Environmental temperatures should range from 18–26°C. Because they lack skin sweat glands, temperatures above 28–29°C will rapidly induce hyperthermia and death in rats and mice. Rats can tolerate cooler temperatures better than mice, due to their lower surface area to body mass ratio and deposits of brown fat beneath the skin. However, temperatures consistently below 10°C will lead to poor health and hypothermia.

Substrate

Wood shavings are well tolerated by rats and mice, but be aware that many pine and coniferous woods contain resins which may cause skin and airway irritation. Alternatively, newspaper or paper towelling may be used. Straw and hay may be used, but again beware that parasites may be introduced from wild rodents inadvertently with these bedding materials.

Cage furniture

As with hamsters, wheels are enjoyed by mice in particular. But these should be solid in construction rather than open wired to avoid damage to limbs. Rats are less keen to use wheels, although they do enjoy climbing and hiding inside cardboard tubes and other enclosed items.

Food and water bowls

As with rabbits, sip feeders are ideal, as they lead to minimal wastage and contamination. Ceramic or stainless steel bowls are preferred to plastic.

Social grouping

Rat

Male rats may be kept with other males, particularly if reared together from an early age, without fighting. Females may also be paired with other females, and seem to benefit from the company. Intersex groups also work well, although care should be taken to neuter the males (which may be performed from 3–4 months of age) if unwanted pregnancies are to be avoided. This may be done from 3–4 months of age. If breeding, male rats may be 'paired' with 1–6 females. The pregnant female should be removed to a separate cage from the male rat 4–5 days prior to parturition to avoid disturbing the female at this sensitive time.

Mouse

Females may be kept in groups, particularly if reared together from a young age. Males however should always be housed singly, as severe fights and even death may result from aggression between sexually mature males. If breeding, male mice may be 'paired' with 1–6 females. It is then advised to remove the pregnant female from the male some 4–5 days prior to parturition.

Behaviour

Rat

Rats are generally docile and rarely do they bite. Female rats are prone to cannibalism of the young if disturbed in the first few days following parturition. Food and water should therefore be provided *prior* to whelping, to last for the following 7–10 days, and the female then left. The female rat builds a relatively poor nest in comparison to other members of the rodent family.

Mouse

Mice are generally relatively docile, although male mice may be more aggressive than females. The latter though will be aggressive in the defence of her young. In addition, although cannibalism towards her young is rare, a female mouse should be left undisturbed for a minimum of 2–3 days post partum. It is advisable to remove the female to a separate tank once mated to allow her to give birth and rear her young undisturbed.

Fostering

It is extremely difficult to rear young rats and mice successfully. Attempts may be made using a 1:1 dilution of evaporated milk to previously boiled water fed every 2 hours for the first 1–2 weeks. Weaning may be performed at 3 weeks. Stimulation of the anogenital area should be performed to encourage urination and defaecation.

GERBIL AND HAMSTER

Varieties

Gerbil

There seems to be one main breed common in captivity, although a separate species known as the fat-tailed gerbil (*Pachyuromys duprasi*) has become more popular recently. There are however several different fur colour types, with albinos, black variants and greys as well as the normal tan colouration now available.

Hamster

There are four main species: Syrian, European, Chinese and Russian. Within these species there are many colour variations, from albino to red to black, with differing fur types such as the fluffy 'teddy bear' version of the Syrian hamster in addition to the more common short-coated varieties.

Cage requirements

Cages and substrates

Gerbil

These enjoy tunnelling through deep litter substrates. It is important that the environment is kept dry, as humid conditions lead to poor fur quality and increased skin and respiratory infections. Shavings are an ideal substrate and should be at least 10–15cm deep. Placing ceramic or cardboard tubes through the substrate can help tunnel formation and provide environmental enrichment. Peat and other soil substrates should however be avoided due because they are more likely to encourage damp. Environmental temperatures are usually kept around 20–25°C if possible.

Hamster

Cages for hamsters are best constructed of solid walls. The Rotastak®-style cage is ideal, with multiple tunnels for the hamster to manoeuvre from enclosed space to enclosed space. Wire cages are not so good, as hamsters have a habit of climbing up the sides, and then hand-over-hand across the roofs of these cages. They will often lose their grip suffer back injuries or compound fractures of the tibia as they land on the cage floor. It is advised to keep housing temperatures between 18–26°C. Lower temperatures than 5–6°C will result in the hamster hibernating. In this state respiration and heart rates slow considerably, making it difficult in many instances to detect if the hamster is still alive. Temperatures above 29–30°C will result in hyperthermia and death.

Cage furniture

Hamsters much enjoy wheels, but these should be of a solid type, rather than the open wire format. This is to prevent the inadvertent damaging or even fracturing of a hind leg if it gets pushed between the wire slats. Tubes are ideal to entertain gerbils as mentioned above.

Food and water bowls

Food bowls for both species are best made of a ceramic material, as these resist gnawing, are easily cleaned and difficult to tip over. Water is usually supplied in the traditional drip feeders, although care should be taken especially with gerbils that the valve is not leaky, as this leads to excessively wet substrate conditions and resultant dermatitis.

Social grouping

Gerbil

Gerbils are best housed singly, as a female pair or a neutered male and female pair. In the wild they will often bond, male to female, for life. Males housed together though will fight, inflicting severe wounds. Female gerbils will rarely cannibalise their young, unlike hamsters, although care should still be taken not to disturb the female and young too much in the first week post partum.

Hamster

Males of the European, Chinese and Syrian species will fight. To a certain extent males of the Russian species will also fight, although this is lessened somewhat if they are reared from a young age together. Females may also be aggressive and so it is advised that hamsters in general are housed individually. For breeding purposes it is better to introduce a male hamster to a female's cage, rather than the other way around, to minimise fighting. A female hamster which has recently given birth should not be disturbed for a minimum of 10 days as the incidence of cannibalism of the young is high. To avoid this, enough food, water and bedding material (too little bedding is another reason for a female hamster killing the young) should be placed in the female's cage a few days prior to parturition and the female left undisturbed for the next 10–14 days.

Behaviour

Gerbil

Gerbils can be difficult to handle if not acclimatised to it from an early age. They will often bite if frightened or roughly handled. They are rarely vocal, but they will communicate their alarm through regular drumming of the floor of the cage with one hind leg, in much the same way as a rabbit will do. Gerbils spend the day dozing and they are most active at night, that is they are nocturnal.

Hamster

Hamsters are frequently accused of being aggressive. They will certainly bite readily if roughly handled, disturbed or frightened. Chinese and Russian species are more aggressive than Syrian and Europeans. Hamsters are also nocturnal and much of the aggression is due to being disturbed from their nest during the day. They therefore really do not make good children's pets. Females may be aggressive towards their young if disturbed.

Fostering

Gerbil

See rats and mice. Young gerbils are extremely difficult to rear artificially.

Hamster

See rats and mice. Young hamsters are extremely difficult to rear artificially. They do not foster well onto another female in any of the species, except perhaps the Russian hamster where a lactating female *may* accept another's young.

GUINEA PIG AND CHINCHILLA

Breeds

Guinea pig

There are several different varieties of domesticated guinea pig: the Abyssinian, which possesses whorls of fur over the body and head; the Peruvian, which is particularly long furred; the English or short-furred variety; the Rex varieties, with short fuzzy fur. Colour variations are many and varied from whole body colours of tan, white and black, through mixtures of two or three colours and albinos.

Chinchilla

There are just two subspecies of chinchilla recognised. *Chinchilla laniger* is the standard domestic long-tailed chinchilla, which comes in a variety of colours from silver, to white, to champagne, to black. Some authorities also recognise a subspecies known as *Chinchilla brevicauda* which is a short-tailed, larger version of the above.

Cage requirements

Guinea pig

A hutch system similar to that outlined above for rabbits is advised, although the whole structure should be on one level. The same substrate and bedding materials are offered. In addition, it is often advised that lengths of tubing, such as drain-pipe, should be offered as bolt holes for the guinea pigs to use when frightened. Access to grazing is useful, and guinea pigs cannot climb or dig so pen requirements are easier to provide than for rabbits. Care should be taken to ensure that any steps or ramps are not so steep that a guinea pig could fall, as their long and fragile backbone is easily damaged. Guinea pigs are expert chewers so, if allowed access to the home, precautions as with rabbits should be observed. Bowls and drinkers for food and water are as for rabbits.

Chinchilla

Space requirements for chinchillas are greater than for guinea pigs as they are extremely active. Recommendations include enclosures in excess of $2\,m^3$. They appreciate vertical space, unlike the ground-dwelling guinea pig. Cage construction should be of wire mesh, with a solid or mesh floor. This is because chinchillas are particularly good at chewing wood, and rapidly destroy wooden hutches. Chinchillas prefer an actual nest box rather than plentiful substrate. This should ideally be $20\,cm^3$ or more in size and can be lined with hay or straw, although the rest of the cage is often left bare. The floor is often a wire grid structure, to prevent any fluid accumulating, as this may lead to damage of the fur. The provision of lengths of drainpipe tubing is also advised, as for guinea pigs, to allow the shy chinchilla to hide from public gaze.

Water can be provided in the traditional drip feeders. Chinchilla fur matts very quickly when wet, so care should be taken to prevent the cage from becoming damp from any leakage. Because of this tendency to matt easily, chinchillas should not be allowed to bathe in water, but instead pro-vided with daily access to a fine, pumice sand and fullers earth mixture as a dust bath. This can be provided in a metal box which may be clipped onto the inside of the cage or in a cat litter tray. The latter is less satisfactory as the chinchilla may chew the plastic. The sand bath should only be provided for short periods each day as otherwise the chinchilla tends to spend all day in the bath! Environmental temperatures should not exceed 20–22°C as heat stress may occur with that thick fur coat.

Social grouping

Guinea pig

Guinea pigs are a social species, and they live a much more contented life in the presence of other guinea pigs. Entire males can fight, although this is less likely if they are reared together from an early age. Even so, males will form a hierarchical system, and subordinate males may be bullied and bitten on a regular basis. Females live happily together, and the sexes may be mixed, although castration of the males (which may be done from 4–5 months of age) is advised to prevent unwanted pregnancies. In addition, females are unusual amongst the species so far discussed in that they will allow the nursing of other young than their own.

Chinchilla

The chinchilla will often form bonded pairs, although they will equally live happily in multi-sex and multi-chinchilla groups. If breeding is to be prevented, one or both of the sexes should be neutered. Males may be castrated from 5–6 months and females from 6–7 months.

Behaviour

Guinea pig

Guinea pigs make good pets for the older child. They are docile and easily handled and rarely bite. Unlike many of the other species discussed here, they are very vocal. Their normal, contented vocal sounds include a series of chirrups and chattering noises which are low pitched. When alarmed though they will emit higher pitched squeaks of warning. They will also run around the perimeter of their enclosure at high speed when stressed, and may flatten any younger guinea pigs in the process!

Chinchilla

Chinchillas are shy and retiring creatures. They are very affectionate and will make chirruping noises when contented. When frightened they will bite, bark and often exhibit fur-slip, where fur will drop out leaving alopecic areas which last for many weeks. When distressed, many chinchillas will urinate at the handler. This includes females who, having a large urinary papilla, can direct their urination as accurately as males!

Fostering

Guinea pig

Use of a foster mother for any orphaned guinea pigs is advisable, even though they are precocious and may start to eat solids from day 3 post partum. Even so, rearing milk formulas are still advised to be fed. Recipes for these include commercial feline weaner formulas, or using a 1:2 mixture of evaporated milk to previously boiled and then cooled water, thickened with a proprietary vegetable baby food powder (Richardson, 1992). This may be given through a kitten-rearing feeder every 2 hours for the first week, but the young should be encouraged to take solids as early as possible as a high incidence of cataracts is noticed in young guinea pigs fed for too long on cat, dog, or cow's milk replacers. For the first 7–10 days the anogenital area of the young guinea pig should be stimulated with damp cotton wool to encourage urination and defaecation.

Chinchilla

Even though young chinchillas are precocious at birth, they can be difficult to rear successfully. A rough guide to a rearing formula is to feed a 50:50 mix of a commercial cat or dog rearing formula added to evaporated milk. Alternatively, a 1:2 mix of evaporated milk with cooled, previously boiled water, thickened with a little fruit or vegetable baby food (Milupa or Farex) may be used. This should be fed through a kitten feeder every 2 hours for the first week, dropping to every 3–4 hours once the young chinchilla starts nibbling small volumes of solid. Chinchillas may be weaned early at 4 weeks if eating sufficient dry foods. Their weight should be measured daily to ensure regular gains. After each meal, the anogenital area should be stimulated with a piece of damp cotton wool to stimulate urination and defaecation, although this is really only necessary for the first 7–10 days.

CHIPMUNK

Species

The two main species seen in captivity are the Siberian chipmunk and, to a lesser extent, the North American species. The coat variations are limited, but the basic pattern is a with a light brown base coat with darker longitudinal stripes. Albinos do exist.

Cage requirements

Cages and substrates

Chipmunks appreciate a combination of cage environments. The enclosure itself resembles more closely an aviary system designed for cage birds, with a wire mesh wall. The most successful combine a deep litter floor, with bark chippings to allow foraging for food for environmental enrichment and roost boxes attached a few feet off the ground. These are constructed along similar lines to bird boxes. The cage may be further enhanced by stringing ropes from side to side to create aerial walkways.

Positioning

It is important not to house chipmunks near any source of electrical radiation in the 50–60 hertz range. This includes television sets and many strip lights and computer terminals. The radiation waves given off by these electrical items cause high degrees of stress to the chipmunks, who will exhibit manic behaviour. This occurs even when they are turned off but still plugged in to the mains socket.

Social grouping

Chipmunks prefer to be grouped together. Males are territorial and will fight during the breeding season, but females will tolerate each other well. In general, family groups are preferred, but the parents will chase away the young when weaned.

Behaviour

Chipmunks are extremely nervous and highly strung creatures. They will bite if handled, and are difficult to tame, even when hand reared. They will chatter excitedly to each other when stressed, and often emit high pitched squeaks. Some will also drum their hind legs as a warning signal. Tail flicking occurs almost continually, but becomes even more excited when stressed.

Fostering

Young abandoned chipmunks are difficult to rear. A rearing formula has been proposed using a mixture of 1 part evaporated milk to 2 parts water, adding vegetable baby foods to this as the chipmunk ages. Minerals and vitamins may then be added, and the whole fed through a kitten rearing feeder every four hours for the first 2 weeks of life, dropping down to every 8 hours from 3 weeks until they are weaned at 5–6 weeks. The young chipmunk should be stimulated to urinate and defaecate with a piece of damp cotton wool rubbed over the anogenital area immediately after feeding.

FERRET

Cage requirements

Cages and substrates

Many ferrets are kept in outside hutches in a fashion similar to rabbits in the United Kingdom.

Increasingly though, ferrets are being kept as house pets in the United Kingdom, and of course have been kept as such in the United States of America for many years now. The problem with wooden hutches is that the often strong-smelling urine of the ferret will penetrate the wood. This is not so bad in ferrets that are kept outdoors, but for indoor ones this may be a considerable downside! The use therefore of steel bottomed and wire upper cages is preferred for indoor ferret keeping, as this type of cage is easily disinfectable. The size of the ferret cage should be a minimum of two ferret lengths in each direction. Ferrets like to make use of vertical space, so the provision of a shelf and raised sleeping quarters are useful. Care should be taken to ensure that the wire mesh is no larger than 2.5 cm square to avoid smaller ferrets escaping. Substrate in the cage may be newspaper, hay, shavings or straw. The nest box is best lined with towelling or a similar material. Ferrets enjoy hiding in plastic tubing and investigating every nook and cranny of a house. It is therefore essential not to allow a ferret access to rooms where there are holes in the walls for pipes, such as the kitchen, as they usually end up disappearing down them!

Social grouping

Female ferrets get on well together, and ferrets in general like company, so it is often advisable to house them together. Male ferrets (hobs) though may fight and so care should be taken when housing multiples. Castration of male ferrets is advised on grounds of reducing odour in any case, and this makes them more malleable and less likely to fight as well. The female ferret is not susceptible to cannibalism of the young if disturbed, although care should be exercised when interfering with the young as the jill will defend them vigorously if she feels threatened.

Behaviour

Ferrets are extremely inquisitive creatures, and will explore everything and anything! They are generally docile when reared in the company of humans, but they can give a ferocious bite when frightened, which may be difficult to disengage from.

Management

Ferrets are currently kept in the United Kingdom mainly as working pets, for hunting, chiefly, of rabbits. Ferrets may be 'trained' to flush out rabbits from their warrens, although this is merely taking advantage of their natural hunting tendency.

Ferrets may be walked on a harness, and they can be litter trained with perseverance.

The odour of ferrets is reduced in the case of the hob by castration. The removal of the anal glands is prohibited as an unnecessary mutilation in the United Kingdom.

Fostering

Care should be taken to ensure correct nursing of the kit after failure of the jill to nurse, produce milk or when mastitis occurs. This is best done by fostering the kits onto another lactating jill, but this is often difficult. If the affected jill is still well enough the kits should be left with her to gain what little milk they may. Supplemental feeding may then be given using a proprietary feline milk replacer enriched with whipping cream to increase the fat content. A rough guide is 2–3 parts feline milk replacer to one part whipping cream. This needs to be fed every 2 hours or so via a nipple feeder, preferably warmed prior to feeding. Weaning may be brought forward to 3 weeks, and the kits trained to drink milk replacer from a saucer. Generally kits cannot manage to survive on solid foods alone until they are over 5 weeks of age. As with neonatal cats and dogs, kits require stimulation of their anogenital areas with damp cotton wool after each feed to encourage urination and defaecation.

References

Okerman, L. (1994) *Diseases of Domestic Rabbits*, p. 117. Blackwell Science, Oxford.

Richardson, V.C.G. (1992) *Diseases of Domestic Guinea Pigs*. Blackwell Science, Oxford.

Further reading

Harkness, J.E. and Wagner, J.E. (2000) *Biology and Medicine of Rabbits and Rodents, 5th edn*. Lea & Febiger, Philadelphia.

Hillyer, E.V. and Quesenberry, K.E. (1997) *Ferrets, Rabbits and Rodents*. W.B. Saunders, Philadelphia.

Meredith, A. and Redrobe, S. (2001) *Manual of Exotic Pets, 4th edn*. BSAVA, Cheltenham.

Chapter 15
Small Mammal Handling and Chemical Restraint

Before attempting to restrain a small mammal patient, we must first be sure that it is necessary. Having decided that it is so there are some general guidelines to follow in order to safeguard the small mammal patient's welfare. Points to be considered include:

- Is the patient severely debilitated and in respiratory distress? Examples include the pneumonic rabbit with obvious oculo-nasal discharge and dyspnoea, or the chronic lung disease so often seen in older rats. Excessive, or rough handling of these patients is contraindicated.
- Is the species a tame one? Examples of the more unusual small mammals which may be kept include chipmunks, marmosets (a form of small primate), pine martens (a wild mustelid from the same family as stoats and weasels) and racoons. All of these are potentially hazardous to handlers and themselves as they will often bolt for freedom when frightened, or turn and fight!
- Is the small mammal suffering from a metabolic bone disease? This is often seen in small primates and young rabbits and, to a lesser extent, guinea pigs. The diet may have been deficient in calcium and vitamin D_3 and exposure to natural sunlight may be absent. Therefore, long-bone mineralisation during growth will be poor leading to easily fractured bones.
- Does the small mammal patient require medication or physical examination, in which case restraint may be essential?

Handling techniques

Because of the wide range of species grouped under the heading small mammal, this section is easier if considered under specific groups and orders. Always approach small mammals from the sides and low levels to avoid mimicking the swooping action of a bird of prey.

Domestic rabbit

The majority of domestic rabbits are docile, but the odd aggressive doe or buck, usually those not used to being handled, does exist. In rabbits, the main dangers are from the claws, which can inflict deep scratches, and the incisors, which can produce deep bites. Aggression is frequently worse at the start of the breeding season in March and April, or when the rabbit is frightened. In addition to the damage they may cause the handler, a struggling rabbit may lash out with its powerful hind limbs and fracture or dislocate its spine. Severe stress can even induce cardiac arrest in some individuals. Rapid and safe restraint is therefore essential.

If aggressive, the lagomorph may be grasped by the scruff with one hand whilst the other supports the hind legs. If the rabbit is not aggressive, then one hand may be placed under the thorax, with the thumb and first two fingers encircling the front limbs, whilst the other is placed under the hind legs to support the back (Plate 15.1).

When transferred from one room to another the rabbit must be held close to the handler's chest. Non-fractious individuals may also be supported with their heads pushed into the crook of one arm, with that forearm supporting the length of the rabbit's body. The other hand is then used to place pressure on or grasp the scruff region.

Once caught the rabbit may be calmed further by wrapping him or her in a towel, similar to the method used for cats, so that just the head and ears protrude. There are also specific rabbit papooses that encircle the rabbit, but leave the head and ears free. This allows ear blood sampling and oral examinations, but controls their powerful hind limbs. It is important not to allow them to overheat in this position, as rabbits do not have significant sweat glands and do not actively pant. They can therefore overheat quickly if their environmental temperature exceeds 23–25°C with fatal results.

Rat and mouse

Mice will frequently bite an unfamiliar handler especially in strange surroundings. First grasp the tail near to the base and then position the mouse on a non-slip surface. Whilst still grasping the tail, the scruff may now be grasped firmly between thumb and forefinger of the other hand.

Rats will rarely bite unless roughly handled. They are best picked up by encircling the pectoral girdle immediately behind the front limbs with the thumb and fingers of one hand, whilst bringing the other hand underneath the rear limbs to support the rat's weight (Fig. 15.1). The more fractious

rat may be temporarily restrained by grasping the base of the tail before scruffing it with thumb and forefinger.

Under no circumstances should mice or rats be restrained by the tips of their tails as degloving injuries to the skin covering them will occur.

Gerbil and hamster

Hamsters can be difficult to handle as, being nocturnal, they do not like being handled during the day. If the hamster is relatively tame, cupping the hands underneath the animal is sufficient to transfer it from one cage to another.

Some breeds of hamster are more aggressive than others, with the Russian hamster (also known as the Djungarian or hairy-footed hamster) being notorious for its short temper. In these cases, the hamster should be placed onto a firm flat surface, and gentle but firm pressure placed onto the scruff region with finger and thumb of one hand. As much of the scruff should then be grasped as possible, with the pull in a cranial direction, to ensure that the skin is not drawn tight around the eyes (hamsters have a tendency to proptose their eyes if roughly scruffed) (Fig. 15.2). If a very aggressive animal is encountered, the use of a small glass or perspex container with a lid for examination and transport purposes is useful.

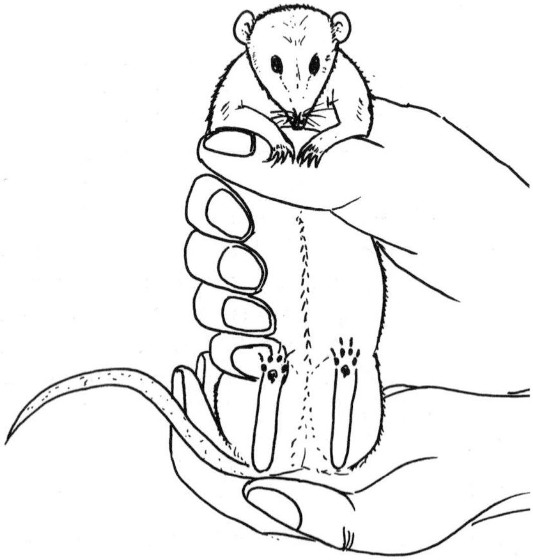

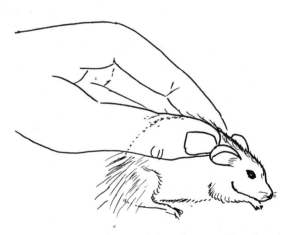

Fig. 15.1 Method of restraining a hand tame rat. Note support of hind quarters with free hand.

Fig. 15.2 Method for restraining a hamster. Note dotted line indicating the large amount of loose skin which must be grasped and the high position at which it is grasped immediately behind the ears to avoid *eye proptosis*.

Gerbils are relatively docile, but can jump extremely well when frightened and may bite. For simple transport they may be moved from one place to another by cupping the hands underneath them. For more rigorous restraint, the gerbil may be grasped by the scruff between thumb and forefinger of one hand after placing it onto a flat level surface. It is vitally important not to grasp a gerbil by the tail. The skin will strip off, leaving denuded coccygeal vertebrae, and the skin will never regrow. Jerds and jerboas are related species and handling techniques are the same.

Guinea pig and chinchilla

Guinea pigs are rarely aggressive, but they are highly stressed when separated from their companions and normal surroundings. This makes them difficult to catch as they will move at high speed around their cages. Dimming the lighting, and reducing noise and other stress can aid in control. Restraint is also easier if the guinea pig is already in a small box or cage, as there is less room for it to escape.

The guinea pig should be grasped behind the forelimbs from the dorsal aspect with one hand, whilst the other is placed beneath the hind limbs to support its weight (Fig. 15.3). This is particularly important as the guinea pig has a large abdomen but slender bones and spine. Without supporting the rear end, spinal damage is risked.

Chinchillas are equally timorous and rarely if ever bite. They too can be easily stressed and reducing noise and dimming room lighting can be useful techniques in limiting stress. When restrained they must not be scruffed under any circumstances as this will result in the loss of fur at the site held. This fur-slip will leave a bare patch which will take many weeks to regrow. Chinchillas may actually lose some fur due to stress of restraint, even if no physical gripping of the skin occurs. Some chinchillas, when particularly stressed, will rear up on their hind legs and urinate at the handler with surprising accuracy! It is therefore essential to pick up the chinchilla calmly and quickly with minimal restraint, placing one hand around the pectoral girdle from the dorsal aspect just behind the front legs, and the other hand cupping the hind legs and supporting

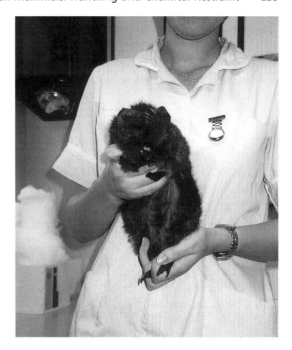

Fig. 15.3   Method for restraining a guinea pig.

the chinchilla's weight (Fig. 15.4). Degus may be handled in a similar fashion, although they are less prone to fur-slip.

Chipmunk

As a species, chipmunks are highly strung, and the avoidance of stress and fear aggression is essential to avoid fatalities. They are difficult to handle without being bitten, unless hand reared, when they may be scruffed quickly, or cupped in both hands. To catch them in their aviary-style enclosures the easiest method is to use a fine-meshed aviary or butterfly net, preferably made of a dark material. The chipmunk may then be safely netted and quickly transferred to a towel for manual restraint, examination or injection or induction of chemical restraint.

Ferret

Ferrets can make excellent house pets and many are friendly and hand tame. However in the United Kingdom the most frequent use for which ferrets are kept is for rabbit hunting, hence many

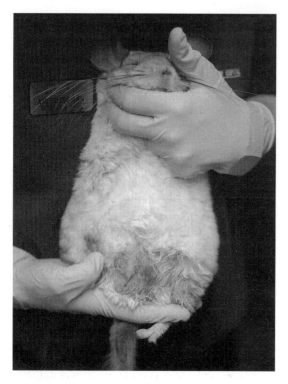

Fig. 15.4 Method for restraining a chinchilla.

ferrets are not regularly handled and so may be aggressive.

For excitable or aggressive animals, a firm grasp of the scruff, high up at the back of the neck is advised. The ferret may then be suspended whilst stabilising the lower body with the other hand around the pelvis. In the case of tamer animals, they may be suspended with one hand behind the front legs, cupped between thumb and fingers from the dorsal aspect, with the other hand supporting the hind limbs. This hold may be varied somewhat in the more lively individuals by placing the thumb of one hand underneath the chin, so pushing the jaw upwards, and the rest of the fingers grasping the other side of the neck. The other hand is then brought under the hind limbs as support.

Aspects of chemical restraint

Chemical restraint may be necessary for a number of reasons in small mammals:

- Sample collection, such as blood testing or urine collection
- For procedures such as radiography
- Oral examinations.

Anaesthetic procedures are now becoming routine for most small mammals. Levels of safety and success in this area have greatly improved in recent years. This has been due mainly to our increased awareness of certain health problems which frequently beset these patients, principally the high prevalence of low-grade respiratory infections.

Is the patient fit enough for chemical restraint?

It is important to make an assessment as to whether or not the patient is fit enough before chemical restraint is attempted. Factors which should be considered prior to the anaesthesia of small mammals are outlined below.

Low-grade respiratory infections

Many of the rodents and lagomorphs suffer from low-grade respiratory infection all of their lives. Many will cope with this on a day-to-day basis, but when anaesthetised the respiratory rate slows and respiratory secretions, already thickened or increased due to chronic infection, become more tenacious. This can cause physical blockage of the airways.

Respiratory system anatomy

The majority of the species considered are nose breathers, with their soft palates permanently locked around the epiglottis. Therefore, if the patient has a blocked nose, whether it be due to pus, blood, tumours or abscesses, then respiratory arrest is made much more likely under anaesthetic.

Hypothermia

Due to their small size and resultant high body surface area to volume ratios, these small mammals are prone to hypothermia during anaesthesia. This is because of the cooling effect of the inhaled gases and reduced muscular activity. It is dangerous, therefore, to anaesthetise a patient that is already hypothermic without first treating this condition.

Dehydration

Respiratory fluid losses during drying gaseous anaesthetic procedures are much greater than in cats, dogs or larger species. Hence putting a severely dehydrated small mammalian patient through an anaesthetic without prior fluid therapy is not advisable.

Pre-anaesthetic management

Weight measurement

It is vitally important to weigh the patient accurately. A mistake of just 10 g in a hamster, say, will lead to an under- or overdosage of 10%! The use of scales which will read accurately down to 1 g in weight is therefore essential.

Blood testing

Blood testing is starting to become much more common in small mammals, and should be considered in every clinically unwell or senior patient where a large enough sample may be obtained. Sites for venipuncture are detailed below.

Rabbit: a 25–27 gauge needle may be used in the lateral ear vein. Prior to sampling, apply a local anaesthetic cream to the site and warm the ear under a heat lamp or with a hot water bottle to allow dilation of the vessel. Alternatively, the cephalic or the jugular veins, may be used. The latter should be used with caution as it is the only source of blood drainage from the eyes, and so, if a thrombus forms in this vessel, ocular oedema and permanent damage or even loss of the eye may occur.

Rat and mouse: the lateral tail veins may be used in rats and mice. These run either side of the coccygeal vertebrae, and are best seen when the tail is warmed as for the lateral ear vein in lagomorphs. A 25–27 gauge needle is required.

Ferret: the jugular vein is probably the easiest to access, but may be difficult in a fractious animal. The positioning adopted for cats is used. One handler holds onto both front limbs with one hand, clamping the body with forearm and elbow, the other hand placed under the chin and raising the head. Towel restraint may also be utilised to papoose the ferret. Cephalic veins may also be used. 23–25 gauge needles suffice.

Guinea pig and chinchilla: the jugular veins are the most accessible. One handler holds both front limbs with one hand and brings the patient to the edge of the table, raising the head with the other hand. The other operator may then take a jugular sample with a 23–25 gauge needle. Lateral saphenous veins may be used in guinea pigs, but chinchillas rarely have any other peripheral vessel large enough to sample.

Gerbil and hamster: these are the most challenging, and blood sampling may not be possible. With care (particularly in gerbils) the lateral tail veins may be used. Frequently cardiac puncture under anaesthetic is often necessary to obtain a sufficient sample.

Chipmunk: jugular blood samples may be taken, but in nearly every case anaesthesia is required first.

Fasting

This again depends on the species considered.

Rabbit: these do not need to be fasted prior to anaesthesia, as they have a very tight cardiac sphincter preventing vomiting. Indeed, starving may actually be deleterious to the patient's health as it causes a cessation in gut contractility and subsequent ileus. It is important, though, to ensure that no food is present in the mouth at the time of induction, hence a period of 30–60 minutes starvation should be ensured.

Rat and mouse: due to their high metabolic rate and likelihood of hypoglycaemia, rats and mice need only be starved a matter of 40–60 minutes (mice) to 45–90 minutes (rats) prior to anaesthetic induction.

Ferret: these may be starved for 2–4 hours. Any more than this will lead to hypoglycaemia, as mustelids have a high metabolic rate, and short gut transit times.

Guinea pig and chinchilla: these may be starved for 3–6 hours prior to surgery to ensure a relatively empty stomach and reduce pressure on the diaphragm. Again, prolonged starvation (>4 hours) will lead to hypoglycaemia and gut stasis and increase the risks of intra- or post-operative mortality.

Gerbil and hamster: as for Muridae, a period of 45–90 minutes is usually sufficient. Any longer than 2 hours and post-operative hypoglycaemia is a real problem.

Chipmunk: periods of fasting of 2 hours have been reported as safe.

Pre-anaesthetic medications

Pre-anaesthetic drugs are used either because they provide a smooth induction and recovery from anaesthesia, or because they ensure a reduction in airway secretions, act as a respiratory stimulant or prevent serious bradycardia.

Antimuscarinics

Atropine is used in some species such as guinea pigs and chinchillas where oral secretions are high and intubation difficult. Doses of 0.05 mg/kg have been used subcutaneously 30 minutes before induction. Atropine also acts to prevent excessive bradycardia which often occurs during the induction phase.

It is not so useful in lagomorphs, as around 60% of rabbits have a serum *atropinesterase* which breaks down atropine before it has a chance to work. Glycopyrrolate, which functions in a similar manner may also be used at doses of 0.01 mg/kg subcutaneously.

Tranquilisers

Tranquilisers are frequently used to reduce the stress of induction, which increases the risks of anaesthetising lagomorphs and hystricomorphs. These species will breath-hold during gaseous induction, to the point where they may become cyanotic. In rabbits, the 'shock' organ is the lungs, and during intense stress the pulmonary circulation can go into spasm, making the hypoxia due to breath-holding even worse, even to the point of collapse and cardiac arrest!

Acepromazine (ACP): ACP can be used at doses of 0.2 mg/kg in ferrets, 0.5 mg/kg in rabbits and 0.5–1 mg/kg in rats, mice, hamsters, chinchillas and guinea pigs. In general it is a very safe premedicant even in debilitated animals. However, it is advised not to use it in gerbils, as acepromazine reduces the seizure threshold, and many gerbils suffer from hereditary epilepsy.

Diazepam: diazepam is useful as a premedicant in some species. In rodents, doses of 3 mg/kg can be used, even in gerbils. In rabbits, the benefits are somewhat outweighed by the larger volumes required. In addition, as the drug is oil based, the intramuscular route is employed and this may be painful.

Neuroleptanalgesics

The fentanyl/fluanisone combination (Hypnorm®) may be used at varying doses as either a premedicant, a sedative or as part of an injectable full anaesthesia. As a premedicant, doses of 0.1 ml/kg for rabbits, 0.08 ml/kg for rats, 0.2 ml/kg for guinea pigs (one fifth the recommended sedation doses) can produce sufficient sedation to prevent breath-holding and allow gaseous induction. These doses are given intramuscularly 15–20 minutes before induction. However, Hypnorm® is an irritant and large doses in one spot may cause post-operative lameness so care must be taken to avoid this. It can be reversed after the operation with butorphanol at 0.2 mg/kg or buprenorphine at 0.05 mg/kg intravenously. Should a vein not be available, both may also be given intramuscularly.

Fluid therapy

Fluid therapy is a vitally important pre-anaesthetic consideration and will be mentioned below and elsewhere in the book.

Induction of anaesthesia

Injectable agents

Table 15.1 outlines some of the advantages and disadvantages of injectable anaesthetics in small mammals.

Propofol

This has some limited use in small mammals. It may be used in ferrets at 10 mg/kg after the use of a premedicant such as acepromazine. However, in rabbits and hystricomorphs, the apnoea can be a problem, and because it must be given intravenously it is difficult to use in the smaller rodents.

Ketamine

Ketamine is a dissociative anaesthetic commonly used in small mammals.

Ferret: ketamine may be used alone for chemical restraint in the ferret at doses of 10–20 mg/kg but, as with cats and dogs, the muscle relaxation is poor and salivation can be a problem. More often, ketamine is combined with other drugs such as the alpha-2 agonists xylazine and medetomidine. In ferrets, 10–30 mg/kg ketamine may be used with 1–2 mg/kg xylazine (Flecknall, 1998), preferably

Table 15.1 Advantages and disadvantages of injectable anaesthetics.

Advantages	Disadvantages
Easily administered	Delay in reversal
Minimal stress	Hypoxia and hypotension common
Prevent breath-holding	Tissue necrosis
Inexpensive	Organ metabolism required

giving the xylazine 5–10 minutes before the ketamine.

Rabbit: ketamine is used at a dose of 15 mg/kg in conjunction with medetomidine at 0.25 mg/kg or with xylazine at 5 mg/kg (Flecknall, 2000). The advantages are a quick and stress-free anaesthetic, but the combination will cause blueing of the mucous membranes due to peripheral shutdown, and this may make detection of hypoxia difficult. Respiratory depression during longer procedures may become a problem and intubation is often advised. The medetomidine may be reversed using atipamazole at 1 mg/kg.

Rat, mouse, gerbil and hamster: ketamine can be used at 90 mg/kg in combination with xylazine at 5 mg/kg intramuscularly or intraperitoneally in rats and 100 mg/kg ketamine with 5 mg/kg xylazine in hamsters (Harkness & Wagner, 1989). Mice require 100 mg/kg of ketamine and 10 mg/kg xylazine (Orr, 2001). These combinations provide 30 minutes or so of anaesthesia.

In gerbils, the dose of xylazine may be reduced to 2–3 mg/kg as they appear more sensitive to the hypovolaemic effects of the alpha-2 drugs, with ketamine doses at 50 mg/kg (Flecknell, 1998).

Ketamine may also be used at 75 mg/kg in combination with medetomidine at 0.5 mg/kg in gerbils (Keeble, 2001) and rats (Orr, 2001). Mice may require as much as 1 mg/kg medetomidine (Orr, 2001). The advantages of the alpha-2 agonists are that they produce good analgesia (which ketamine does not) and that they may be quickly reversed with atipamazole at 1 mg/kg. Their disadvantages include their severe hypotensive effects, and that, in common with all injectable preparations, once administered it is more difficult to control than a gaseous anaesthetic. Alpha-2 agonists also increase diuresis and may exacerbate renal dysfunction.

Guinea pig and chinchilla: ketamine at 40 mg/kg in conjunction with xylazine at 5 mg/kg can be used in guinea pigs to produce a light plane of anaesthesia (Mason, 1997). Ketamine at 40 mg/kg may also be used with medetomidine at 0.5 mg/kg for guinea pigs (Flecknell, 2001), or ketamine at 30 mg/kg with medetomidine at 0.3 mg/kg for chinchillas (Mason, 1997). These doses may be reversed with 1 mg/kg atipamazole. The response to both of these combinations may be improved after an acepromazine premedication of 0.25 mg/kg. Alternatively, for chinchillas, a ketamine (40 mg/kg) and acepromazine (0.5 mg/kg) combination can be used (Morgan *et al.*, 1981). Induction with these drugs takes 5–10 minutes and typically lasts for 45–60 minutes, but recovery may take 2–5 hours for the non-reversible acepromazine combination, hence reducing the dose of this drug and using the reversible alpha-2 antagonists may be beneficial, but should be weighed against the greater hypotensive effects of the alpha-2 drugs.

Fentanyl/fluanisone (Hypnorm® Janssen)

This drug combination is a neuroleptanalgesic licensed for use in rats, mice, rabbits and guinea pigs. Fentanyl is a morphine/opioid derivative, and fluanisone is the neuroleptic. It is mentioned here particularly because it is specifically licensed for use in rabbits, rats and mice and guinea pigs in the United Kingdom.

Rabbit: sedation is produced at doses of 0.5 ml/kg intramuscularly (*see data sheets*). This produces sedation and immobilisation for 30–60 minutes, but the analgesic effect from the opioid derivative fentanyl will persist for some time longer. It may however be reversed with 0.5 mg/kg butorphanol intravenously, or 0.05 mg/kg buprenorphine, both of which will counteract the fentanyl and its analgesia and substitute their own pain relief.

Alternatively, to provide anaesthetic depth fentanyl/fluanisone may be combined with diazepam at a dose of 0.3 ml Hypnorm® to 2 mg/kg diazepam given intraperitoneally or intravenously (but in separate syringes as they do not mix). It may also be combined with midazolam (0.3 ml Hypnorm® to 2 mg/kg midazolam) and given intramuscularly or intraperitoneally in the same syringe. Hypnorm® may also be given intramuscularly first and then followed 15 minutes later by midazolam given intravenously into the lateral ear vein. These two combinations provide good anal-

gesia and muscle relaxation with a duration of anaesthesia of 20–40 minutes.

The fentanyl part may be reversed with buprenorphine or butorphanol given intravenously. In emergencies, naloxone at 0.1 mg/kg intramuscularly or intravenously may be given, but this provides no substitute analgesia.

Fentanyl/fluanisone combinations are well tolerated in most rabbits, but they can produce respiratory depression and hypoxia.

Rat and mouse: Hypnorm® may be used as sedation only on its own at a dose of 0.01 ml/30 g body weight in mice and 0.4 ml/kg in rats. This produces sedation and immobilisation for 30–60 minutes and may be reversed with buprenorphine or butorphanol as above.

Alternatively, it may be combined with diazepam (mice 0.01 ml/30 g Hypnorm® with 5 mg/kg diazepam intraperitoneally; rats 0.3 ml/kg Hypnorm® with 2.5 mg/kg diazepam intraperitoneally). In this case the diazepam and Hypnorm® are given in separate syringes as they do not mix. Midazolam is miscible with Hypnorm® and for rodents the recommendation is that each drug is individually mixed with an equal volume of sterile water first. These solutions are then mixed together in equal volumes. Of this stock solution, mice receive 10 ml/kg and rats 2.7 ml/kg as a single intraperitoneal injection. These two combinations provide anaesthesia for a period of 20–40 minutes.

Guinea pig and chinchilla: Hypnorm® may be used for sedation only on its own at a dose of 1 ml/kg intramuscularly. This may be problematic in guinea pigs as large volumes are required. Hypnorm® is an irritant and may cause lameness when the whole dose is placed in one spot – multiple sites are therefore preferred.

Alternatively, it may be combined with diazepam (1 ml/kg Hypnorm® and 2.5 mg/kg diazepam) in separate syringes and given intraperitoneally, or with midazolam by making the stock solution as described above for rats and mice, and then administering 8 ml/kg of this solution intraperitoneally. Hypnorm® may be reversed with the partial opioid agonists buprenorphine and butorphanol, or with the full antagonist naloxone.

Gaseous agents

Table 15.2 gives some advantages and disadvantages of gaseous anaesthetics in small mammals.

Halothane

In general, induction concentrations should not exceed 3% and anaesthesia can usually be maintained with 1.5%.

Halothane has two main disadvantages. The first is that it can induce cardiac arrhythmias. This is a particular problem in lagomorphs, which are also some of the worst breath-holders. These factors may lead to apnoea and cardiac arrest. The second disadvantage is that it is metabolised by the liver. Its use in small mammals with hepatic disease should be avoided, therefore. In addition, premedication with acepromazine rather than Hypnorm® is preferred as Hypnorm® also requires hepatic metabolism.

Methoxyflurane

Methoxyflurane has often been quoted as the gas of choice for rodents and rabbits. Face-mask gaseous induction is relatively straightforward, although guinea pigs and rabbits are renowned for breath-holding, making the use of a pre-anaesthetic sedative or tranquiliser advisable. Maintenance may be combined with nitrous oxide as a 1:1 mixture with oxygen with 1% methoxyflurane levels being an average level.

Its advantages include excellent analgesia and rapid induction. Its disadvantages include hepatic metabolism and greater risks for operators as well as longer recovery times than isoflurane.

Isoflurane

Isoflurane is now becoming the most widely used gas for maintenance and indeed induction. Usually a premedication is used with analgesia as its analgesic effects and rapidity of knock-down are less than methoxyflurane. Its outweighing advantage, though, is in its safety for the debilitated patient. Only <0.3% of the gas is metabolised hepatically, the rest merely being exhaled for recovery to occur. Recovery is therefore rapid.

Induction levels vary at 2.5–4% and maintenance usually is 1.5–2.5% assuming adequate analgesia. Breath-holding can still be a problem, even with premedication, but the practice of supplying 100% oxygen to the patient for 2 minutes prior to anaesthetic administration helps minimise hypoxia. Isoflurane is then gradually introduced, first 0.5% for 2 minutes, then, assuming regular breathing, increased to 1% for 2 minutes and so on until anaesthetic levels are reached. This allows a smooth induction.

Maintenance of anaesthesia

Intubation

As with all gaseous anaesthetics, the placement of an endotracheal tube for maintenance after induction is to be recommended whenever possible. This is relatively straightforward in ferrets, being much the same procedure as for cats.

In rabbits, the use of a number 1 Wisconsin flat-bladed paedeatric laryngoscope and a 2–3 mm tube is advised. The rabbit is first induced either with an injectable anaesthetic or with an inhalational one. It is then placed in dorsal recumbency, allowing the larynx to fall dorsally and into view. A rabbit mouth gag aids visibility at this stage, and the laryngoscope and endotracheal tube are inserted. A guide wire may first be passed through

Table 15.2 Advantages and disadvantages of gaseous anaesthetics.

Advantages	Disadvantages
Faster alteration of depth of anaesthesia possible	Increased drying effect on respiratory membranes
Recovery times shorter	Hypothermic effect from drying
Less organ metabolism	Difficulty in some species which breath-hold

the laryngeal opening, and, once in, the endotracheal tube is threaded over the top and the wire withdrawn.

Alternatively the rabbit may be intubated blindly. This is performed in sternal recumbency, after initial induction. The head is lifted vertically off the table and the endotracheal tube inserted orally in the midline until slight resistance and a cough is elicited. It is then advanced slowly, and air passage through the tube checked to ensure correct placement.

Intubation is a specialised procedure for rodents such as rats and mice where rigid guide tubes and wires and smaller scopes are used to guide the tube into the larynx.

In rabbits and ferrets it is helpful to use xylocaine spray on the larynx to reduce laryngospasm and aid intubation.

Intermittent positive pressure ventilation (IPPV)

IPPV may be necessary in some individuals who breath-hold during induction. The patient should receive ventilation at their resting respiratory rate. If intubation is not possible then three options are available:

(1) Ensure a tight-fitting face-mask and use an Ayres T-piece, Mapleson C or modified Bain circuit with half litre bag attached to attempt ventilation.
(2) Place a nasopharygeal tube, via the medial meatus of the nose, into the pharyngeal area. Then supply 4 litres or so of oxygen (to combat the resistance of the small diameter tubing of 1–2 mm) via this route. This cannot be done in mammals smaller than a young guinea pig.
(3) Perform an emergency tracheostomy with a 25–27 gauge needle attached to the oxygen outlet, placing the needle between the supporting C-shaped laryngeal cartilages ventrally.

Anaesthetic circuits

Most of the small mammals described here are less than 2 kg in weight. For this reason an Ayres

T-piece, modified Bain or Mapleson C circuit are the best ones to use, as they provide the minimum of dead space (Fig. 15.5). For larger rabbits, an Ayres T-piece is usually sufficient.

Supportive therapy during and after anaesthesia

Recumbency

For most surgical procedures the positioning for restraint or recumbency will be dependent upon the area being operated on. Frequently, this necessitates the patient being placed in dorsal recumbency. Because small herbivores rely on their gut flora to aid digestion, most of them have developed an enlarged hindgut. This means that when they are in dorsal recumbency there is a lot of weight on the diaphragm, and so more resistance to inspiration. During lengthy surgical procedures this may lead to apnoea and hypoxia. Therefore, place the patient with its cranial end elevated above the caudal when in dorsal recumbency. This allows gravity to draw the intestine away from the diaphragm.

Maintenance of body temperature

Maintenance of core body temperature is vitally important in all patients to ensure successful

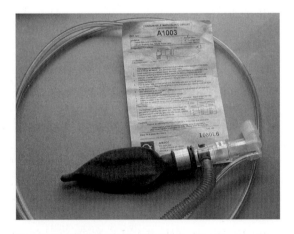

Fig. 15.5   A Mapleson C circuit with a 0.25 l rebreathing bag is deal for smaller species.

recovery from anaesthesia, but is particularly important in small mammals. This is primarily due to their increased surface area to volume ratio, allowing more heat to escape per gram of animal. To help minimise this the following actions may be taken:

- Perform minimal surgical scrubbing of the site, and minimal clipping of fur from the area. Do not use surgical spirit as this rapidly cools the skin.
- Ensure the environmental room temperature is at the warm end of comfortable.
- Place the patient onto either a water circulating heat pad, or use latex gloves or hot water bottles filled with warm water grouped around the patient (making sure that the containers are not in direct contact with the patient as skin burns may ensue).
- Administer warmed isotonic fluids subcutaneously, intravenously or intraperitoneally prior to and during surgery.

It is also worth noting that anaesthetic gases have a rapidly cooling effect on the oral and respiratory membranes, and so patients maintained on gaseous anaesthetics will cool down quicker than those on injectable ones. This effect will worsen as the length of the anaesthesia increases.

These precautions will prevent hypothermia setting in and so improve anaesthesia success rates. It is worth noting however that *hyperthermia* may be as bad as *hypothermia*. Small mammals generally have few or no sweat glands, and so heat cannot be lost via this route. In addition, very few actually pant to lose heat, so if overwarmed the core body temperature rises and irreversible hyperthermia will occur. A rectal thermometer is useful to monitor body temperature. Normal body temperature ranges are given in Table 15.3.

Fluid therapy

Intra-, pre- and post-operative fluid therapy is very important in small mammals, even for routine surgery. The small size and relatively large body surface area in relation to volume of these patients means that they will dehydrate much faster, gram for gram, than a larger cat or dog.

Table 15.3 Normal body temperatures for selected small mammals.

Species	Normal body temperature range (°C)
Rabbit	37–39.4
Guinea pig	37.2–39.5
Chinchilla	37.8–40
Rat	38 (average)
Mouse	37.5 (average)
Gerbil	37.4–39
Hamster	36.2–37.5
Chipmunk	38 (average)

Studies have shown that the provision of maintenance levels of fluids to small mammals during and immediately after routine surgery improved anaesthetic safety levels by as much as 15% in some cases, with higher levels if the surgery was being performed on severely debilitated animals.

It is therefore to be strongly recommended that all small mammal patients receive fluids during and after an anaesthetic whether it be routine or not. For further information see pages 285–294.

Monitoring anaesthesia

Monitoring anaesthesia becomes more and more difficult as the size of the patient decreases. No one factor will allow you to assess anaesthetic depth. Indeed, in small mammals many of the useful techniques used in cats and dogs are irrelevant. Eye position for example should not be used to assess depth of anaesthesia in small mammals. Instead a useful method is to assess the response to noxious stimuli such as pain.

Initially, the first reflex lost is usually the righting reflex – the animal is unable to return to ventral recumbancy.

The next reflex to be lost, for example in rabbits and guinea pigs is the swallow reflex, however this may be difficult to assess. Palpebral reflexes (the response of blinking when the eye surface is lightly touched) are generally lost early on in the course of anaesthetic, but rabbits may retain this reflex until well into the deeper planes of surgical anaesthesia. The palpebral reflex is also affected by the anaesthetic agent used. Most inhalant gaseous anaesthetics cause loss of the reflex early on, but it is maintained with ketamine.

The pedal withdrawal reflex is useful in small mammals, with the leg being extended and the toe firmly pinched. Loss of this reflex suggests surgical planes of anaesthesia, but again rabbits will retain the pedal reflex in the forelimbs until much deeper (and often dangerously deep!) planes of anaesthesia are reached. Other pain stimuli such as the ear pinch in the guinea pig and rabbit are useful. Loss of this indicates a surgical plane, as does the loss of the tail pinch reflex in rats and mice.

Monitoring of the heart and circulation may be done in a conventional manner, with stethoscope and femoral pulse evaluation, or, in the larger species, an oesophageal stethoscope may be used. As with cats and dogs, increases in the respiratory and heart rates can indicate lightening of the plane of anaesthesia. More sophisticated monitoring equipment, such as pulse oximeters, may also be used to monitor heart rate and haemoglobin saturation. As with cats and dogs, the aim is to achieve 100% saturation, and levels below 90% would indicate hypoxaemia and the initiation of assisted ventilation. The ear artery is useful for this in rabbits, using the clip-on probe, while the linear probes may be used successfully on the ventral aspect of the tail in most other species. Other forms of cardiac monitoring include the ECG, which is frequently adapted to minimise trauma from the alligator forcep attachments by substituting fine needle probes for these, or by blunting the alligator teeth.

An extremely useful monitoring device is the Doppler probe which can detect blood flow in the smallest of vessels up to the heart itself. The Doppler probe converts blood flow into an audible signal, which is transmitted through a speaker device. This can then be assessed by the anaesthetist during surgery for changes in strength of output and heart rate.

Respiratory monitors may also be used if the patient is intubated and many pulse oximeters have outlets for these allowing assessment of respiratory rates. Obviously they are not useful for patients that are being maintained on face-masks or on injectable anaesthetics.

Recovery and analgesia

Recovery from anaesthesia is improved with the use of suitable reversal agents if available. Examples include the use of atipamazole after medetomidine anaesthesia or sedation, and the use of naloxone, butorphanol or buprenorphine after opioid or Hypnorm® anaesthesia or sedation. Gaseous anaesthesia, particularly with isoflurane, tends to result in more rapid recovery than the injectable anaesthetics, but recovery from all forms of anaesthesia is improved by ensuring adequate maintenance of body temperature and fluid balance during and after anaesthesia.

Most small mammals will benefit from a quiet, darkened and warm recovery area. Subsequent fluid administration the same day is frequently beneficial, as many of these creatures will not be eating as normal for the first 12–24 hours.

Analgesia is vitally important to a quick and smooth recovery process. The time taken to return to normal activity such as grooming, eating, drink-

Table 15.4 Analgesics used in small mammals (information adapted from Flecknell, 1998 and Mason, 1997).

Drug	Ferret	Rabbit	Rodent	Chinchilla	Guinea pig	Chipmunk
Butorphanol	0.3 q4h	0.3 q4h	1–5 q4h	2 q4h	1–2 q4h	1–5 q4h
Buprenorphine	0.01–0.03 q8–12h	0.01–0.05 q8–12h	0.01–0.05 q12h	0.05 q8–12h	0.05 q8–12h —	0.01–0.05 q8–12h
Carprofen	4 q24h	4 q24h	5 q24h	5 q24h	5 q24h	4 q24h
Flunixin	1 q24h	1.1 q24h	2.5 q12h	2.5 q24h	2.5 q24h	2.5 q24h
Meloxicam	0.2 q24h	0.2 q24h	0.2–0.4 q24h	0.2 q24h	0.2 q24h	0.2 q24h

Values are in mg/kg body weight.
q4h = 'every 4 hours', q8h = 'every 8 hours', and so on.

ing etc. has been shown to be considerably shortened following adequate analgesia.

Dosages for analgesics frequently used in small mammals are given in Table 15.4.

As with cats and dogs (and, indeed, humans), the administration of analgesia *prior* to the onset of pain makes for the most effective control. Analgesics are therefore now frequently being used as part of premedication injections.

Choice of analgesic depends on the level of pain and other factors, such as concurrent disease processes. Flunixin, for example, is not a good analgesic to use in dehydrated animals or those with renal disease and opioids depress respiration and so may be contraindicated in cases of severe respiratory disease. Buprenorphine requires twice daily administration, while carprofen and meloxicam has been shown to be useful when given only once daily.

References

Flecknell, P.A. (1998) Analgesia in small mammals. *Seminars in Avian and Exotic Pet Medicine*, **7** (1), 41–47. W.B. Saunders, Philadelphia.

Flecknell, P.A. (2000) Anaesthesia. In *Manual of Rabbit Medicine and Surgery*. BSAVA, Cheltenham.

Harkness, J.E. and Wagner, J.E. (1989) *The Biology and Medicine of Rabbits and Rodents*, 3rd edn, pp. 61–67. Lea and Febiger, Philadelphia.

Keeble, E. (2001) Gerbils. In *Manual of Exotic Pets* 4th edn (Meredith, A. and Redrobe, S., eds), pp. 34–46. BSAVA, Cheltenham.

Mason, D.E. (1997) Anaesthesia, analgesia and sedation for small mammals. In *Ferrets, Rabbits and Rodents* (Hillyer, E.V. and Quesenberry, K.E., eds), pp. 378–391. W.B. Saunders, Philadelphia.

Morgan, R.J., Eddy, L.B., Solie, T.N. and Turbe, C.C. (1981) Ketamine–acepromazine as anaesthetic agent for chinchillas (*Chinchilla laniger*). *Laboratory Animals* **15**, 281–283.

Orr, H. (2001) Rats and mice. In *Manual of Exotic Pets*, 4th edn (Meredith, A. and Redrobe, S., eds), pp. 13–25. BSAVA, Cheltenham.

Further reading

Beynon, P.H. and Cooper, J.E. (1991) *Manual of Exotic Pets*, 3rd edn. BSAVA, Cheltenham.

Flecknell, P.A. (2001) Guinea pigs. In *Manual of Exotic Pets*, 4th edn (Meredith, A. and Redrobe, S., eds), pp. 52–64. BSAVA, Cheltenham.

Chapter 16
Small Mammal Nutrition

Classification

One way of classifying small mammals is according to their diet. There are three main categories of the commonly seen small mammals as defined by their diet:

- **Carnivores**

  The main carnivore seen in small mammal practice is the ferret, which, like the cat, is totally carnivorous. To cope with this diet, the ferret has developed sharp shearing teeth and powerful crushing jaws. In addition, because its diet consists of highly digestible fats and proteins, if has a very short gastrointestinal tract.

- **Herbivores**

  A variety of species, from lagomorphs to hystricomorphs, are herbivores. Their teeth are grinding in nature. Some species have continually growing molars and incisors, and their gastrointestinal tracts are long and often sacculated. This increases their volume and allows the bacterial fermentation that assists digestion of the relatively indigestible cellulose, which forms a large part of their diet in the wild.

- **Omnivores**

  Some rodents will eat a mixed diet. Rats and chipmunks will consume meat and eggs if offered, but both species are primarily herbivorous by preference, and true omnivores, such as humans, are uncommon amongst the small mammals seen routinely.

Individual species have become highly evolved to cope with certain types of food. In addition to the above generalisations we also know that many of these creatures, in the wild, have a changing food supply throughout the year.

General nutritional requirements

Water

Maintaining good water quality is important. Many small mammals will dunk food in their water supply or, if the water feeders are poorly situated in bowls rather than in sip-feeders, some animals may actually defaecate in their water bowls. This can cause massive bacterial population explosions which may lead to gastroenteritis. Enriching the water with mineral and vitamin supplements will also allow rapid bacterial growth.

The amount of water an individual small mammal consumes will obviously depend on the diet being offered and the species considered. On dry biscuit or seed-based diets, water consumption will be much higher than for small mammals such as rabbits and guinea pigs, which consume large amounts of fruit and vegetables. A gerbil, for example, is a desert, seed-eating rodent and may only drink 5–10 ml of water in a 24-hour period whereas an average 2 kg rabbit may drink 200 ml or more.

Maintenance energy requirements (MER)

Every species has a level of energy consumption per day that is needed to satisfy basic maintenance requirements. It is the energy used purely to maintain current status under minimal activity and hence is frequently the lowest energy requirement during that mammal's life. As with other species a formula has been derived as MER is dependent on the basal metabolic rate (BMR = the energy requirement when at complete rest) and metabolic body weight as follows:

$$MER = constant (k) \times (body weight)^{0.75}$$

The constant, k, varies with family groups, and has been estimated at 100 for adult rabbits, going up to 200 for growth and 300 for lactation (Carpenter & Kolmstetter, 2000). Other small mammals are similar, having much higher metabolic rates than their larger dog and cat counterparts.

Energy requirements give a guide to what a small mammal must consume per day in order to continue to maintain good health and body weight. Hence, if the foods offered are so low in energy content that the small mammal has to eat more of it than will fit into its digestive system in 24 hours, the animal will rapidly lose condition.

An example is that of meat based foods such as rodent prey which have an energy content of 19–21 kJ/g dry matter (6.3–7.5 kJ/g real or wet weight), whereas high water-content vegetable foods such as lettuce have a lower energy density of 12.5 kJ/g dry matter (0.75 kJ/g real or wet weight). The latter is therefore unlikely to meet the requirements of a high-energy-demanding ferret (irrespective of the fact it is a carnivore!) which has a requirement of 837–1255 kJ ME/kg/day (Carpenter and Kolmstetter, 2000).

Conversely, many pet small mammals will continue eating until their digestive tracts are full. If all they are offered are the energy-dense seed types (the all sunflower seed diet) then they will rapidly achieve their MER and then exceed it, so leading to obesity.

Protein and amino acids

The ten essential amino acids required by birds and reptiles are also needed by the small mammals considered here, and the concept of biological value of a protein is just as applicable. In addition, it is known that an extra supplement of the amino acid glycine is required for diets low in the amino acids methionine or arginine.

For small mammals, levels of dietary protein required have been shown to vary from maintenance to reproductive needs (Hillyer *et al.*, 1997), and from species to species:

- 35% for ferrets
- 14–20% in rodents

- 18–20% in guinea pigs
- 15–18% in rabbits as dry matter
- 16–20% for chinchillas and guinea pigs.

The majority of this protein in granivorous rodent diets seems to come from seeds. Some seeds are very high providers of certain amino acids. Sunflower seeds, white millet and rape seed for example provide high levels of the sulphur-containing amino acids methionine and cystine, useful when moulting. In rabbits and other grazing herbivores, the majority of the proteins are from plant sources such as clover, alfalfa hay and good quality grass hays.

Deficiencies in amino acids have been shown to cause certain diseases. An example of this is urolithiasis seen in ferrets that are fed on plant protein sources, which are deficient in several essential amino acids. In addition, the lack of arginine in plant proteins will cause the young growing ferret to develop hyperammonaemia and neurological signs such as fitting (Bell, 1993).

Fats and essential fatty acids (EFAs)

Fats provide high concentrations of energy, but also supply the small mammal with essential fatty acids. These are required for cellular integrity and as the building blocks of internal chemicals such as prostaglandins, which play a part in reproduction and inflammation.

Fats also provide a carrier mechanism for the absorption of fat-soluble vitamins such as vitamin A, D, E and K.

The primary EFA for small mammals is linoleic acid, as it is for larger mammals, with the absolute dietary requirement being 1% of the diet. If the diet becomes deficient, a rapid decline in cellular integrity occurs. This is manifested clinically by the skin becoming flaky and dry and prone to recurrent infections. Fluid loss through the skin is also increased, even to the extent of causing polydipsia. It is, however, unlikely that any seed-eating small mammal will be deficient in linoleic acid as it is widely found in sunflower seeds and safflower seeds amongst others. It is also present in the animal protein fed to ferrets.

The latter species has a requirement for arachidonic acid as well, similar to cats, without which they will develop a number of problems such as skin diseases, including intense pruritus. Ferrets have an overall fat requirement of 20–30% of dry matter fed. Rabbits require no additional dietary fat other than the 2–5% provided in their vegetable-based diet, similar to the rodent, chinchilla and guinea pig families.

Another essential fatty acid which is thought to be important for rodents is alpha-linolenic acid which is necessary for some prostaglandin and eicosanoid synthesis.

The problem of overconsumption of fats in small mammals which are not exercising regularly is well known, and high-fat oil seeds are the prime culprits in this. Obesity can also be a problem for overfed, underworked ferrets, fed overweight laboratory rats for example. Saturated animal fats provide cholesterol, often in excessive amounts, to ferrets, and hepatic lipidosis can be the result. Because rodents and rabbits have a much lower requirement for fat, excess plant fats can also cause severe hepatic lipidosis and, in rabbits, atherosclerosis in the aorta. Sources of sunflower and other high-fat oil-based seeds are often the culprits.

Carbohydrate

Carbohydrates are primarily used for rapid energy production. This is particularly important for herbivorous small mammals which constantly demand rapid supplies of energy for their often hyperactive and high-metabolic-rate lives. Small mammals that are debilitated in some way will particularly benefit from the supply of high carbohydrate foods. Ferrets have no requirement for carbohydrates (similarly to cats) with blood glucose being provided by hepatic gluconeogenesis from amino acid sources.

Fibre

Dietary fibre does not seem to be important for ferrets. Indeed their extremely short gastrointestinal tract and minimal bacterial microflora show an inability to cope with any fibre at all. Herbivorous small mammals, particularly the guinea pig, the chinchilla and the rabbit, rely more heavily on fibre. Fibre in these species is important for a number of reasons.

First it provides a source of abrasive food, as most of the fibre-providing foods, such as grasses, contain silicates, which wear down the teeth. This is important as these species have open-rooted or continually-growing teeth, which need to be kept in check (Figs 16.1 and 16.2).

Second, the fibre is essential to stimulate gut motility. These species are hind-gut fermenters and rely on the microflora of the hind gut to digest food by breaking down the cellulose. Fibre is converted by the intestinal microflora into volatile

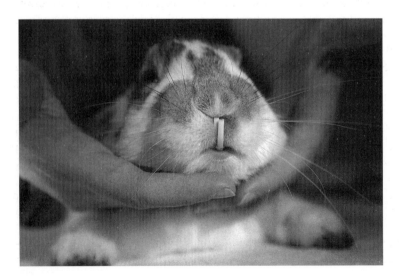

Fig. 16.1 Incisor malocclusion in a rabbit may be due to inappropriately low levels of fibre in the diet, leading to molar over growth. This forces the mouth open so that the incisors do not wear against each other and so overgrow.

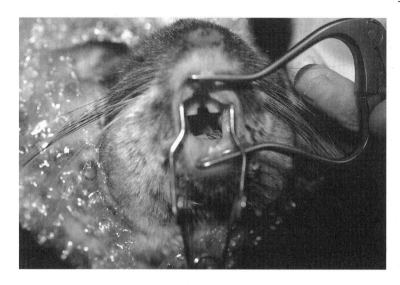

Fig. 16.2 A chinchilla showing cheek tooth elongation leading to mouth ulcers and anorexia.

fatty acids, which decrease the pH of the caecum and large bowel, so preventing bacterial overgrowth and minimising enteritis problems. Without sufficient fibre, the hind gut fermenting species develop a mucoid enteropathy, with intermittent constipation, diarrhoea and colic.

Rabbits may also be inclined to overgroom themselves, consume large volumes of fur as a 'fibre source' and so develop fur balls (*trichobezoars*) which may completely block the stomach. Rabbits have a requirement for 12–16% crude fibre, which is similar to guinea pigs, but chinchilla dietary fibre levels have been quoted as varying from 15–35% (Hoefer, 1994). The high levels for chinchillas is explained by their natural diet, which is chiefly composed of poor-quality, highly abrasive and fibrous grasses in the arid and high altitude Andes mountains of South America. The lack of such fibre in pet diets may well account for the chinchilla's appalling susceptibility to molar malocclusion problems. It is recommended that chinchillas and rabbits are fed good quality hay, dried grass or dried grass pellets as 30–50% of their diet as a minimum. The sole feeding of pelleted and dry mix foods currently available leads to a major fibre shortage which leads to lack of dental wear, gastrointestinal upsets and obesity.

Unlike rabbits and other species, guinea pigs do not eat until their calorific requirements are satisfied and then stop, but instead eat until their digestive system is full, irrespective of how diluted the energy of the diet is by increased fibre. Recommended minimum crude fibre levels for guinea pigs are 10%, with an average of 13% being routinely offered (Hillyer *et al.*, 1997).

Vitamins

Fat-soluble vitamins

Vitamin A: in small herbivores the diet frequently contains only the vitamin A precursors, as carotenoid plant pigments, whereas in ferrets vitamin A itself is obtained from animal proteins and does not need to be synthesised. In small herbivores, the most important form of these precursors in terms of how much vitamin A can be produced from it is beta-carotene. Because it is fat soluble, vitamin A can be stored in the body, primarily in the liver.

Hypovitaminosis A is an uncommonly seen problem in small mammals. This is because green vegetables are good providers of the beta-carotenes. A problem can arise with rodents that develop an addiction to seeds such as sunflower seeds and peanuts. Hypovitaminosis A in rabbits can cause infertility, foetal resorption, abortion, stillbirth and neurological defects such as hydrocephalus. In ferrets it can cause infertility, poor coat and fluid retention (anasarca). Recommendations for dietary levels include 7000 IU/kg for rabbits (Carpenter & Kolmstetter, 2000). The low levels may be met by as little as 200 g of carrot per day for a 2 kg rabbit, but would require 70 kg of oats to provide the same levels!

Hypervitaminosis A rarely occurs naturally, but may be induced by overdosing with vitamin A injections at 1000 times or more the daily recommended doses. If this occurs, acute toxicity develops with mucus membrane and skin sloughing, liver damage and frequently death within 24–48 hours. It may also be seen in ferrets fed predominantly the livers of prey items. In these cases excess bony production may occur similar to the syndrome seen in cats.

Vitamin D: this vitamin is primarily concerned with calcium metabolism. Cholecalciferol is manufactured in the small mammal's skin, a process enhanced by ultraviolet light. Small mammals kept-indoors therefore produce much less of this compound, and this can lead to deficiency. Cholecalciferol must then be activated in the liver and kidneys before it can function in calcium metabolism. Once formed into its active metabolite it acts in concert with parathyroid hormone to increase reabsorption of calcium at the expense of phosphorus from the kidneys, to increase absorption of calcium from the intestines and to mobilise calcium from the bones, all of these functions increasing the blood's calcium levels.

Hypovitaminosis D_3 causes problems with calcium metabolism and leads to rickets. This is exacerbated by low-calcium-containing diets, a typical sufferer being an indoor kept small mammal, fed an all seed diet in the case of a rodent or an all meat and no calcium supplement diet for a ferret. This leads to well-muscled, heavy rodents or ferrets, with poorly mineralised bones, flaring of the epiphyseal plates at the ends of the long bones and concomitant bowing of the limbs, especially the tibiotarsal bones. Recommended minimum levels are 3.5–9 IU/g of feed for rodents and lagomorphs (Wallach & Hoff, 1982).

Hypervitaminosis D_3 occurs due to over supplementation with D_3 and calcium and leads to calcification of soft tissues, such as the medial arterial walls, and the kidneys, creating hypertension and causing organ failure. Recommended maximum levels are 2000 IU/kg dry matter of food fed for most small mammals (Wallach & Hoff, 1982).

Vitamin E: this compound is found in several active forms in plants, the most active being alpha-tocopherol. It is used as an anti-oxidant and in immune system function.

Hypovitaminosis E in ferrets results in a yellow discolouration in body fat deposits, haemolytic anaemia and a progressive paresis of the limbs. In addition, a series of firm swellings underneath the skin in the inguinal area may be seen. In rabbits a similar disease is seen with hind limb paresis and white muscle degeneration. In hamsters, deficiencies have been reported as causing muscular weakness, ocular secretions and death, often due to cardiac muscle damage. Hypovitaminosis E may occur due to a reduction in fat metabolism or absorption as can occur in small intestinal, pancreatic or biliary diseases, or due to a lack of green plant material, the chief source of the compound, in the diet. Recommended levels for rabbits are 40 mg/kg dry matter of food offered (National Research Council, 1978).

In addition, feeding diets high in unsaturated fats (such as oily fish) may use up the body's reserves of Vitamin E and so induce signs of hypovitaminosis E. This has occurred in ferrets and mink fed such a diet.

Hypervitaminosis E is extremely rare.

Vitamin K: because of its production by bacteria, it is very difficult to get a true deficiency of Vitamin K, although absorption will again be reduced when fat digestion or absorption is reduced, as in, for example, biliary or pancreatic disease.

Ferrets eating prey which has been killed by warfarin will show signs of deficiency. Rabbits and guinea pigs eating large amounts of sweet clovers can also experience a relative deficiency. The signs of disease that are seen are due to increased internal and external haemorrhage, but vitamin K also has some function in calcium/phosphorous metabolism in the bones and this may also be affected.

Water-soluble vitamins

Vitamin B₁ (thiamine): hypovitaminosis B_1 is uncommon, but may be seen in ferrets fed raw salt-water fish which contain thiaminases. When a relative deficiency occurs, neurological signs such as opisthotonus, weakness and head tremors are seen. Ferrets can suffer from a condition known as Chastek syndrome. The symptoms may include salivation, paralysis, incoordination, pupillary dilation and easily-induced convulsions, which are characterised by strong ventral flexion of the neck. Evidence of dilated cardiomyopathies is seen at post mortem. The recommended minimum level for most small mammals is around 6–7 mg/kg of diet dry matter (Wallach & Hoff, 1982).

Vitamin B₂ (riboflavin): hypovitaminosis B_2 is very rare and produces growth retardation, roughened coat, alopecia, excess scurf and cataract formation.

Niacin: rodents fed a high proportion of one type of seed such as sweetcorn, can become deficient in niacin. They exhibit blackening of the tongue (known as *pellagra*) and oral mucosa, retarded growth, poor coat quality and scaly dermatitis. Rats may also have anaemia and porphyrin-encrusted noses.

Biotin: deficiency may occur in animals fed large amounts of unfertilised, raw eggs, the whites of which contain the antibiotin vitamin, *avidin*. This can be seen in ferrets and chipmunks when greater than 10% of the diet is composed of raw egg. Deficiency produces exfoliative dermatitis, toes may become gangrenous and slough off and ataxia may be observed. The recommended minimum requirement is 0.12–0.34 ppm food as dry matter for small mammals (Wallach & Hoff, 1982).

Folic acid: deficiency occurs mainly because of the folic acid inhibitors that are present in some foods such as cabbage and other brassicas, oranges, beans and peas. The use of trimethoprim sulphonamide drugs also reduces gut bacterial folic acid production. Deficiency causes a number of problems, such as failure in reproductive tract maturation, macrocytic anaemia due to failure of red blood cell maturation and immune system cellular dysfunction.

Choline: because of their interactions, the need for choline is dependent on levels of folic acid and vitamin B_{12}. That is, a deficiency may be caused if the latter are deficient, as may occur in an animal fed a diet high in fats. Deficiency causes retarded growth, disrupted fat metabolism and fatty liver damage. Recommended minimum requirements for small mammals are 880–1540 mg/kg food as dry matter.

Vitamin C there is no direct need for this vitamin in small mammals other than the guinea pig, as vitamin C may be synthesised from glucose in the liver. The guinea pig lacks the enzyme L-gluconolactone oxidase and therefore cannot convert glucose to ascorbic acid, so has a dietary requirement for vitamin C. However, during disease processes, particularly those conditions that affect liver function, it may be beneficial to the recovery process in all species to provide a dietary source of vitamin C.

Vitamin C is required for the formation of elastic fibres and connective tissues and is an excellent anti-oxidant, similar to vitamin E. Deficiency leads to 'scurvy'. Signs of scurvy include poor wound healing, increased bleeding due to capillary-wall fragility, gingivitis and bone alterations. These include the swelling of long bones close to joints (the *epiphyseal plates*), which become very painful. In addition, crusting occurs at mucocutaneous junctions such as the eyes, mouth and nose, as well as loosening of the teeth due to periodontal ligament weakening.

Vitamin C also helps in the absorption from the gut of some minerals, such as iron.

The daily recommended requirement for guinea pigs is 10 mg/kg body weight for maintenance, increasing to 30 mg/kg body weight during gestation, although treatment of scurvy recommends levels of 50–100 mg/kg until resolution of clinical signs (Harkness & Wagner, 1995). This may be given by injection, or soluble human vitamin C tablets may be placed in the drinking water each day if the guinea pig is still drinking adequately. In addition, fresh fruit and vegetables as well as a specific supplemented guinea pig diet, should always be fed. Many deficiencies occur due to guinea pigs being housed with rabbits and therefore fed only dry rabbit food which has no supplemental vitamin C.

Minerals

Macro-minerals

Calcium: calcium has a wide range of functions, the two most obvious being its role in the formation of the skeleton and mineralisation of bone matrix, and its use in muscular contraction. The active form of calcium in the body is the ionic double-charged molecule Ca^{2+}. Low levels of this form, even though the overall body reserves of calcium may be normal, lead to hyperexcitability, fitting and death.

Calcium levels in the body are controlled by vitamin D_3, parathyroid hormone and calcitonin.

The ratio of calcium to phosphorus is very important. As one increases the other decreases and vice versa. A ratio therefore of 2:1 calcium to phosphorus is desirable in juvenile and lactating small mammals, and 1.5:1 for adults. Excessive dietary calcium (>1%) though reduces the use of proteins, fats, phosphorus, manganese, zinc, iron and iodine. In rabbits, this is exacerbated by their unique method of calcium control, in that they have no ability to reduce calcium absorption from the gut, as do other species. Instead all available calcium is absorbed from the diet, and any excess must then be excreted through the kidneys. This leads to excess calcium excretion into the urine, the formation of calcium carbonate crystals and urolithiasis. In addition, as rabbits are herbivorous, their urine pH is alkaline, and as calcium carbonate (limestone) is less soluble in alkaline environments it precipitates more readily in the urine, forming crystals. Levels of calcium >4% dry matter for rabbits will lead to soft tissue mineralisation in sites such as the aorta and kidneys.

Phosphorus: like calcium, phosphorus is used in bone formation, but it is also used in cell structure and energy storage. It is widespread in plant and animal tissues, but in the former it may be bound up in unavailable form as phytates. Levels of phosphorus are controlled in the body as for calcium, the two being in equal and opposite equilibrium with each other. Therefore, if dietary phosphorus levels exceed calcium levels appreciably (a maximum of twice the calcium levels on average) the parathyroid glands become stimulated to produce more parathyroid hormone in an effort to restore the balance. This causes nutritional secondary hyperparathyroidism which leads to progressive bone demineralisation and then renal damage due to the high circulating levels of parathyroid hormone. High dietary phosphorus also reduces the amount of calcium which can be absorbed from the gut, as it complexes with the calcium present there. This can be a big problem for ferrets that are fed pure meat diets with no calcium or bone supplement, and in rodents that are predominantly seed eaters, as cereals are high phosphorus/low calcium foods. Feeding green vegetables or supplementation with calcium powders may therefore be necessary. In the case of ferrets a standard ferret complete diet, or whole rodent prey, should be fed to avoid this.

Potassium: as with larger mammals, this is the major intracellular positive ion. Rarely is there a dietary deficiency. Severe stress can cause hypokalaemia due to increased kidney excretion of potassium due to elevated plasma proteins, as can persistent diarrhoea. Hypokalaemia can lead to cardiac dysrhythmias, muscle spasticity and neurological dysfunction. Other symptoms are stunted growth, ascites, abnormally short hair and reduced appetite. Potassium is present in high amounts in certain fruits, such as bananas. It is controlled in equilibrium with sodium by the adrenal hormone aldosterone which promotes sodium retention and potassium excretion.

Sodium: this is the main extracellular positive ion and regulates the body's acid–base balance and osmotic potential. In conjunction with potassium, it is responsible for nerve signals and impulses. Rarely does a true dietary deficiency occur, but hyponatraemia may occur due to chronic diarrhoea or renal disease. This disrupts the osmotic potential gradient in the kidneys and water is lost leading to further dehydration. Excessive levels of sodium in the diet (>10 times recommended) lead to poor coat, polyuria, hypertension, oedema and death.

Chlorine: this is the major extracellular negative ion and responsible for maintaining acid–base balances in conjunction with sodium and potassium. Deficiencies are rare, but if they do occur, retarded growth and kidney disease are commonly seen.

Micro-minerals (trace elements)

Copper: copper is used in haemaglobin synthesis, collagen synthesis and in the maintenance of the nervous system. Copper toxicosis has been reported in ferrets in the United States as a possible hereditary storage disease. The symptoms are of liver disease, as seen in Bedlington Terriers (Brown, 1997). Deficiency has been reported in hamsters as a cause of poor coat quality and generalised alopecia. Minimum recommended levels are 13–20 ppm (Wallach & Hoff, 1982).

Iodine: iodine's sole function is in thyroid hormone synthesis, which affects metabolic rate. Deficiency causes goitre, and has knock-on effects on growth causing stunting, stillbirths and neurological problems. It is a relatively uncommon finding in small mammals but may occur in species such as rabbits that are fed large volumes of goitrogenic (iodine inhibiting) plants such as cabbage, kale, Brussels sprouts etc.

Iron: this is essential, as with larger mammals, for the formation of the oxygen carrying part of the haemoglobin molecule. Absorption from the gut is normally relatively poor, as the body is very good at recycling its own iron levels.

Manganese: deficiency has been reported as causing poor bone growth, with limb shortening as a consequence. Recommended daily requirements are from 40–120.7 ppm with the higher dosages for guinea pigs (Wallach & Hoff, 1982).

Selenium: the main role of selenium is as part of the anti-oxidant enzyme glutathione peroxidase,

with which vitamin E is also involved. Its functions are therefore similar to those of vitamin E in that it helps keep peroxidases from attacking polyunsaturated fats in cell membranes. A general deficiency in both selenium and vitamin E will lead to liver necrosis, steatitis and muscular dystrophy. The selenium content of plants is dependent on where they were grown and the levels of selenium in the soil. Recommended minimum requirements are still not clearly defined for small mammals in general.

Zinc: zinc this is a vital trace element for wound healing and tissue formation, forming part of a number of enzymes. Deficiencies can occur in young rapidly growing guinea pigs and chinchillas fed on plant material high in phytates such as cabbage, wheat bran and beans etc. In addition, high dietary calcium decreases zinc uptake. Deficiency produces retarded growth and poor skin quality with increased scurf and hyperirritability. Zinc deficiency alopecia is particularly seen at about day 50 of gestation in chinchillas with hair regrowth occurring 2–3 weeks after parturition (Smith *et al.*, 1977). Minimum recommended requirements are 20–122 ppm for small mammals (Wallach & Hoff, 1982). Zinc toxicosis has been reported in ferrets, with anaemia, lethargy and hind limb paresis, and was associated with feeding from zinc galvanised buckets (Donnelly, 1997).

Requirements for young and lactating small mammals

Rabbit

Neonatal rabbits nurse for only 3–5 minutes at a time once or twice in a 24-hour period and are totally dependent on their mother's milk up to day 21 post partum (Okerman, 1994). At this time they should be weighed, as solid foods offered will be increasingly consumed, and weight losses may be seen if they do not eat enough of this. The doe may be offered increasingly more pelleted dry foods before weaning, as her energy demands increase to 3.5× maintenance by peak lactation. Ad-lib dry food is therefore often advocated for the doe at this stage. It should be noted though that levels of food for the doe should not start to be dramatically increased until 5–7 days after parturition. Early overfeeding can cause excessive milk production, and mastitis will result if the kits do not have enough appetite to empty the mammary glands at each sitting. For hand-rearing formulas, see page 225.

Growing kits require higher levels of vitamin D_3 and calcium than their adult counterparts. To ensure that this is received, a balanced diet should be offered, combining pelleted food, good quality grass hay and some greens. Dry foods should be carefully chosen. Many are balanced nutritionally, but only if the rabbit consumes all parts equally. Rabbits are concentrate selectors (that is they will preferentially pick out those foods containing the highest calories in their environment and eat them first). Therefore, if offered one of the 'muesli'-type diets, it will eat all of the fatty, carbohydrate foods first, and, if provided ad lib, they will not get around to eating the high fibre, calcium-containing grass pellets. Hence it is advised either to use a homogenous pelleted diet where all of the pellets are exactly the same, or to feed enough in 24 hours so that the bowl is completely emptied before offering more. Access to unfiltered natural sunlight is also advised, even if for only 15–20 minutes per day, to ensure sufficient vitamin D_3 synthesis. Lactating does will also have higher calcium requirements, and so their consumption of pelleted diet and grass products (both high in calcium) will increase.

Ferret

Young ferrets have a higher calorific requirement than adults, as do lactating jills, needing 1.5–2× maintenance adult calorie levels. The protein requirement is a minimum of 35% in young growing ferrets and lactating jills with a fat level of a minimum of 25% as dry matter (Kupersmith, 1998). For rearing formulas see page 232

Rodents, chinchilla and guinea pig

The guinea pig sow when lactating has a requirement for vitamin C which increases from 10 mg/kg per day to 30 mg/kg per day. She also has the usual increases in calcium, energy and protein demands. The demands for increased calories are particularly important as the long gestation of the guinea pig (average 63 days) and the frequent litter size of 3–4 piglets, place huge stresses on the sow. If these increased requirements are not met, then a condition known as pregnancy toxaemia, or ketosis ensues. This is when a lack of available calories leads to increased fat mobilisation. If this is combined with a glucose deficit the fats are converted into chemicals known as ketones. These produce metabolic acidosis in addition to the hypoglycaemic state. Death can follow within 24 hours. Prevention is geared towards avoiding obesity and sudden dietary change, both of which set up the condition.

Young guinea pigs are frequently not hungry for the first 12–24 hours after birth because they have brown fat reserves. They should not be force-fed during this time. Young chinchillas and guinea pigs are eating solid foods practically from day one after parturition. It is important therefore to ensure high-fibre foods are offered preferentially at this stage so as to avoid them developing into fussy eaters in later life.

Rodents such as rats and gerbils have been quoted as needing a dietary protein level of 20–26% during and prior to pregnancy and lactation as opposed to their more usual 16–18%.

For rearing formulas see page 230.

Requirements for debilitated small mammals

In general, requirements for debilitated animals will vary from 1.5–3 times maintenance levels, with the lower levels being for mildly injured or infected animals and the upper levels for burns victims and cases of serious organ damage or septicaemia.

Fluid therapy as additional support is essential, particularly for the herbivorous mammals, which have very high maintenance requirements when compared with cats and dogs (average 80–100 ml/kg/day). Also, herbivore gut contents are voluminous and need to be kept fluid. For further details see pages 285–294.

Rabbit

The debilitated rabbit may be supported with nasogastric or oral syringe feeding of vegetable-based baby foods (lactose free varieties), or, for preference, with a gruel composed of ground dry rabbit pellets and water as this will supply a better fibre level for gut stimulation. Amounts suggested to feed at any one sitting vary from 3–15 ml four to six times daily.

A nasogastric tube (more correctly a naso-oesophageal tube as the tubing must not allow reflux of acid stomach contents into the oesophagus) is placed after first spraying the nose with lignocaine spray. A 3–4 French tube is pre-measured from the extended nose to the seventh rib or caudal end of the sternum and then inserted. Sterile water should be flushed through the tube before and after feeding to ensure it is correctly placed and does not become blocked. The tube may then be glued, taped or sutured to the dorsal aspect of the head and a bung inserted when not in use. It may be necessary to put an Elizabethan collar on the rabbit to prevent removal.

The use of cisapride at a dose of 0.5 mg/kg orally every 8–24 hrs (Smith & Bergmann, 1997) is to be advocated in rabbits to stimulate large bowel activity, and encourage a return of normal appetite.

Older rabbits often do better on lower protein (14%) and higher fibre (18%) diets as these reduce the risk of obesity, kidney and liver damage.

Ferret

The debilitated ferret may be supported with nasogastric or oral syringe feeding of meat-based baby foods, or commercially prepared liquid meat-based formulas designed for cats and dogs such as Reanimyl® and Hill's a/d. Amounts suggested to be fed at any one sitting vary from 2–10 ml three to six times daily. It is vitally important that no debilitated ferret goes longer than 4 hours without nutritional support, as they will become rapidly hypoglycaemic.

A feline 3 French nasogastric tube can easily be placed via the nostril after first spraying the area with lignocaine spray. The tube should be pre-measured to extend from the nose tip to the level of the seventh rib (i.e. it is really a naso-oesophageal tube, to avoid the acid contents of the stomach refluxing and causing an oesophagitis) and cut to this length. It may then be secured with tissue glue, or taped or sutured to the skin over the forehead. It is advised to fit an Elizabethan collar to prevent the ferret removing the tube. The tube should be flushed with sterile water before and after feeding to ensure the tubing is in the correct position and does not block.

Rodents, chinchilla and guinea pig

Syringe feeding orally or using a straight avian crop tube to administer liquid food directly into the oesophagus are advised. The latter may be stressful, as the rodent must be scruffed prior to administration. Volumes suggested vary from 0.5 ml for a mouse up to 2.5 ml for a rat at any one sitting, the dose to be repeated 6–8 times daily to ensure correct calorie administration. Diets such as dry rodent pellets ground in a coffee grinder and then added to water to form a gruel, or the use of vegetable-based, lactose-free baby foods may be used. Guinea pigs and chinchillas benefit from the use of oral cisapride to stimulate gut motility, as well as the use of gruels made from higher-fibre chinchilla or rabbit pellets. Naso-oesophageal tubes can be attempted for the larger individuals of these two species.

Probiotics

The use of oral probiotics is to be advocated for small herbivores, to encourage normal digestive function by providing enzymes and to encourage normal pH conditions. Probiotics are best added to the drinking water but may be added to the syringed food to ensure consumption.

References

Bell, J. (1993) Ferret nutrition and diseases associated with inadequate nutrition. *Proceedings of the North American Veterinary Conference*, pp. 719–720. Orlando, Florida.

Brown, S.A. (1997) Basic anatomy, physiology and husbandry. In *Ferrets, Rabbits and Rodents: Clinical Medicine and Surgery* (Hillyer, E.V. and Quesenberry K.E., eds), pp. 3–13. W.B. Saunders, Philadelphia.

Carpenter, J.W. and Kolmstetter, C.M. (2000) Feeding small exotic mammals In *Hill's Nutrition*, pp. 943–960. Mark Mervis Institute, Marceline, Missouri.

Donnelly, T.M. (1997) Basic anatomy, physiology and husbandry. In *Ferrets, Rabbits and Rodents: Clinical Medicine and Surgery* (Hillyer, E.V. and Quesenberry, K.E., eds), pp. 147–159. W.B. Saunders, Philadelphia.

Harkness, J.E. and Wagner, J.E. (1995) *The Biology and Medicine of Rabbits and Rodents*, 4th edn, p. 230. Lea & Febiger, Philadelphia.

Hillyer, E.V., Quesenberry, K.E. and Donnelly T.M. (1997) Biology, husbandry and clinical techniques In *Ferrets, Rabbits and Rodents: Clinical Medicine and Surgery* (Hillyer, E.V. and Quesenberry, K.E., eds), pp. 243–259. W.B. Saunders, Philadelphia.

Hoefer, H.L. (1994) Chinchillas. *Veterinary Clinics North American Small Animal Practice* **24**,103–111.

Kupersmith, D.S. (1998) A practical overview of small mammal nutrition. *Seminars in Avian and Exotic Pet Medicine* **7** (3), 141–147.

National Research Council (1978) *Nutrient Requirements of Laboratory Animals*. National Academy Press, Washington, D.C.

Okerman, L. (1994) *Diseases of Domestic Rabbits*, 2nd edn. Blackwell Science, Oxford.

Smith, J.C., Brown, E.D. and Cassidy, W.A. (1977) Zinc and vitamin A: Interrelationships of zinc metabolism. In *Current Aspects in Health and Disease*. Alan R. Liss, Inc., New York.

Smith, D.A. and Bergmann, P.M. (1997) Formulary. In *Ferrets, Rabbits and Rodents: Clinical Medicine and Surgery* (Hillyer, E.V. and Quesenberry K.E., eds), pp. 392–403. W.B. Saunders, Philadelphia.

Wallach, J.D. and Hoff, G.L. (1982) Nutritional diseases of mammals In *Noninfectious Diseases of Wildlife* (Hoff, G.L. and Davis, J.W., eds), pp. 133–135 and 143–144. Iowa State University Press, Iowa.

Further reading

Richardson, V.C.G. (1992) *Diseases of Domestic Guinea Pigs*. Blackwell Science, Oxford.

Chapter 17
Common Diseases of Small Mammals

DISEASES OF THE DOMESTIC RABBIT

This section will consider the diseases of the domestic rabbit, *Oryctolagus cuniculus*.

Skin disease

Causes of mammalian skin problems may be separated into the following categories: ectoparasitic, bacterial, viral, fungal and managemental.

Ectoparasitic

Mites

Cheyletiella parasitivorax: Cheyletiella parasitivorax is from the same family as the cat and dog *Cheyletiella* spp and produces similar signs of dense, white scurf, chiefly along the dorsum, usually starting around the nape of the neck and spreading outwards and caudally. The fur drops out and new fur regrows rapidly. The condition may not appear pruritic, although in severe cases rabbits will self-traumatise. *Cheyletiella parasitivorax* appears as a large mite, with an obvious waist, under the microscope. The mouthparts have claws, and the ends of the legs possess combs rather than suckers. Owners may be bitten by this mite in the classical pattern of three bites (breakfast, lunch and dinner!).

Psoroptes cuniculi: This mite lives chiefly in the external ear canal of the rabbit, where it irritates the lining of the canal making it weep serum. The serum dries in brown crusts within the ear canals and in severe cases may obliterate the lumen completely. Infestation can lead to serious secondary bacterial ear infections which can cause vesti-bular disease. The mites are large enough to be seen with the naked eye. They have a classical *Psoroptes* spp form with pointed mouthparts and conical suckers to the ends of the legs.

Leporarcus (Listrophorus) gibbus: This is a non-pathogenic fur mite of rabbits. It has recently changed its name from *Listrophorus* to *Leporarcus* so some texts still have the former. It is an oval mite with short legs, and so may be distinguished from the above two mites on the clinical signs and the absence of a 'waist'. It has conical suckers and combs on the end of its legs.

Neotrombicula autumnalis: This mite is the harvest mite. It is not a true parasite, but the juvenile (six legged as opposed to the adult eight legged) bright orange-red mite may irritate the skin of rabbits which have access to the hay or straw which it infests. It causes irritation of the skin surface chiefly over the palmar/plantar aspect of the feet, the face and ears. Its typical orange-red colour is visible to the naked eye, and its six-legged form distinguishes it from other mites.

All of the above mites are surface-dwelling, rather than burrowing mites. They may therefore be harvested for identification using a flea comb, or Sellotape® strip applied to the affected area and then stuck to a microscope slide for examination.

Burrowing mites are uncommonly found in rabbits, the two main ones being *Sarcoptes scabei* and *Noetedres* spp. They appear similar to the forms found in other mammals such as cats and dogs, with intensely pruritic skin lesions, and are diagnosed after skin scrapings and microscopical examination.

Lice

Haemodipsus ventricosis is an uncommon louse in domestic rabbits, and belongs to the sucking (Anoplura) family. It is slender and often blood filled, and may cause significant anaemia in young kits.

Fleas

The rabbit flea is *Spillopsyllus cuniculi* and is the chief vector for myxomatosis. It tends to concentrate around the ears of the rabbit and may be distinguished from the cat and dog flea by the presence of obliquely arranged *genal ctenidium*. These are the fronds which line the mouthparts of the flea, and which are horizontal in the cat and dog fleas.

Blow-fly

Blow flies cause a condition called *myiasis* ('fly strike').

This horrible condition is common in outdoor rabbits that have perineal soiling due to urine scalding or diarrhoea. It is caused by flies including the blue, black and green bottle families. These are the primary instigators of the disease, laying their eggs on the skin of the rabbit. In warm conditions these eggs hatch into larvae within 2 hours, and these immediately start to burrow into the rabbit away from the light.

Other parasites

Another parasite known as *Coenurus serialis*, which is the intermediate host for the adult tapeworm of dogs *Taenia serialis*, may form large, fluid-filled cysts in subcutaneous sites containing the scolices of the tapeworm.

Viral

Myxomatosis

In rabbits with some immunity, myxomatosis may produce crusting nodules on the skin of the nose, lips, feet and base of the ears (Fig. 17.1). In some rabbits, death will still occur up to 40 days after the initial signs, but many will recover. The acute

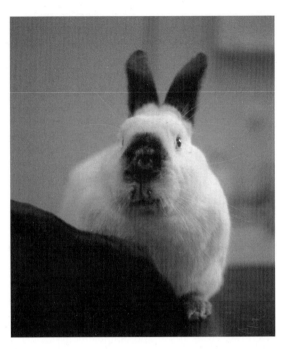

Fig. 17.1 Myxoma lesions on the nose of a rabbit with partial immunity to myxomatosis.

form of myxomatosis causes oedema of the periocular region, the base of the ears and the anal and genital openings. The virus attacks internal organs as well, and in the unvaccinated domestic rabbit is almost invariably fatal, running a course of 5–15 days.

The myxomatosis virus is a member of the pox virus family, and is transmitted by biting insects, chiefly fleas, but mosquitos and lice may also provide a source of infection.

Bacterial

Rabbit pus is thick and often inspissated, so they form firm abscesses. These are common in the head region, where they are invariably associated with dental disease. The bacteria involved are often *Pasteurella multocida* and *Staphylococcus aureus* although, after prolonged antibiotic treatment, many anaerobic bacteria will flourish.

'Blue fur disease' is caused by the bacteria *Pseudomonas aeruginosa*. The bacteria produces a blue pigment, which stains the fur, and is common in outdoor rabbits, or those kept in damp conditions. It will infect damaged skin, such as occurs in the dewlap area of many lop breeds, where wet skin chafes.

Rabbit syphilis, caused by the bacteria *Treponema cuniculi*, affects the anogenital area, the nose and lips, producing brown crusting lesions. These may progress over the face. The bacteria is thought to be passed from doe to young during parturition, and may be sexually transmitted from buck to doe and vice versa. It is not infectious for humans.

Fungal

The two commonly seen fungal forms are the cat and dog ringworm *Microsporum canis*, which will fluoresce under the ultraviolet Wood's lamp light, and the environmental *Trichophyton mentagrophytes*, which does not. The lesions are dry, scaly, often grey plaques appearing over the head initially, but then spreading to the feet and the rest of the body. Culturing brushings of the lesions on dermatophyte medium is advised for definitive diagnosis.

Managemental

Rabbits are as prone to neglect as any other species. Particular problems occur in the fine- and long-haired breeds such as the Angoras. This breed has especially fine fur which mats easily, particularly when the animal is bedded on straw, hay or shavings. Owners of these breeds will need to be advised to keep them on paper or wire mesh, and to groom their rabbit once or even twice daily. Even then, when the Angora moults in the spring and autumn, the chances are the coat will become matted. This can lead to dermatitis underneath the matted areas.

Overgrown claws are another common feature in rabbits, particularly hutch-kept rabbits with little access to the outside. Claws should be regularly assessed and, if necessary, trimmed on a 4–6 week basis. Overgrown claws can lead to lateral twisting of digit joints and deformity of the foot.

Perineal soiling is a common condition in pet rabbits. It may be due to faecal soiling from diarrhoea, or inability or lack of desire to consume the caecotrophs which are softer than the faecal pellet. Urine scalding is also common. Older rabbits may have spinal arthritis, which prevents them from positioning correctly to urinate, and lop breeds have excessive folds of skin around the urogenital area. For mild cases, provision of absorbent bedding underneath a deep layer of straw is advised. Attention to cage and rabbit hygiene on a daily basis are essential to prevent blow fly strike and secondary bacterial skin infections. In severe cases, in addition to treating any underlying condition, housing the rabbit on a suspended mesh floor so the urine and faeces drop through should be considered.

Digestive disease

Oral

Dental disease is one of the most commonly seen conditions in rabbits in the United Kingdom. Dental disease problems may present with salivation and anorexia, through to jaw bone swellings from root elongations of cheek teeth, to full-blown abscesses. Overgrown teeth may be obvious, as with incisor malocclusions, or may be hidden from external view, as with cheek teeth malocclusions. Dental problems may affect other parts of the head, creating abscesses behind the globe of the eye, or affecting the lumen of the tear duct as it runs over the cheek teeth and maxillary incisor roots, causing pus to appear at the eye or nares.

Causes of dental disease can be hereditary defects (Netherland dwarf and lops, Plate 17.1), due to a shortened rostrocaudal length of skull and abnormal bite (Fig. 17.2), or dietary deficiencies. The two most commonly cited dietary deficiencies include a lack of suitable abrasive foodstuffs for dental wear, and a lack of calcium and vitamin D_3 for proper jawbone mineralisation.

Rabbits have adapted over thousands of years to survive on a diet consisting of 85% grass, and 15% leafy herbage. Grass, of the meadow variety, is very high in silicates. These are abrasive compounds of silica, the chief mineral in sand, and are naturally very wearing. Rabbits' dental growth has therefore evolved to cope with this. Even if

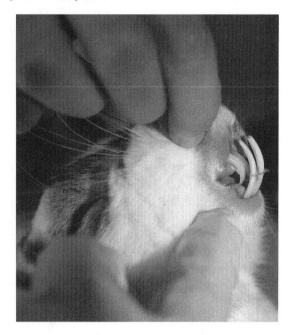

Fig. 17.2 Brachygnathism is hereditary and may be a cause of malocclusion in rabbits.

the rabbit is not wearing its teeth down they continue to grow at several millimetres per week. In addition, with a reduced abrasive diet, what chewing is done can be less vigorous. As the rabbit's mandible is narrower than its maxilla, the only way the whole surface of the opposing sets of cheek teeth will wear evenly, is by the lateral movement of the mandible across the maxilla. In less abrasive, easier-chewed diets, this happens less effectively, and so the outer or buccal edges of the mandibular cheek teeth wear, and the inner or lingual edges of the maxillary cheek teeth wear, causing sharp points to form on the tongue side of the mandibular teeth and the cheek side of the maxillary. These points grow, the teeth tilt, and the mandibular teeth then cut into the tongue, and the maxillary teeth into the cheeks leading to deep ulcers, pain and anorexia.

In addition, the roots of the cheek teeth may grow back into the jaws as they elongate, due to a lack of space inside the mouth and continued growth. The roots then push through the ventral aspect of the mandible, and may be felt as a series of lumps underneath the angle of the lower jaw. In the maxilla, the roots of the last two cheek teeth can push into the orbit of the eye, causing ocular pain and watering of the eye. All of the maxillary cheek tooth roots can cause blockage or strictures of the tear duct which runs in the bone above them.

Incisors may overgrow due to elongation of the molars pushing the mouth open wider. The maxillary incisors are tightly curved, whereas the mandibular incisors are more gently curving. If the mouth is forced slightly open, the maxillary incisors no longer close rostral to the mandibular ones, and overgrowth ensues. The maxillary incisors curl back and into the mouth like ram's-horns, the mandibular incisors grow up in front of the nose. Root elongation may also occur with incisors, with maxillary root elongation causing constriction of the tear duct which bends around them. This leads to dacrocystitis or infection of the tear duct. The duct then dams back and a milky white discharge appears at the eye. This is often misdiagnosed as a primary conjunctivitis (Plate 17.2).

Other causes of dental disease include physical trauma to the head and inappropriate 'clipping' of the teeth with nail clippers. This often twists and cracks the tooth root causing further deformity and predisposing to infection of the root and abscess formation.

Hairballs

Some rabbits will overgroom and this may lead to an abnormal build-up of fur in the stomach. The resultant *trichobezoar* may be palpated in the cranial abdomen, and may cause a decrease in gut motility due to poor stomach emptying. Causes of overgrooming include parasitic skin conditions, dental disease and intestinal discomfort or disease.

Gastrointestinal

Dietary

Dietary causes, such as a sudden change in diet, as with the feeding of an excess of leafy greens to a rabbit previously fed dry formulas, will lead to a temporary diarrhoea. Other dietary factors include the type of food fed. Spoiled foods and foods such as part-fermented grass cuttings will inevitably lead to diarrhoea.

Iatrogenic

Iatrogenic causes include the administration of certain antibiotics, such as many penicillins and the macrolide family. These destroy the normal flora of the gut, leaving bacteria such as *Clostridia spiriformae* to flourish. This bacteria is found in small quantities in the normal gastrointestinal flora of the rabbit, but once it achieves a critical threshold level, it can release an iota toxin which is absorbed across the gut wall into the bloodstream and causing toxaemia, with hepatic and renal necrosis.

Bacterial

Bacteria such as the *E. coli* family, which are particularly common in young weaner rabbits, are a cause of sudden death, due to the release of another form of toxin known as an enterotoxin. Death may occur before any signs of diarrhoea.

Parasitic

Parasitic causes of diarrhoea include the coccidial parasites *Eimeria* spp. These are single-celled protozoal parasites which destroy the lining of the small intestine, causing diarrhoea and death in heavy infestations. In mild cases it may simply cause poor growth and stunting in young rabbits. The coccidia *Eimeria stiediae* is of particular importance in rabbits as it will also infest and damage the liver. Coccidial oocysts may be detected in the faeces by direct smears or sugar solution flotation methods, as for cats and dogs.

Other parasitic causes of diarrhoea and digestive upsets include the stomach worm *Graphidium strigosum* and the small intestinal worm *Trichostrongylus retortaeformis*. These are usually only found in rabbits with access to the outside where they may pick up the eggs of these worms directly from wild rabbits' faeces or indirectly via passive spread from wild birds etc. A large intestinal pinworm, *Passalurus ambiguus*, is commonly seen, but rarely causes disease. All of these worms' eggs may be detected in the faeces by flotation methods.

Mucoid enteropathy

This is a catch-all term for a condition commonly affecting 4–14 week old rabbits which pass thick mucus instead of faeces. These animals are dull, lethargic and in abdominal pain. The caecal and large intestinal contents are often dried out and impacted. The causes of this condition are not well identified, but the feeding of a highly fermentable low fibre diet does predispose many rabbits to this. In addition, some evidence now suggests that a primary gut dysautonomia may be responsible for some cases.

Respiratory disease

Pasteurellosis

The bacteria most commonly involved in rabbit respiratory disease is *Pasteurella multocida* and it causes 'rabbit snuffles'. It is commonly found in the airways of apparently healthy rabbits, but it can lead to severe upper airway disease, with a purulent oculonasal discharge, and the characteristic wet, matted fur of the fore paws. It can develop into pneumonia. Poor housing, with damp, ammonia-laden bedding can irritate the airways and allow rapid infection to occur. Dental disease and myxomatosis are other factors. Similarly, overcrowded hutches and concurrent disease elsewhere in the body may lower immunity.

Viral haemorrhagic disease (VHD)

This is a calici virus and has been in the United Kingdom since 1992. It does not cause respiratory disease exclusively, as it will attack all organs within the body, particularly the lungs, digestive system and liver. It is spread via contact, and is

100% fatal, often causing death with no obvious clinical disease. Post-mortem examination reveals widespread internal haemorrhage. Young, weaned rabbits are most at risk.

Cardiovascular disease

Arterial wall calcification is seen in rabbits fed excess amounts of vitamin D_3 and calcium in their diets. The calcium becomes deposited in the walls of the major blood vessels, reducing their elasticity and leading to increased blood pressure.

Urinary tract disease

Urolithiasis and cystitis

Cystitis and urolithiasis are common problems in rabbits, due to their unusual method of controlling calcium levels in the body. They absorb all of the calcium they can from their diet, and then excrete any excess into the urine via the kidneys. The commonest urolith to form is the calcium carbonate crystal. This forms readily in the rabbit's alkaline urine, and is radio-dense, being seen to fill the bladder outline on radiography. Secondary bladder infections are common with calcium carbonate urolithiasis, as the crystals irritate the lining of the bladder, and secondary, often *E. coli*, infections result.

Haematuria

The presence of red-coloured urine in the rabbit does not necessarily indicate haematuria. Many red porphyrin pigments from the diet (particularly some leafy greens such as beetroot) will be excreted in the urine. Causes of haematuria include cystitis, uterine tumours, aneurysms and kidney infections.

Encephalitozoonosis

Infection of the kidneys with *Encephalitozoan cuniculi*, a single-celled protozoal microsporidian parasite, can cause severe scarring and damage. This parasite may also be responsible for various neurological symptoms (see below).

Reproductive tract disease

Uterine

Uterine adenocarcinoma

This is a common condition seen in does over the age of four years. Some authors have put the incidence at nearly 80%. The condition is fatal if not detected early as the tumour readily metastasizes, primarily to the lungs. Radiography of the chest is therefore advised if the condition is suspected, to determine if spread has occurred.

Venereal spirochaetosis

This is rabbit syphilis, which is caused by the bacteria *Treponema cuniculi*. The condition is self-limiting, but produces crusting of the anogenital area, the nose and lips.

Pyometra

Uterine infections do occur in older does, and are often due to *E. coli* infections of hyperplastic endometrial tissues.

Mammary gland

Mastitis is seen following a pregnancy when the kittens are lost or in phantom pregnancy. The unused milk can easily become infected, particularly if the hutch or other environmental conditions are poor. Many of the coliform type of bacteria involved will release endotoxins into the bloodstream causing rapid toxaemia, fever and death of the doe. Others may just cause severe mastitis with abscess formation.

Musculoskeletal disease

Splayleg

Splayleg is an inherited congenital disease wherein the kit cannot position one or more hind limbs underneath itself. Instead the affected limb sticks out awkwardly. There is no treatment for this condition.

Fractured or dislocated spine

This is a common condition in indoor-reared, poorly-fed rabbits. The close confinement leads to weakening of the bones and muscles due to disuse atrophy, and the absence of sunlight can exacerbate a vitamin D_3 and calcium deficiency in a poor diet. Osteoporosis occurs, with spontaneous fractures, often located in the lumbosacral area.

Neurological disease

Encephalitozoonosis

The microsporidian intracellular parasite *Encephalitozoan cuniculi* is common in many domestic rabbits. It is passed from rabbit to rabbit in the urine gaining access via the oral or mucocutaneous route. It may be transferred from mother to young at the time of birth. It affects the kidneys and the central nervous system, and may remain latent for years, producing no clinical signs. Alternatively, paralysis of the hind limbs, fitting, head tilt or other vestibular symptoms and blindness may be seen. Diagnosis is difficult to make in the live rabbit, as the only test so far available involves detecting the antibodies to the infection, therefore a negative result is a definite negative, but a positive result in an otherwise healthy rabbit could merely suggest that the rabbit has been exposed to the parasite, but is not currently infected. Alternatively, the rabbit may be permanently infected.

Vestibular disease

One cause of vestibular disease is Encephalitozoonosis. Others include tumours or infarcts of the hind brain, and more commonly *Pasteurella multocida* infection of the middle and inner ear. The bacteria gain access to the middle ear via the Eustachian tube, or via a perforated ear drum such as are seen in ear mite infestations. The balance centres in the inner ear and/or the hind brain are affected and the rabbit exhibits a head tilt, of varying severity which often worsens when stressed or handled, and nystagmus. Many are unable to stand. Prognosis in these cases is poor and euthanasia should be considered.

DISEASES OF THE RAT AND MOUSE

Rat and mouse diseases are relatively similar as they are so closely related. Therefore the following will detail the diseases of both species highlighting any differences as they arise.

Skin disease

Ectoparasitic

Mites

The mite *Myobia musculi* tends to affect the head of mice causing intense pruritus in many cases, inducing self-mutilation. Some mice may be asymptomatic carriers of this mite, but equally some may be so severely affected as to die of secondary bacterial infection (Plate 17.3).

Myocoptes musculinus causes disease over the body of the mouse. It may produce intense pruritus, but does not tend to induce the large areas of ulceration which form the feature of *Myobia musculi* infection.

In the rat the commonly seen fur mite is *Radfordia ensifera*. In the tropics the blood sucking mite *Liponyssus bacoti* can cause anaemia and general debilitation.

Notoedres muris is a burrowing mite of rats and causes crusting lesions on the ear tips and tail which may then spread to the rest of the body. It appears to be extremely pruritic in the rat and secondary bacterial infections are common.

Diagnosis of these mites is based on the clinical signs and discovering them on skin scrapings of affected lesions.

Lice

The common sucking louse seen in both rats and mice is *Polyplax spinulosa*. This seems to be mildly pruritic in both species, but if present in sufficient numbers (the louse may be seen with the naked eye) it can cause anaemia.

Fleas

In most pet households which also contain cats or dogs, infestation of pet rats and mice with either

Ctenocephalides felis or *Ctenocephalides canis* is possible. These may cause significant anaemic states to develop. The flea *Xenopsylla cheopis* is the main transmissal agent of the bacteria *Yersinia pestis* which is the cause of bubonic plague. It is not found in the United Kingdom, but in certain parts of the world the wild rat population is infested with this flea and the disease (e.g. parts of Africa, China, South America and the western states of the USA).

Viral

Both species may be affected by their own form of pox virus. These are rarely seen in general practice, although the mouse pox virus (known as *ectromelia*) can cause problems in laboratory situations.

Sialodacryoadenitis virus infection is a coronaviral disease affecting the tear glands and periorbital areas of both rats and mice. It causes some local swelling and excess tears to be produced. The tears contain porphyrin pigments making the them red (*chromodacryorrhoea*) and mimicking dried blood. The disease is not treatable, but is generally self-limiting, although red tears may reappear in rats at times of stress.

Bacterial

Generalised bacterial skin problems are common as a sequel to any self-induced trauma. The infections are commonly due to bacteria such as *Staphylococcus aureus* and *Streptococcus* spp although infections with commensal or environmental bacteria such as *Pseudomonas* spp are also seen.

Pododermatitis

This is not so much a primary bacterial skin problem as a secondary one. Sores commonly develop on the hocks of older, overweight rats. These occur as pressure sores, with the blood supply to the pressure points being compromised, allowing secondary infections to occur. Causes include osteoarthritis, excessive weight carriage and poor bedding.

Fungal

As with rabbits, the main fungal skin infection that is seen is that due to ringworm organisms. In rats and mice it is relatively uncommon and usually due to the fungus *Tricophyton mentagrophytes*. This produces lesions on the head and neck, with a typical scaling and dry crust. The tail may also be affected, and the lesions do not appear to be pruritic. This ringworm does not fluoresce under Wood's lamp.

Miscellaneous

Barbering

Barbering of the whiskers and fur is very common in male mice kept together. The whiskers and fur is chewed short by the companion(s) and may proceed to more serious injuries. For this reason male mice should not be kept together.

Ringtail

Ringtail is seen in rats when circular constrictions of the skin covering the tail occur stopping the blood supply and causing skin sloughing. It is thought to be due to a reduction in the relative humidity of the cage or environment of the rat. Levels of humidity below 40–50% have been associated with this problem.

Atopy

Atopy is hypothesised to exist in rats. This is an allergic skin condition similar to that seen in dogs, and can occur due to contact with any potential allergen in their environment. Classically, the rat is pruritic and is covered in scabs. There is no evidence of mites on skin scrapings, and no response to ivermectin medication.

Digestive disease

Oral

Dental disease is uncommon in rats and mice. Their cheek teeth grow very slowly and so the classical overgrowth problems seen in rabbits and chinchillas are not seen in rats and mice.

Gastrointestinal

Endoparasitic

Worm infestations with species of pinworms such as *Syphacia obvelata* (chiefly in mice), *Syphacia muris* (chiefly in rats) and *Aspiculuris tetraptera* (chiefly in mice) are common. They may cause no disease at all, but the characteristic asymmetrical eggs may be found in the faeces, or around the anus, where the *Syphacia* spp may cause irritation. Diarrhoea, if present, is generally mild, but severe infestations may cause rectal prolapses.

Protozoal

These include infections with *Entamoeba muris*, *Trichomonas muris* and *Giardia muris*. All can cause a mild diarrhoea, but many may cause no disease signs at all when present in low numbers.

Bacterial

Salmonellosis: salmonellosis is also a not uncommon problem and mice and rats, which may remain subclinical carriers of the bacteria for years. Diarrhoea is not always seen, treatment is difficult as clearing a rat or mouse of *Salmonella* spp is almost impossible, and therefore euthanasia is often advised due to the human health risk.

Transmissible murine colonic hyperplasia (TMCH): TMCH is an infection of mice caused by the environmental bacteria *Citrobacter freundii*. It causes progressive thickening of the mucosa of the large intestine, causing diarrhoea, abdominal pain, anorexia and sometimes rectal prolapse, particularly in young mice, 2–4 weeks of age. Death occurs in a small number of cases. The more common outcome is stunting of the mouse. It is highly infectious, and poor cage hygiene allows rapid spread through a colony.

Tyzzer's disease: this is an infection by a bacteria known as *Clostridium (Bacillus) piliformis*. It is common in rats, where it can cause sudden death, or watery diarrhoea, perineal staining, heart and liver disease. It is highly infectious and spread in the faeces.

Viral

Rotavirus: rotavirus infection is seen in rats and mice before weaning. Chronic infections, yellow diarrhoea and stunted growth are common.

Mouse hepatitis virus (MHV): MHV is a highly pathogenic corona virus mainly affecting suckling mice. It causes rapid deterioration, a yellow diarrhoea, muscle tremors, fitting and death in infected individuals, and is spread via the respiratory and faecal–oral routes.

Respiratory disease

Respiratory disease is extremely common in rats and mice, particularly the former where it makes up the most frequently seen problem in rats in general practice.

Mycoplasma pulmonis

The bacteria *Mycoplasma pulmonis* is widespread in the rat and mouse population. It is carried, in asymptomatic individuals, in the upper airways and the reproductive tract. Transmission is by close contact between male and female at mating, mother and young during nursing and by aerosol spread from individual to individual over greater distances. It is highly infectious.

Signs of disease include snuffles, head tilts due to inner and middle ear infections, dyspnoea, hyperpnoea and death from advanced bronchopulmonary disease. The course of the infection can be chronic, with affected individuals suffering repeated bouts of bronchitis and pneumonia. They will exhibit poor body condition, a dull staring coat, secondary red tear production due to stress and anorexia and lethargy. Another form of the disease affects the reproductive tract and causes infertility, reduced fertility and early abortions.

Some factors will encourage rapid onset of the infection and these include any concurrent illness, other respiratory tract infections, the Sendai virus (see below) and unsanitary conditions. Particularly implicated is urine soiling which leads to a build up of ammonia gas which then leads to respiratory tract irritation and infection.

Sendai virus

Sendai virus is a paramyxovirus type 1 which may be transmitted by sneezing, by direct contact, via food bowls or fomites. It is commonest in recently weaned mice as younger mice are protected by maternal antibodies. Signs of disease include dullness, dyspnoea, chattering of the teeth, weight loss, anorexia and a dull coat. In young mice the mortality rate may be high.

Other respiratory infections

Streptococcus pneumoniae (a common cause of pneumonia and meningitis in older humans and therefore a potential zoonosis), *Pasteurella pneumotropica, Bordetella bronchiseptica, Corynebacterium kutscheri* and the cilia-associated respiratory bacillus (CAR) may all occur in respiratory disease in rats and mice. Clinical signs produced are variations on those seen above, with respiratory disease and often reproductive disease occurring.

Cardiovascular disease

Cardiovascular disease is uncommon in mice and rats, except when caused by association with Tyzzer's disease where myocardial microabscesses may be seen.

Urinary tract disease

Chronic progressive nephrosis

Chronic progressive nephrosis is a common condition in ageing rats and mice. The kidneys become progressively more damaged by protein deposits in the tubular lumens. In certain strains of mice an autoimmune factor is seen. In rats a high protein, low potassium diet has been implicated, with males more susceptible than females. Recurrent disease processes equally may have a role to play. An increase in thirst and urination may be seen, with progressive weight loss and dehydration. Blood samples showing increased levels of urea and creatinine with low blood albumin are suggestive of this condition.

Urolithiasis

This is common in older rats and mice, especially males, where uroliths may block the narrower urethra proximal to the os penis. The composition of the uroliths varies, but is frequently of calcium carbonate, ammonium phosphate or calcium oxalate. There is often a secondary cystitis.

Reproductive tract disease

Uterine

Dystocias are uncommon in rats and mice. Uterine infections do occur infrequently, with pyometras being the most common in rats (Plate 17.4).

Mammary gland

The mammary glands are commonly affected by cancer in both rats and mice.

In rats, the cancer which occurs most frequently is the fibroadenoma. This is a benign, but rapidly growing tumour, and can occur in any of the mammary tissue which extends from cranially at the forelimbs to the inguinal region. The masses are well defined and easily removed surgically, although the predisposition appears to be hereditary, and the likelihood of further tumours occurring is high. Fibroadenomas can occur in male rats as well as females. Adenocarcinomas do occur in 10% of cases and may spread to the rest of the body.

In mice, the mammary cancer most commonly seen is malignant and caused by an RNA virus, the

Bittner agent, which, in a susceptible strain of mouse, causes a mammary adenocarcinoma. Surgery is often unsuccessful in curing this condition due to the aggressive nature of the cancer.

Testicular

A form of testicular cancer, a Leydig cell adenoma, is seen in old male rats. It is benign and causes a soft swelling, and may be accompanied by some hair loss over the body.

Musculoskeletal disease

Spondylosis is common in older rats, and may be responsible for incontinence and reduction of function of the hind limbs. Typically, the lumbosacral area is affected by the osteoarthritis, reducing mobility, causing pain and irritating spinal nerve function.

Ocular disease

The virus causing red tears has been mentioned above, and will infect rats, mice, hamsters and gerbils. Chronic infections may cause permanent reduction in tears, leading to keratitis sicca. Conjunctivitis may occur secondary to this, or to the presence of finely chopped or dusty bedding, creating a foreign body reaction.

Cataracts are occasionally seen, often associated with a hereditary deformed eye seen as microphthalmia.

Many young rats and mice have a persistent hyaloid artery which may bleed into the vitreus humour and appear as haemorrhages at the front of the eye.

Albino rats and mice must be given shelter from light as their retinas are very prone to the damage this can cause. Even normal-coloured rats and mice require a shelter that is light proof.

Neurological disease

Vestibular disease

Head tilts are common in rats. Some causes include infections due to *Mycoplasma pulmonis* and *Streptococcus pneumoniae*, which can cause inner ear disease or hind brain abscesses and so affect the balance centres. Other causes of vestibular disease are tumours, with pituitary tumours reported as commonly occurring in older female rats on high calorie/protein diets.

Lymphocytic choriomeningitis

This condition is mainly seen in wild mice. It is a virus, which is shed in the urine and saliva, and affected mice may show no symptoms, or they may show neurological signs such as head tilts, fitting and death. It is a zoonotic disease and can cause a meningitis which may be fatal to humans and other primates. Thankfully it is rare in animals in captivity.

DISEASES OF THE GERBIL

Skin disease

Ectoparasitic

The only mite of any note in gerbils is *Demodex merioni*, and it rarely causes disease. It has a typical cigar shape under microscopy of skin scrapings. Other mite infestations are rare, although cases of *Notoedres muris* and *Sarcoptes scabei* have been reported.

Storage mites have been reported as causing a problem in gerbils, amongst other rodents. The mites, which live on cereal products, may contaminate food and bedding material and cause irritation to the nose and facial area which is in contact with food.

Bacterial

Staphylococcus aureus infections of the nose and face occur secondary to wet substrate conditions such as peat or earth. Another cause of the condition is the *sialodacryoadenitis* virus infection of the tear glands, which causes excessive tear production. This may lead to a wet dermatitis in the perinasal area, which allows *Staphylococcus aureus* to create a pyoderma.

Fungal

As with rats and mice, the ringworm *Trichophyton mentagrophytes* is the commonest seen, causing areas of hyperkeratosis with grey scaling of the skin, particularly in the head region. Diagnosis is made on microscopy and culture.

Skin tumours

The commonest seen cancer of gerbils is the ventral scent gland adenocarcinoma which develops from 2 years of age onwards and is most commonly seen in the male gerbil.

Other skin tumours, such as the melanoma, are seen, particularly on the extremities. Squamous cell carcinomas of the ears and nose are also seen.

Endocrine

Cystic ovarian disease (see below) has been associated with symmetrical hair loss over the flanks of female gerbils, along with a swollen abdomen.

Miscellaneous

Tail skin degloving injuries are common in gerbils that have been roughly handled or restrained by the end of the tail. The denuded vertebrae will die off later on, and the tail never regrows.

Digestive disease

Oral

This is relatively uncommon in the gerbil, although traumatic damage to the incisors leading to fractures and overgrowth may occur.

Gastrointestinal

Bacterial

Tyzzer's disease – Clostridium (Bacillus) piliformis: Tyzzer's disease causes an enteritis, but rarely diarrhoea and often spreads to the liver and heart. The disease lasts for 1–4 days and may produce sudden death or a more lingering disease with dullness, lethargy, a hunched posture, scant or soft faeces and a dull staring coat.

Proliferative ileitis: proliferative ileitis is thought to be caused by the intracellular bacteria *Lawsonia intracellularis* which is the pathogen causing wet-tail in hamsters. It is passed from gerbil to gerbil via the faecal–oral route, and causes thickening of the ileum. This prevents it from absorbing nutrients and water, causing weight loss, debilitation and diarrhoea producing the classical 'wet tail' of matted damp fur around the rear. The condition is much less common in gerbils than hamsters, but can nonetheless be a serious and fatal condition.

Endoparasitic

Gerbils may suffer from the mouse pinworm *Syphacia obvelata* and the rat pinworm *Syphacia muris* eggs of which may be found in the faeces. Rarely do these cause clinical disease and treatment is as for rats and mice.

The zoonotic cestode *Hymenolepis nana* can be found and is discussed in hamsters.

Respiratory disease

The gerbil is affected by more or less the same respiratory conditions as the rat and mouse, although in general, gerbils are not affected as commonly as rats and mice.

Cardiovascular disease

Tyzzer's disease may cause myocarditis, otherwise cardiovascular disease is uncommon.

Urinary tract disease

Gerbils are moderately prone to ageing changes involving gradual scarring of renal tissue and the nephrotic syndrome, but the incidence of this is much less than in the rat or mouse.

Reproductive tract disease

Uterine infection

Uterine infections are uncommon in gerbils.

Ovarian cysts

Ovarian cysts are common. The cysts may be quite large and cause distension of the abdomen. The condition is hereditary and bilateral and causes disruption of the oestrus cycle. The follicle cyst secretes low levels of oestrogens which may have an effect on fur growth, causing mild alopecia over the flanks of the gerbil.

Uterine and ovarian neoplasia

After cancer of the adrenal gland, cancer of the ovaries and the female reproductive tract are considered the most common tumours in the gerbil. Uterine cancers may cause bleeding from the reproductive tract entrance, or abdominal swelling. Diagnosis may be made on clinical signs, or ultrasound and radiographical examination.

Musculoskeletal disease

Fractures are uncommon in gerbils, as are other musculoskeletal problems other than the degloving tail injuries mentioned above.

Neurological disease

Vestibular disease

Vestibular disease is common in gerbils and is usually due to inner ear disease of a bacterial nature, often *Mycoplasma pulmonis*, *Pasteurella pneumotropica* or *Streptococcus pneumoniae*, which gain access from the oropharynx via the Eustachian canals and the middle ear. Pus may be observed at the external ear canal in some cases.

Epilepsy

Epilepsy in gerbils appears to be of a hereditary nature, and it is advised not to keep susceptible individuals in rooms with strip lighting, television sets or computer terminals as these all emit electromagnetic radiation of around 50–60 Hz which may induce a fit.

DISEASES OF THE HAMSTER

Skin disease

Ectoparasitic

The mites *Demodex criceti* and *Demodex aurati* both infest hamsters and can cause clinical disease. Under the microscope, *D. criceti* is shorter and rounder, whereas *D. aurati* is longer and more like *D. canis*. The clinical disease is manifested by alopecia over the dorsum caudally and intense white scurf. The lesions are mildly pruritic. Diagnosis is made on positive skin scrapings.

Fungal

The fungus *Trichophyton mentagrophytes* is often found as a secondary cause of skin disease in hamsters, usually as a sequel to mange or mycosis fungoides (see below).

Bacterial

Bacterial skin disease is uncommonly seen in hamsters. The main bacteria isolated from wounds inflicted by other hamsters include *Pasteurella pneumotropica* and *Staphylococcus aureus*.

Skin tumours

The commonest skin tumour in the hamster is a form of T-cell leukaemia known as *mycosis fungoides*. This infiltrates the epidermis producing chronic thickening of the skin, and is pruritic. Alopecia is seen due to the obliteration of the hair follicles. The cancer eventually spreads internally.

Melanomas affecting the head, ears and flank scent glands are also seen. These are usually pigmented, relatively fast growing and occur more frequently in males than females.

Endocrine

Cushing's syndrome can produce bilaterally symmetrical hair loss over the flanks, which may spread to the rest of the body. The disease is due to a chromophobe adenoma in the pituitary gland. This secretes excessive levels of ACTH which causes bilateral adrenal gland hyperplasia and hence increased body levels of cortisol. This causes the classical signs of Cushing's syndrome, i.e. polydipsia, polyuria, symmetrical alopecia, increased appetite and thinning of the skin.

Irritant

Skin irritation has been reported in hamsters kept on cedar pine chips. These are highly resinous and can cause intense skin irritation, particularly over the ventrum and nasal areas. Removal of the hamster from these shavings produces improvement within days.

Digestive disease

Oral

Cheek pouch impaction

Impaction of the cheek pouch with food may occur for a number of reasons. The hamster may have been so enthusiastic in filling the cheek pouch that it becomes too full to empty. Alternatively, the hamster may have filled the pouch and become ill before emptying it. Because the hamster uses his hind limb to empty the pouch, losing a hind leg may also lead to impaction on that side.

Cheek pouch prolapse

Prolapse may occur after the hamster has emptied the cheek pouch. The sac, now everted, may not return to normal and protrudes as a pink mass from the mouth.

Gastrointestinal

Proliferative ileitis ('wet-tail')

Wet-tail is caused by the bacteria *Lawsonia intracellularis* which produces hypertrophy of the ileum, reducing digestion and absorption which leads to diarrhoea. Some hamsters die within 24 hours of contracting the disease without showing any obvious signs.

Salmonellosis

Salmonellosis is uncommon, but does occur in hamsters. The bacteria *Salmonella enteritidis* is the most frequently reported and this is a zoonotic disease. Signs include sudden death, frequently before any diarrhoea is produced. Younger animals seem more susceptible.

Parasitic

Hymenolepis nana is a dwarf tapeworm which is potentially transmissible to humans. It appears to cause little or no disease in hamsters. A diagnosis may be made by finding cestode egg sachets in the faeces, or by seeing the cream coloured, 1–2 mm long egg packet wriggling on the perianal fur!

Miscellaneous

Examples of other causes of diarrhoea include the sudden introduction of fresh fruit and vegetables to a previously all-dry diet. Any dietary changes should be made gradually, as the initial mild diarrhoea may allow secondary bacterial pathogens to cause more serious disease. Certain foods should be avoided altogether, including foods containing lactose, such as many dairy products. In addition, over-sugary fruit such as grapes, kiwi fruit and bananas should be fed in moderation if at all, as they can induce diarrhoea or colic.

Respiratory disease

Hamsters suffer from pulmonary thromboembolisms from atrial thrombotic lesions (see below) which may prove fatal, and are a cause of sudden death.

Cardiovascular disease

Atrial thromboses form mainly in the left atrium as a result of a cardiomyopathy. If the right side is affected, thrombosis may induce pulmonary thromboembolisms which can prove fatal. In any case the thromboses often start a chain of coagulation events. Clinical signs of cardiomyopathy include tachypnoea, cyanosed membranes and extremities and lethargy. The incidence is higher in female hamsters and castrated males suggesting that the presence of testosterone has some protective effect. Diagnosis is based on the signs and the demonstration of an enlarged heart on radiography and ultrasound examination. The latter are often able to show the thrombi in the atria.

Urinary tract disease

Kidney

Hamsters are prone to chronic progressive nephropathy in much the same way as mice and rats. They are also prone to amyloidosis. This is a condition wherein proteins of immunoglobulin origin are deposited within various organs of the body, such as the kidneys, affecting their function. The cause of the condition is not known. Clinical signs vary, but may include weight loss, lethargy, polydipsia and polyuria with or without proteinuria.

Bladder

Like mice and rats, hamsters can suffer from cystitis and urolithiasis. Calcium oxalate and calcium carbonate are the two commonly seen uroliths.

Endocrine disease

Cushing's syndrome

See above under the discussion of skin diseases.

Diabetes mellitus

In the Chinese hamster diabetes mellitus is a hereditary condition. Clinical signs include polydipsia (drinking often in excess of 50 ml of water per day) and polyuria, cystitis, lethargy and weight loss. Glucosuria of 2% is common and blood glucose is often in excess of 25–30 mmol/l.

Reproductive tract disease

Uterus

Pyometra is a not uncommon condition in hamsters, but may be mistaken for the normal reproductive tract discharge seen during the oestrus cycle. Pyometras, however, persist, and smell much worse! Closed pyometras are more difficult to diagnose due to the absence of a discharge, but the hamster is often lethargic, anorectic, polydipsic, dehydrated and has a tender, swollen abdomen.

Ovaries

Cystic ovaries are relatively common in female hamsters over the age of 8 months. The condition is often bilateral, and may be accompanied by some mild symmetrical alopecia of the flanks.

Ocular disease

Chinese hamsters are prone to cataract development as a result of diabetes mellitus.

Musculoskeletal disease

Compound fractures of the tibia are the commonest, especially from hamsters falling from the roof or sides of wire cages up which they have climbed, and leg amputation may be required (Plate 17.5). Other fractures commonly seen are fractures of spinal vertebrae, or more commonly vertebral subluxations, usually in the lumbar area, again due to falls. These will present as bilateral hind limb paresis or paralysis.

Neurological disease

Lymphocytic choriomeningitis generally produces little or no clinical signs in the hamster.

It is excreted in the urine and saliva. It is relatively rare in captive hamsters, being found more commonly in wild mice, but it is a serious zoonotic disease causing meningitis in man.

DISEASES OF THE GUINEA PIG

Skin disease

Ectoparasitic

Mites

The scabies mite *Trixicara caviae* is a source of intense pruritus and distress for guinea pigs. The affected individual may scratch itself deeply, creating multiple areas of alopecia and open sores over the dorsum, and may be so severe as to cause abortion in heavily pregnant females. Diagnosis is made on the clinical signs and demonstration of this sarcoptid mite on skin scrapings under the microscope.

Another mite, *Chirodiscoides caviae*, is seen in guinea pigs. This is a fur mite and seems to cause little trouble.

Lice

Gliricola porcelli and *Gyropus ovalis*, both of which are members of the Mallophaga and hence live off cellular debris, are found in guinea pigs, but rarely cause disease.

Bacterial

Cervical lymphadenitis

Cervical lymphadenitis is a disease of the cervical lymph nodes caused by the bacteria *Streptococcus zooepidemicus*. It is found in the airways and mouth of the average healthy guinea pig, but seems to cause a problem when the mucosa of the oropharynx becomes abraded by rough food particles. This leads to local lymphadenitis, with subcutaneous abscessation. The disease may gain access to the bloodstream and so cause a septicaemia which is rapidly fatal.

Pododermatitis

Pododermatitis is commonest in overweight, elderly guinea pigs, who will spend more time resting, and walk on the flat of the hock. Bacteria involved in the pressure sores include members of the *E. coli* family, *Staphylococcus aureus* and *Streptococcus* spp.

Fungal

Ringworm due to *Microsporum canis* and *Trichophyton mentagrophytes* is not uncommon in guinea pigs. Lesions are typical and cover the head, paws and rear with brittle hairs, grey crusts and some scabs. Diagnosis is as for rats and mice.

Skin tumours

Guinea pigs get a skin tumour that causes a *lymphosarcoma* that affects the superficial lymph nodes. It is caused by a retrovirus similar to the one that causes feline leukaemia. It also produces a blood-borne leukaemia and affects the spleen and the liver. The course of the disease lasts only 3–4 weeks, with rapid deterioration, weight loss, increased secondary infections and organ failure. Treatment with chemotherapeutic agents is frequently unsuccessful.

The benign *trichofolliculoma* appears as a solid, cyst-like structure, often over the lumbosacral area dorsally.

Hormonal

Bilateral, non-pruritic hair loss in female guinea pigs is commonly seen in association with cystic ovarian disease. This resolves on treatment of the cystic ovaries.

Miscellaneous

Guinea pigs may barber each other in the same way as rats and mice, particularly boar guinea pigs kept in cramped conditions. It is advised to increase fibre in the cage and provide more space and tubing or other hides so that they can escape from sight of each other. *Cheilitis* is common, and may be due to lack of vitamin C, although a pox virus and *Candida* spp yeasts have also been found.

Digestive disease

Oral

Dental disease is less common in guinea pigs than in rabbits or chinchillas, but probably more common than in other rodents.

Gastrointestinal

Salmonellosis

The bacteria *Salmonella enteritidis* and *Salmonella typhimurium* can both cause enteritis in guinea pigs. The young and debilitated are most at risk. Diarrhoea is uncommon, instead a dull staring coat, weight loss, and abortion are the most commonly seen signs.

Other bacterial disease

Yersinia pseudotuberculosis is a bacteria which can produce intestinal abscesses, in much same way as the real tuberculosis organism, *Mycobacterium tuberculosis*, *Listeria monocytogenes* and *Clostridium perfringens* can cause intestinal disease. As with rats, mice, hamsters and gerbils, guinea pigs are prone to Tyzzer's disease, which is caused by *Clostridium (Bacillus) piliformis*.

Endoparasitic

Balantidium coli may potentially cause disease in humans and causes large intestinal inflammation and profuse diarrhoea in an immunocompromised or debilitated individual. A coccidial organism, *Eimeria caviae*, may also cause problems.

Faecal impaction

This is a not uncommon problem in older guinea pigs, particularly males. It occurs when excessive folds loose skin around the anogenital opening trap faecal pellets. This can create serious constipation problems, and localised infection.

Respiratory disease

Lung infections are common in guinea pigs that are housed with rabbits, as the latter often carry the bacteria *Bordetella bronchiseptica* asymptomatically. This bacteria causes a severe bronchopneumonia in guinea pigs. Other pathogenic bacteria include *Streptococcus pneumoniae*, which is zoonotic. Guinea pigs are often severely affected by respiratory tract disease, becoming dyspnoeic and cyanotic, and the prognosis is frequently guarded. Diagnosis can be made on history, clinical signs, auscultation of the harsh-sounding chest and, if necessary, radiography showing consolidation of the lungs and bronchioalveolar patterns.

Pulmonary adenoma, a form of lung cancer, has been commonly recorded in guinea pigs. The tumour is slow growing and does not metastasise but causes a reduction in functional lung volume. It may be discovered on radiography or may cause clinical dyspnoea in conjunction with a respiratory pathogen.

Cardiovascular disease

Pericarditis has been recorded in conjunction with respiratory tract infection involving *Streptococcus pneumoniae* and may cause heart failure and death.

Urinary tract disease

Kidney

Chronic progressive interstitial nephritis may be a sequel to diabetes mellitus and staphylococcal pododermatitis. Clinically the guinea pig is polyuric and polydipsic and loses weight. Blood parameters may indicate elevated urea and creatinine levels, often with low blood albumin due to urinary protein losses. Urinalysis may detect cystitis, and commonly reveals proteinuria.

Bladder

Calcium oxalate or calcium carbonate crystals are commonly found in the bladder. Older boars may experience urethral obstruction due to dried accessory sex gland secretions, as well as being more susceptible to urolith blockage of the urethra at the os penis.

Secondary, or primary bacterial cystitis is often seen, the former due to irritation of the bladder by the uroliths, the latter leading to clumps of bacteria around which uroliths form. Clinically the affected guinea pig is often dull, lethargic, makes intermittent squeaks of discomfort and may periodically strain, passing small volumes of blood-stained urine. Diagnosis may be made on these signs, along with examination of the sediment of a centrifuged urine sample. Radiography is also helpful, although calcium oxalate crystals are less radio-dense than struvite.

Reproductive tract disease

Cystic ovarian disease

Cystic ovarian disease is common in female guinea pigs over the age of 15 months. It is often bilateral with the cysts such an enormous size, that they cause a swollen abdomen (Plate 17.6). There is frequently bilateral symmetrical alopecia over the flanks.

Reproductive tract tumours

Ovarian granulosa cell tumours often follow on from cystic ovaries. Other forms of reproductive tract cancer include benign leiomyomas, and uterine adenocarcinomas, which are malignant. Diagnosis is made on palpation of an enlarged womb, radiographical or ultrasonographic evidence of enlargement of the tract, or reproductive tract discharge, which may be haemorrhagic.

Dystocia

Dystocia is common in sows mated for the first time when they are over 12 months of age. If a sow has not given birth before this time, the fibrocartilaginous ligament which holds the two sides of the pubis and ischium together will become mineralised and fuse. This ligament normally stretches just before parturition under the influence of the hormone relaxin. If it does not, it significantly narrows the birth canal, and this will lead to dystocias. Any maiden sow older than 7–8 months of age should not be mated.

Pregnancy toxaemia

This is a common condition in late pregnancy and early lactation in overweight first-time mothers. It is most likely to happen in the presence of concurrent disease, such as *Trixicara caviae* mange, which may reduce the sow's appetite. A rapid mobilisation of body fats occurs, producing ketones. These cause a ketoacidosis that is rapidly fatal. Blood glucose levels are very low (below 3 mmol/l) and there is an increase in the acidity of the blood. The urine develops a pH of nearly 5 when it should be 8–9. The sow becomes dull, lethargic and hyperpnoeic and then collapses and becomes comatose. Death can occur within two days, the sow fitting and convulsing towards the end.

Mammary gland tumours

Mammary gland adenomas are common in older sows. They are slow growing but may reach appreciable sizes. In 20–30% of cases the tumour may be a malignant adenocarcinoma.

Mastitis

Poor hygiene predisposes the guinea pig to this condition, with the mammary glands quickly becoming hot and swollen. The bacteria involved (such as *E. coli*) may release endotoxins into the bloodstream which can rapidly cause endotoxic shock.

Musculoskeletal disease

Scurvy

The daily requirement for vitamin C is 10 mg/kg. If the guinea pig is fed non-vitamin-C-containing dry foods, such as rabbit food, and no fresh fruit and vegetables, then it will develop scurvy within 4–5 days. Clinical signs include a staring coat, dental malocclusions, anorexia, slobbers, diarrhoea and immobility due to painful, swollen joints. The guinea pig is in constant pain and clinical signs and history are enough to make a diagnosis. Radiographically though, it can be seen that the epiphyses of the long bones and the costochondral junctions of the ribs are flared laterally, hence younger, still-growing guinea pigs are more susceptible.

Fractures

Fractures of the spine are not uncommon in guinea pigs that are housed with rabbits. The rabbit has tremendously strong hind legs and one well-placed kick can produce a lot of damage to the long and fragile guinea pig backbone. Clinically there is paresis or paralysis of the rear limbs, urinary incontinence etc. depending on the severity of the lesion. This may be confirmed as a fracture or subluxation on radiography. The prognosis is poor.

Ocular disease

Hypovitaminosis C can cause flaking of the skin of the eyelids and periocular area, as can the fungal infection ringworm.

Conjunctivitis is often seen in guinea pigs kept on deep shavings or fine-chopped straw. Traumatic damage to the conjunctiva may be severe, and grass awns can become jammed behind the third eyelid, causing intense damage. These lesions may become secondarily infected with bacteria such as *Pasteurella* or *Streptococcus* spp.

A primary cause of conjunctivitis is *Chlamydophila psittaci*, which cause crusting of the lids, reddening of the conjunctiva, increased tear production and a white-green tinged mucus discharge.

Other ocular problems include hereditary and diabetic cataracts, and a condition known as 'pea eye' where subconjunctival fat accumulates, usually in the ventral fornix area, making the tissue protrude.

Neurological disease

Pregnancy toxaemia

See page 274 for details.

Spinal trauma

See pages 271–2 for details.

DISEASES OF THE CHINCHILLA

Skin disease

Fur slip

Stress and rough handling will cause clumps of fur to fall out spontaneously. This will regrow, but often not for some time.

Fur ring

In male chinchillas, a ring of fur can become wrapped around the penis inside the prepuce. This must be removed before it constricts the blood supply to the end of the penis. Males should be checked monthly, but more frequently during the breeding season – every 2–3 days – as there is evidence that the condition is caused by mounting behaviour.

Fur matting

This is common if a chinchilla's fur is allowed to become damp. They should never be washed, shampooed or allowed to live in damp environmental conditions. Fine pumice sand and Fuller's earth should be provided once or twice daily as a dust bath for fur hygiene and grooming.

Barbering

This is a common problem in chinchillas housed in pairs or groups. The fur of the tail and the whiskers are the most commonly chewed parts, and this increases when environmental stresses such as overcrowding are high, and when the diet is lacking in fibre or when dental disease is present.

Fungal disease

The ringworm organism *Trichophyton mentagrophytes* can cause alopecia in chinchillas, particularly over the nose and pinnae where non-pruritic grey crusts form.

Digestive disease

Oral

Dental disease is probably the most commonly seen ailment of captive chinchillas. The problem is predominantly cheek tooth malocclusion. The latter occurs, as with rabbits, usually due to a lack of abrasive foods in the diet, and possibly combined with a lack of calcium and vitamin D_3 during growth. There is probably a hereditary component to the disease. Elongation of the *crowns* of the maxillary cheek teeth occurs laterally, so that they penetrate the cheek mucosa, with the crowns of the mandibular cheek teeth flaring medially, impinging on the tongue.

In addition, elongation of the *roots* of the third and fourth maxillary cheek-teeth can be a serious cause of pain and discomfort, as they may then penetrate the ocular orbit causing increased tear production and ocular pain. The first and second cheek teeth of the maxilla push up into the floor of the nasal passages and sinuses causing sneezing and nasal discharge. The mandibular cheek teeth roots penetrate the ventral aspect of the jaw and can be felt as a series of bumps along its lower border.

When the molars overgrow, gaps form between individual molars. These allow food particles to become wedged between the molars, which decays, creating periodontal disease and eventually abscesses.

Diagnosis of these problems can be made on clinical signs and radiography. Clinically, the chinchilla is often seen to be drooling saliva (the so-called 'slobbers'). It may also be anorectic, have lost weight and started consuming softer fresh foods rather than the harder dry pellets.

Gastrointestinal

Colic

Colic is often due to feeding sugary food items such as banana. When it has colic, the chinchilla is often dull, and droppings may be reduced or smaller than normal. There may be teeth grinding and a hunched appearance.

Caecocolic disease

Caecocolic disease occurs rarely in chinchillas, but is more likely if the chinchilla is suffering from severe diarrhoea. The caecum or proximal colon may become involved in an intussusception or a torsion. This is an acute crisis. The chinchilla is presented in severe pain, usually extremely dull and hunched in posture, often grinding its teeth and drooling saliva, and occasionally rolling around the cage. History of previous diarrhoea, and a lack of faecal pellet production should alert one to the possibility of caecocolic disease. Loops of bowel in the caudal and ventral portions of the abdomen, grossly swollen with gas, are seen on radiograph. The prognosis for these cases is poor, and immediate surgery is required.

Constipation

Constipation is occasionally seen, most commonly as a sequel to: dental disease; obesity; late stage pregnancy; intestinal or abdominal surgery; sudden change in diet to a less fibrous, higher protein (such as an all-seed diet) diet. The chinchilla may produce scant, small faecal pellets for a number of days, and then none at all. It may continue to strain to pass faeces during this time, even prolapsing the rectum in the process. Chinchillas so affected are often uncomfortable, and may sit hunched with tucked in abdomens.

Diarrhoea

Surprisingly, diarrhoea is less common in the chinchilla than constipation.

Bacterial: any of the bacteria mentioned in the section on guinea pigs may cause diarrhoea, with the *E. coli* and *Salmonella* spp families appearing high up on the list. *Clostridia* spp enterotoxaemia will occur if inappropriate antibiotics are used (see page 295).

Endoparasitic: Giardia is a single-celled protozoal parasite is found in healthy and sick chinchillas alike, and therefore its role in disease is not fully understood. It is however a potential hazard to humans as giardiasis is a zoonotic disease. It is currently thought that poor diet, stress or concurrent disease allows the normally present *Giardia* spp parasite to multiply up to sufficient numbers in the large bowel to cause diarrhoea. There is often the presence of soiled fur around the rear, and a generally dull chinchilla. Diagnosis is by finding the motile, single-celled organisms on microscope examination of fresh faeces samples suspended in isotonic saline. They have an oval outline with a characteristic 'face' of two dark spots for eyes and a dark line beneath for a 'mouth'. They have eight flagellae.

Hepatic lipidosis

Many chinchillas are overweight. They may then go on to develop dental problems or other conditions which may cause anorexia. Fat reserves are mobilised and the liver becomes swamped in fat compounds to the point at which it can no longer perform its job satisfactorily. The chinchilla may then go into liver failure, with dullness and anorexia being the two most commonly seen non-specific signs. Very rarely jaundice occurs. Diagnosis is made on finding elevated bile acid levels in conjunction with elevated AST (aspartamine transferase) and often GGT (gamma glutamyl transferase) levels in the blood, and an enlarged liver shadow on radiography.

Respiratory disease

Pneumonia is frequently found in chinchillas housed in damp and drafty conditions, but it may occur in any individual. The pathogens chiefly involved are bacteria such as *Bordetella bron-*

chiseptica, Streptococcus pneumoniae, Pasteurella pneumotropica, and *Pseudomonas* spp. Diagnosis and treatment is as for guinea pigs.

Cardiovascular disease

Heart murmurs have been associated with valvular defects and dilated cardiomyopathies. The chinchilla may be asymptomatic or show signs of lethargy and weakness.

Urinary tract disease

Urinary crystalline deposits have been seen in chinchillas and resemble those found in guinea pigs. Diagnosis and treatment is as for guinea pigs.

Reproductive tract disease

Dystocia occurs infrequently. There appears to be no associated significant separation of the pelvis as is seen in the guinea pig, and therefore age at first breeding is not so critical.

Musculoskeletal disease

Fractures are relatively common in chinchillas, and tend to occur in the longer, slender bones such as the tibia and femur.

Ocular disease

Conjunctivitis presents as dampened fur around the eyes, with tear overflow. It may be due to excessive dust bathing with resultant foreign body irritation, or to the bacteria *Chlamydophila psittaci*. Alternatively, dental disease, such as that described above, may be present, so the problem may not be a true conjunctivitis.

Neurological disease

Several causes of fitting have been described in chinchillas. These include the virus which causes *lymphocytic choriomeningitis* (see page 267), as well as the bacteria *Listeria monocytogenes*, which may be spread by rodents.

DISEASES OF THE CHIPMUNK

Skin disease

Ectoparasitic

Chipmunks may be susceptible to burrowing mites such as *Notoedres muris* as well as the more common *Sarcoptes* spp. In addition they may become infested with the opportunist harvest mite *Neotrombicula autumnalis* as well as the avian red cage mite *Dermanyssus gallinae*. The latter can cause anaemia and is commonly found where birds nest and roost.

Bacterial

Bacteria such as those described above for rats and mice are commonly isolated from the skin of chipmunks and their associated abscesses. Abscesses are common in chipmunks housed in groups as they frequently fight amongst themselves.

Digestive disease

Oral

Overgrown incisors are common due to trauma to one or more incisors from a fall etc. Periodontal disease may occur as a sequel to fracture of an incisor, or due to foreign body impaction when gnawing. Overgrowth or damage of the incisors may cause them to impinge on the floor of the nasal passage. The chipmunk often shows signs of a runny nose with a copious discharge.

Gastrointestinal

Chipmunks suffer diarrhoea from similar bacterial causes as are seen in rats and mice, with *Yersinia pseudotuberculosis* and *Salmonella* spp being commonly seen. Tyzzer's disease (*Bacillus piliformis*), which may cause liver damage, is also seen.

Respiratory disease

Pneumonia is frequently of a bacterial nature, and often occurs after periods of stress such as re-homing and handling. In addition, it is thought that the human influenza virus may be transmissible to chipmunks.

Cardiovascular disease

Chipmunks are highly-strung creatures and care should be taken to handle them little, if at all, and to do so carefully and in dimmed lighting. Rough handling and high levels of stress can lead to fitting and cardiac arrest.

Urinary tract disease

Because chipmunks are more omnivorous than most rodents, struvite crystals are seen, along with the more common calcium oxalate. *E. coli* bacterial cystitis is frequently seen at the same time. Since they have a longer urethra and an os penis, urolithiasis causes more problems for males than for females. The chipmunk often strains to pass urine and may squeal at the same time. Haematuria may be seen, and a swollen penis found on close physical examination. The calculi may be demonstrated radiographically and in urine samples.

Reproductive tract disease

Hypocalcaemic paralysis

Hypocalcaemic paralysis can occur soon after parturition, particularly if the chipmunk is on a poor-quality all-seed diet. The female appears lethargic, often is not suckling the young and may become unconscious.

Uterine disease

Uterine infections such as pyometras are often seen in chipmunks. There may be a vulval discharge, sometimes tinged with blood, and the female chipmunk is often anorectic, lethargic and sometimes polydipsic. Metritis may be seen shortly after parturition, with the female presenting as collapsed and weakened with a swollen abdomen and signs of peritonitis.

Mammary gland disease

Mastitis is uncommon, but bacteria such as *E. coli*, *Klebsiella* spp and *Staphylococcus* spp have been isolated. More commonly seen are mammary gland tumours. They are usually fibroadenomas as in rats. They are benign and rapidly growing.

Musculoskeletal disease

Fractures are very common in chipmunks and often involve the spine. Chipmunks are very acrobatic creatures and falls from ropes and the sides or roof of the wire cage are common. If a spinal fracture is suspected, radiography may be performed with the chipmunk conscious and restrained in a perspex box, or under sedation, to confirm it. The prognosis is poor and euthanasia is advised in these cases.

Neurological disease

Fitting is a common problem in chipmunks housed in rooms with television sets, computer terminals and other items of electronic equipment which emit radiowaves on the 50–60 Hertz wavelength. In addition, there is some evidence that some chipmunks may be prone to hereditary epilepsy. Finally, bacteria such as *Listeria monocytogenes* and *Streptococcus pneumoniae*, protozoa such as *Toxoplasma gondii*, as well as viruses such as the cause of *lymphocytic choriomeningitis* may also cause central nervous system disease whose signs include seizures, coma and death.

DISEASES OF THE FERRET

Skin disease

Ectoparasitic

Mites

The commonly seen *Otodectes cynotis*, or ear mite, causes intense ear irritation, and the production of copious black wax. This may lead on to otitis externa, ofitis interna and vestibular syndrome with loss of balance control. It may spill over on to the side of the face creating a traumatised area and pyoderma. Diagnosis is made by finding the typical mites on wax samples, the closed apodemes of the *Otodectes* family being diagnostic.

Less commonly seen is the burrowing mite *Sarcoptes scabei* which can cause intense pruritus over the head, ears, paws and tail. It may however be totally confined to the feet, although this form is uncommon. Diagnosis is made on skin scrapings of the affected areas and finding the rounded, adult mite.

Fleas

The domestic cat and dog fleas *Ctenocephalides felis* and *canis* may be found in a domestic situation. Many ferrets are used in the United Kingdom for hunting, and therefore the rabbit flea *Spilopsyllus cuniculi* or the 'stick tight' flea *Echidnophaga* spp may also be seen, the former commonly found more on the ears of the ferret.

Ticks

The presence of ticks such as *Ixodes ricinus* are commonly found in ferrets used for hunting.

Bacterial

Ferrets kept together will often play fight or worse, and ferrets' mouths are not the cleanest of places! Abscesses frequently develop, particularly in the cervical area. Commonly isolated bacteria include *Streptococcus* spp, *Staphylococcus* spp, *Actinomyces pyogenes*, *Pasteurella* spp, and *E. coli*. The swellings these abscesses produce may be massive in size but the ferret generally remains bright as they are well walled off. *Actinomyces pyogenes* infections often produce a copious green-coloured pus, and may be associated with immunosuppressive conditions.

Fungal

Ringworm due to *Microsporum canis* or *Trichophyton mentagrophytes* is relatively uncommon in the ferret.

Viral

Canine distemper virus (CDV), a paramyxovirus, may affect the skin about a week after infection. A rash appears over the chin and ventrum followed by brown crusts, particularly around the eyes and chin. A nasal discharge may be present. Eventually the cornified layer of the foot pads increases, giving canine distemper its other name of 'hard pad'. Unfortunately, unless vaccinated, most ferrets will die from canine distemper between 7–21 days after contracting the virus.

Skin tumours

Squamous cell carcinomas are the most frequently reported skin neoplasm in ferrets, occurring on the head, along the nose and ear tips in particular. They tend to be rapidly spreading and malignant tumours in ferrets. Sebaceous epitheliomas and basal cell tumours are commonly seen on the head, neck and shoulders and are well defined, benign tumours, but may ulcerate. Fibrosarcomas have been reported in response to injection site reactions as is seen in cats.

Hormonal

Hyperadrenocorticism is the most commonly seen cause of non-pruritic alopecia in the ferret (although some may be pruritic!). Hair loss is mainly over the dorsum and flanks initially. Secondary signs of hyperadrenocortical disease are also present. These include pendulous abdomen, thinning of the skin, weight gain etc.

   In male ferrets, other hormonal causes of skin abnormalities include. Leydig/interstitial cell tumours producing excess testosterone and Sertoli cell tumours producing excess oestrogens. In females, granulosa cell tumours of the ovaries have been associated with hair loss, as has the common hyperoestrogen condition of unmated entire females.

Digestive disease

Oral

Dental disease is extremely common in ferrets over 18 months of age that have been fed on tinned diets. Severe tartar or calculus accumulation and periodontal disease are easily recognisable by reluctance to eat, enlarged local lymph nodes, foul breath and bleeding gums.

Gastric

Gastric ulceration is a common problem in ferrets and is associated with *Helicobacter mustelae* infection. This is a member of a family of bacteria known for its ability to cause ulcers in humans. Gastric tumours and renal disease may also lead to gastric ulcer development, as will gastric foreign bodies.

   The clinical signs vary from a dull ferret, with abdominal pain and salivation, to a ferret which vomits, sometimes with melaena present in the vomitus. Alternatively melaenic faeces may be passed. Further tests involve blood tests for renal disease, radiographs, both plain and barium studies, which may highlight peptic and duodenal ulcers as well as foreign bodies and ultimately gastric biopsy to demonstrate *Helicobacter mustelae*. Culturing techniques for this bacteria are complicated and the bacteria often does not survive transport to the laboratory.

Intestinal

Proliferative ileitis

Proliferative ileitis is similar to the 'wet tail' seen in hamsters and is due to *Lawsonia intracellularis*. It is passed from one ferret to another, often, during the suckling period, from dam to offspring. The bacteria causes thickening of the lining of the ileum and proximal colon, which results in a green, mucoid, bloody diarrhoea and weight loss in the affected ferret. Diagnosis is made on the clinical signs primarily which are unlike almost any other condition. Biopsy of the ileum may be performed under general anaesthetic to demonstrate the bacteria and the loss of structure of the ileum.

Intestinal lymphoma

This condition is relatively uncommon, but lymphoma of the mesenteric lymph nodes and the liver are commonly seen in older ferrets. This may present as vague gastrointestinal signs, such as constipation, liver disease or even as apparently acute liver failure with jaundice.

Endoparasitic disease

Coccidiosis and giardiasis have both been described as causes of lethargy, diarrhoea and dehydration. Nematode and cestode parasites are rarely seen, although hunting individuals are more likely to be exposed to these parasites, with *Toxocara* spp and *Toxascaris* spp being the most commonly seen. Rarely do they cause clinical disease.

Viral disease

Ferrets suffer from a form of parvovirus known as Aleutian disease. This is particularly lethal to mink, but in ferrets it produces an unpleasant diarrhoea, although it is rarely fatal. It may produce melaenic faeces, fever, loss of weight and a number of other immune-system mediated symptoms.

Canine distemper can produce gastrointestinal signs such as diarrhoea. In addition, the influenza virus C may also be responsible for mild diarrhoea.

A member of the rotavirus family can cause diarrhoea in young, unweaned and recently weaned ferrets.

Other bacterial causes of diarrhoea

Salmonellosis due to *Salmonella typhimurium* has been reported. As it poses a zoonotic risk to handlers, it is fortunate that the incidence is very low.

Liver disease

The liver is commonly affected by lymphoma, although primary cancer of the liver is uncommon. Hepatic lipidosis has been recorded in persistently anorectic ferrets. In all of these cases the ferret may simply appear to be vaguely unwell, jaundice being a relatively uncommon feature. Blood results may suggest a rise in ALT (alanine aminotransferase) levels above 275 IU/l (Hillyer & Quesenberry, 1997), but it often requires ultrasonographic and biopsy tests to make a diagnosis.

Respiratory disease

Viral

The most serious pathogen of the ferret's respiratory system is canine distemper virus (CDV). This is a paramyxovirus, in the same family group as measles. The virus is spread by aerosol from one infected ferret or canid to another, when they sneeze or breathe. It may also be transmitted on a handler's hands and clothing. The virus gains access through the upper airways and incubates inside the ferret for 7–10 days, spreading throughout the body via the bloodstream.

The first signs of the disease occur on the chin and ventrum of the ferret where an erythematous rash appears, followed by brown, crusting lesions around the lips. The ferret may be feverish and may have a serous oculonasal discharge. Later in the course of the disease the foot pads may thicken to create the classical 'hard pad'. It is the secondary bacterial infections of the lungs on top of widespread immunosuppression which is often the reason for the death of an infected ferret. Towards the end of the disease fitting, nystagmus and generalised incoordination are all seen. The condition is fatal in nearly all cases of unvaccinated ferrets. Diagnosis is made on clinical signs, demonstration of viral antigens in the bloodstream and/or mucus secretions of the ferret.

Another viral respiratory condition is the human influenza C virus, an orthomyxovirus. This is transmissible from human to ferret and back again. It causes a mainly upper airway disease with a systemic phase producing pyrexia for 3–4 days.

Bacterial

Bacterial lung infections are not so common a problem, although they do often follow as secondary invaders after viral infections. Diagnosis is made on lung radiographs, lung washes and isolation of the bacteria, clinically harsh-sounding lungs, often pyrexia and occasionally a cough.

Cardiovascular disease

Cardiomyopathy

Dilated cardiomyopathy is the most commonly seen, with signs of congestive cardiac failure including lethargy, fluid respiratory noises, weight loss, polydipsia, ascites and audible systolic murmurs on auscultation of the chest. In the ferret the heart normally occupies the space bounded by the sixth to the seventh or eighth ribs. The area of heart sound may also be enlarged. Diagnosis is made on radiographic signs of lung congestion, occasionally pleural effusion and an enlarged cardiac shadow, ECG changes and ultrasonographic demonstration of heart-wall thinning and valvular incompetence. Hypertrophic cardiomyopathy is rarely seen.

Endocardiosis

Endocardiosis is increasingly recognised in ageing ferrets. The presenting signs are similar to those seen in dogs with the same condition, with productive coughs, lethargy and, in more serious cases, heart failure with ascites and blue, congested membranes. Diagnosis is by auscultation, clinical signs and ultrasonographic demonstration of valvular incompetence and thickening.

Urinary tract disease

Kidney

Cystic kidney disease appears to be inherited in ferrets. These are often asymptomatic and go unnoticed in the majority of cases.

Bladder

Urolithiasis is a particular problem in pregnant female ferrets and is mainly due to the build up of struvite or magnesium ammonium phosphate crystals. The problem is seen in ferrets that are fed protein from a plant source as well as animal, such as is found in dog food. This creates an alkaline urine pH and allows these salts to precipitate. The provision of solely animal proteins in the diet leads to acidic urine and dissolution of the calculi. Pregnant jills are susceptible as they are mobilising large volumes of minerals from their bones for foetal development and milk production.

Male ferrets may experience obstruction at the os penis if large enough calculi form. They may present as dull ferrets, straining to urinate and sometimes prolapsing the rectum in the process. The prepuce is often swollen, the abdomen tense and occasionally crystals may be seen on the hairs around the prepuce. Radiography will confirm the diagnosis.

Endocrine disease

Adrenal

Hyperadrenocorticism is one of the prime causes of non-pruritic alopecia in the ferret (see above). Other clinical signs include enlargement of the prostate and urethral blockage in male ferrets, and enlargement of the vulva in female ferrets. Unusually, for a hormonal condition, pruritus may be seen, usually between the shoulder blades, where an erythematous rash may appear. Diagnosis is made based on clinical signs and ultrasonography of the adrenal glands showing enlargement. ACTH stimulation and dexamethasone suppression tests do not seem to work in ferrets.

Diabetes mellitus

Diabetes mellitus is uncommon in ferrets, but presents as a disease similar to that seen in cats.

Hypoglycaemia

Hypoglycaemia may occur due to prolonged fasting (ferrets should not1 be fasted for more than 4–6 hours due to their high metabolic rates), over-dosage with insulin in a diabetic case or due to an insulinoma (an insulin secreting pancreatic tumour). These are extremely common in ferrets in the United States of America, where considerable line breeding of ferrets for the pet trade has led to a narrowed gene pool, but in the United Kingdom this condition is so far uncommon.

Hyperoestrogenism

For details see below.

Reproductive tract disease

Pregnancy toxaemia

Pregnancy toxaemia is a condition similar to that seen in the guinea pig. It occurs in late gestation, often in a first time mother, who experiences a period of anorexia due to disease, food withdrawal or change etc. The result is mobilization of body fats and the production of ketones which reduce the pH of the bloodstream. A toxaemia develops, leading to dullness, lethargy, vomiting, dehydration, alopecia, neurological signs, abortion and death of the jill.

Dystocia

Dystocia is relatively uncommon in the ferret. It is more common in jills carrying a small litter. Corticosteroid hormone production by the foetal kits is the trigger for labour. If there is insufficient hormone produced, the jill may go overdue. If she exceeds day 43 of gestation, the kits will almost certainly die and labour may need to be induced.

Mastitis

Mastitis may occur as an acute illness immediately after parturition. The mammary gland becomes swollen and painful, and a potentially fatal toxaemia may develop if the mammary gland becomes gangrenous. The bacteria commonly present in these cases are *Streptococcus* spp and *E. coli* family members.

A more chronic condition is seen due to the bacteria *Staphylococcus intermedius*. This form of mastitis is highly infectious between jills and destroys much of the mammary tissue, leaving scar tissue and pockets of infection.

Pyometra and metritis

Metritis occurs, as in many species, immediately after parturition and may cause an acute toxic reaction in the jill. The uterus may enlarge and fill with infected bloody discharge. The jill may be very dull and pyrexic at this stage, and have no milk production.

Pyometra occurs at any stage, and is manifested by a dark, foul-smelling vulval discharge, polydipsia and sometimes toxaemia. This is due to the *E. coli* type bacteria that is often present. Occasionally, a closed pyometra with no external discharge may occur. The jill may present as dull, polydipsic, lethargic and occasionally vomiting. Palpation of the abdomen reveals a swollen uterus in the caudal dorsal abdomen. The diagnosis may be confirmed with radiography or ultrasonography.

Hyperoestrogenism

It is well known that an entire female will remain in oestrus for the whole of the breeding season (March–October), unless she is mated or chemically brought out of oestrus. This chronic, long-term exposure to oestrogen results in often fatal anaemia from bone marrow suppression. The jill presents as tachypnoeic, with pale, petechiated mucous membranes, lethargic and collapsed. Early signs though are gradual, and the jill is seen with a prominently swollen vulva, symmetrical alopecia of the flanks, and often a vulval discharge.

Prostatic disease

Prostate cysts are particularly common in ferrets with an actively secreting adrenal gland tumour. The prostate is so shaped in the ferret that it will obstruct the urethra, and therefore signs of an inability to pass urine may be observed.

Musculoskeletal disease

Fractures in ferrets are uncommon, although the spine is the most commonly affected. Posterior paresis or paralysis is often associated with vertebral fractures, but may also be a sign of cardiovascular disease, hypoglycaemia or anaemia (see above). Diagnosis is by radiography and tests listed above.

Ocular disease

Ophthalmia neonatorum, a failure of the kits' eyes to open, is often due to bacteria from the *Staphylococcus* and *Streptococcus* families.

Other ocular problems include crusting and weeping associated with canine distemper virus, photophobia associated with the influenza virus, conjunctivitis, night blindness and cataracts associated with hypovitaminosis A. Corneal ulcers due to trauma and local infections are common in ferrets.

Neurological disease

Fitting may be seen towards the end stages of canine distemper virus infection, and may be seen in the hypoglycaemic syndrome, as well as in severe anaemia. Posterior paresis may be associated with spinal trauma, cardiovascular disease, hypoglycaemia, anaemia and canine distemper virus.

References and further reading

Beynon, P.H. and Cooper, J.E. (1991) *Manual of Exotic Pets, 3rd edn*. BSAVA, Cheltenham.

Harkness, J.E. and Wagner, J.E. (1995) *The Biology and Medicine of Rabbits and Rodents, 4th edn*. Lea and Febiger, Philadelphia.

Hillyer, V.E. and Quesenberry, K.E. (1997) *Ferrets, Rabbits and Rodents: Clinical Medicine and Surgery*. W.B. Saunders, Philadelphia.

Meredith, A. and Redrobe, S. (2001) *Manual of Exotic Pets, 4th edn*. BSAVA, Cheltenham.

Okerman, L. (1994) *Diseases of Domestic Rabbits, 2nd edn*. Blackwell Scientific Publications, Oxford.

Richardson, V.C.G. (1992) *Diseases of Domestic Guinea Pigs*. Blackwell Science, Oxford.

Chapter 18

An Overview of Small Mammal Therapeutics

FLUID THERAPY

Maintenance requirements

In most small mammals there is very little water lost as sweat, as rodents, and lagomorphs have little or no skin sweat glands, and most do not pant either. Increased metabolic rates, and the fact that their size is small in most cases, leads to a large lung surface area in relation to volume. Hence large amounts of fluids are lost during normal respiration. In addition, glomerular filtration rates are higher, due to the higher metabolic rates seen in small mammals. This makes their daily maintenance fluid requirement per kg nearly double those seen in larger mammals. Some values are given in Table 18.1.

The effect of disease on fluid requirements

With any disease, the need for fluids increases, even if no obvious fluid loss occurs. Respiratory disease is not an uncommon finding in small mammals, especially rabbits, rats and mice. In these animals often chronic levels of lung infection are present, with increased respiratory secretions being the result. Fluid loss can therefore be appreciable via this route.

Individuals suffering from diarrhoea will experience fluid loss and often metabolic acidosis due to the prolonged loss of bicarbonate.

Another, less obvious, route of fluid and electrolyte loss is through skin disease. Rabbits (in particular those kept in wet or unsanitary conditions) will contract skin infections from environmental bacterial organisms such as *Pseudomonas* spp. These produce lesions which resemble

chemical or thermal burns, and leave large areas of weeping, exudative skin causing further fluid loss.

Post-surgical fluid requirements

Surgical procedures are being performed more and more frequently on small mammals in both routine and emergency situations. These may cause intrasurgical haemorrhaging, necessitating vascular support with an aqueous electrolyte solution or, in more serious blood losses (>10%), colloidal fluids or even blood transfusions. Even if surgery is relatively bloodless there are inevitable losses via the respiratory route due to the drying nature of the gases used to deliver the anaesthetics.

In addition, many patients are not able to drink immediately after surgery. Some forms of surgery, such as incisor extraction in rabbits suffering from malocclusion, will lead to inappetance for a period of time. Dehydration will result, as many rabbits gain the majority of their fluid intake from their vegetable diets.

Electrolyte replacement

Electrolyte replacement can be necessary in cases of chronic diarrhoea such as in coccidiosis in rabbits or wet-tail in hamsters. Here gut pathology leads to maldigestion and/or malabsorption and loss of food, water and electrolytes to waste. The main electrolyte losses are bicarbonate and potassium leading to metabolic acidosis.

Small herbivores, particularly rabbits, rarely vomit and so electrolyte loss by that note is unlikely to occur. However exceptions are ferrets which can regurgitate food, or may have more serious problems with stomach ulceration due to bacteria such as *Helicobacter mustelae*. In these cases metabolic alkalosis may result.

Fluid types used in small mammal practice

A number of fluid types are commonly used in small mammal practice (Fig. 18.1).

Lactated Ringer's/Hartmann's

As with cats and dogs, lactated Ringer's solution is useful as a general purpose rehydration and maintenance fluid. It is particularly useful for small mammals suffering from metabolic acidosis, such as those described above with chronic gas-trointestinal problems, but can also be used for fluid therapy after routine surgical procedures.

Glucose/saline combinations

Glucose/saline is useful for small mammals, as they may have been through periods of anorexia prior to treatment, and therefore may well be borderline hypoglycaemic. Glucose/saline combinations are also useful for cases of urethral obstruction, such as ferret urolithiasis.

Protein amino acid/B vitamin supplements

Protein and vitamin supplements are useful for nutritional support. Such products as Duphalyte® may be used at the rate of 1 ml/kg/day. These supplements are particularly good in cases where the patient is malnourished or has been suffering from a protein-losing enteropathy or nephro-pathy. It is also a useful supplement for patients with hepatic disease or severe exudative skin diseases.

Colloidal fluids

These are of use in rabbits, guinea pigs and chin-chillas, and even rats which may be given an intra-venous bolus. They are used when a serious loss of blood occurs in order to support central blood

Table 18.1 Maintenance fluid values for selected small mammals.

Species	Fluid maintenance values
Rabbit	80–100 ml/kg/day
Guinea pig	100 ml/kg/day
Chinchilla	100 ml/kg/day
Rodent	90–100 ml/kg/day
Ferret	75–100 ml/kg/day

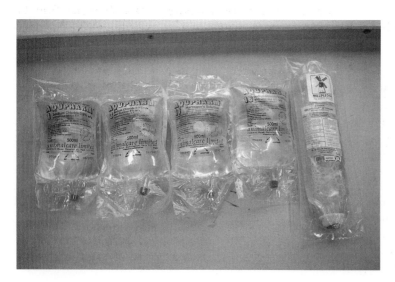

Fig. 18.1 Fluid types used in small mammal practice.

pressure. This may be a temporary measure whilst a blood donor is selected, or, if none is available, the only means of attempting to support such a patient.

Blood transfusions

Blood transfusions are sometimes performed if packed cell volume (PCV) levels start to drop below 20%. They are best performed by direct, same species to species transfers (i.e. rat to rat, and guinea pig to guinea pig). The donor may have 1% body weight in blood removed without any deleterious effects, assuming it is healthy. The sample is best taken directly into a pre-heparinised syringe, or use citrate acid dextrose if available at 1 ml of anticoagulant to 5–6 ml of blood, and immediately transfer it in bolus fashion to the donor. The use of intravenous catheters is advised, as administration should be slow, giving 1 ml over a period of 5–6 minutes. Therefore sedation, or good restraint, is required. Very little information is currently available about cross-matching blood groups of small mammals, although ferrets, it seems, do not have detectable groups. Intraosseous donations may be made if vascular access is not possible.

Oral fluids and electrolytes

Oral fluids may be used in small mammal practice for those patients experiencing mild dehydration, and for home administration. The most useful products contain probiotics which aid the return to normal digestive function.

Calculation of fluid requirements

A lot of fluid is normally taken in as food i.e. in the form of fresh vegetation. This is difficult to take into consideration when calculating fluid needed, and therefore it is safer to assume that the debilitated small mammal will not be eating enough for it to matter. Once it is appreciated that maintenance for most small mammals is double that required for the average cat or dog, then deficits may be calculated in the same manner. Assume that 1% dehydration equates with

needing to supply 10 ml/kg fluid replacement, in addition to maintenance requirements.

Then estimate the percentage of dehydration of the patient as follows:

- 3–5% dehydrated – increased thirst, slight lethargy, tacky mucous membranes
- 7–10% dehydrated – increased thirst, anorexia, dullness, tenting of the skin and slow return to normal, dry mucous membranes, dull corneas
- 10–15% dehydrated – dull to comatose, skin remains tented after pinching, desiccating mucous membranes.

Alternatively if a blood sample may be obtained, a 1% increase in PCV, associated with an increase in total proteins, may be assumed to equate to 10 ml/kg fluid deficit (see Table 18.2).

These deficits may be large and difficult to replenish rapidly. Indeed, it may be dangerous to overload the patient's system with these fluid levels all in one go. Therefore the following protocol is worth following to ensure fluid overload, renal shutdown and pulmonary oedema are avoided:

- **Day one:** Maintenance fluid levels +50% of calculated dehydration factor
- **Day two:** Maintenance fluid levels +50% of calculated dehydration factor
- **Day three:** Maintenance fluid levels

If the dehydration levels are so severe that volumes are still too large to give at any one time, it may be necessary to take 72 rather than 48 hours to replace the calculated deficit.

Table 18.2 Comparison of normal packed cell volume (PCV) and total proteins for selected small mammals. (*NB* the range given for hamsters is an average of Syrian and Russian hamster values.)

Species	PCV range l/l	Total protein g/l
Ferret	0.44–0.6	51–74
Rabbit	0.36–0.48	54–75
Guinea pig	0.37–0.48	46–62
Chinchilla	0.32–0.46	50–60
Rat	0.36–0.48	56–76
Mouse	0.39–0.49	35–72
Gerbil	0.43–0.49	43–85
Hamster	0.36–0.55 average	45–75 average

In addition, in those species such as ferrets, which can vomit, the fluid lost in vomitus expelled should be considered, assuming 2 ml/kg per vomit.

In other species such as the small herbivores, where diarrhoea only is the norm, it is much more difficult to make estimations, although fluid losses may approach 100–150 ml/kg per day.

Equipment for fluid administration

Because the creatures involved are small, the equipment needed is correspondingly small in size. The blood vessels available for intravenous medication, for example, are often 30–50% smaller than their cat and dog counterparts.

Catheters

The catheters that are most useful for small mammals are the series of butterfly catheters available, often adapted from human paediatric medicine. It is advisable to flush it with heparinised saline, prior to use, to prevent clotting. 25–27 gauge sizes are recommended and will cope with venous access for rabbits, guinea pigs, chinchillas and ferrets. Occasionally a 28 or 29 gauge catheter may be needed to catheterise a lateral tail vein in a rat or mouse, although 27 gauge catheters often suffice (Fig. 18.2).

Hypodermic or spinal needles

Hypodermic and spinal needles are useful for the administration of intraosseous, intraperitoneal and subcutaneous fluids. The intraosseous route may be the only method of giving central venous support in very small patients, or patients where vascular collapse is occurring. The proximal femur, tibia or humerus may be used. Entry can be gained by using hypodermic or spinal needles. Spinal needles are preferable because they have a central stylet to prevent clogging of the needle lumen with bone fragments after insertion. 23–25 gauge spinal needles are usually sufficient.

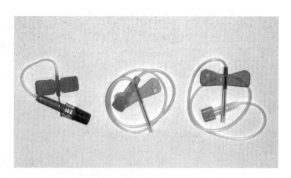

Fig. 18.2 A selection of butterfly catheters for intravenous use in small mammals.

Hypodermic needles may be used for the same purpose, although the risks of blockage are higher. Hypodermic needles may also be used of course for the administration of intraperitoneal and subcutaneous fluids. Generally 23–25 gauge hypodermic needles are sufficient for the task.

Nasogastric tubes

Nasogastric tubes are often used in small mammals in order to provide nutritional support in as stress-free a manner as possible. They are also useful as a route for fluid administration. It should be noted though that in severely dehydrated individuals, there is no way that all of the fluid deficits may be replaced via this route alone. This is due to the limited fluid capacity of the stomach of these species, as well as the real possibility that gut pathology may exist. This route is therefore restricted for use in facilitating fluid replacement, and is used mainly for nutritional support and rehydrating the gut microflora.

Syringe drivers

For continuous fluid administration, such as is required for intravenous and intraosseous fluid administration, syringe drivers are being used more and more (Fig. 18.3). Their advantage is that

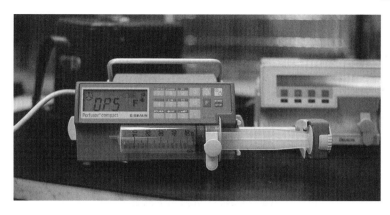

Fig. 18.3 A typical syringe driver used for cat and dog medicine may be adapted for small mammal use.

small volumes, such as a fraction of a millilitre may be administered accurately per hour. An error of 1–2 ml in some of the species dealt with over an hour could be equivalent to an overperfusion of 50–100%! In addition, it is almost impossible to keep gravity fed drip sets running at these low rates.

Intravenous drip tubing

Particular fine drip tubing is available for attachment to syringes and syringe-driver units. It is useful if these are luer locking, as this enhances safety and prevents disconnection when the patient moves. It may be necessary to purchase a sheath, such as is available for protecting household electrical cables, to cover drip tubing, as most of the small herbivores are experts at removing or chewing through plastic drip tubing!

Elizabethan collars

It may be necessary to place some of the small herbivores into an Elizabethan-style collar as they are the world's greatest chewers! These can be purchased as cage bird collars and adapted to fit even the smallest of rodents.

Routes of fluid administration

As with cats and dogs the same medical principles broadly apply, and there are five main routes of administration available to the clinician or veteri-nary nurse. These routes all have their advantages and disadvantages, given in Table 18.3.

Oral

Rabbit

The oral route is not a very good route for seriously debilitated rabbits, but it is useful for those with naso-oesophageal feeding tubes in place (see page 255). It may also be useful for mild cases of dehydration where owners wish to home treat their pet. This route though is restricted to small volumes, with a maximum of 10 ml/kg administered at any one time.

Rat, mouse, gerbil and hamster

Gavage (stomach) tubes or avian straight crop tubes can be used to place fluids directly into the rodent oesophagus. The rodent needs to be firmly scruffed to adequately restrain it and to keep the head and oesophagus in a straight line. This method is often stressful but the alternative is to syringe fluids into the mouth, which often does not work as rodents can close off the back of the mouth with their cheek folds. Maximum volumes which can be given via the oral route in rodents vary from 5–10 ml/kg. Naso-oesophageal or gastric tubes are not a viable option in rodents due to their small size.

Guinea pig and chinchilla

Naso-oesophageal or gastric tubes may be placed and doses of 10 ml/kg may be administered at any

Table 18.3 The advantages and disadvantages of various fluid therapy routes in small mammals.

	Advantages	Disadvantages
Oral	• Reduced stress • Well accepted • Physiological route • Minimal tissue trauma • Rehydrate gut flora (useful for herbivores)	• May increase stress in guinea pigs • Risk of aspiration pneumonia in ferrets • Not useful in gut diseases • Slow rates of rehydration • Maximum volume is 10 ml/kg in most species
Subcutaneous	• Large volumes may be given, reducing dosing frequency and stress • Minimal risk of organ puncture	• Guinea pigs react badly to scruff injections, fur slip is a problem in chinchillas • Slow rehydration rates • May impede respiration due to pressure on chest wall • Hypotonic or isotonic fluids only
Intraperitoneal	• Large volumes may be given • Uptake faster than subcutaneous • Minimal discomfort	• Risk of organ puncture (particularly large intestines and caecum in herbivores) • Stressful positioning (dorsal recumbancy) • Pressure on diaphragm may increase respiratory effort needed • Isotonic or hypotonic fluids only
Intravenous	• Rapid central venous support • Maybe used for continuous perfusion • Can be used for colloidal fluids, hypertonic glucose (for pregnancy toxaemias in ferrets and guinea pigs) and blood transfusions	• Minimal peripheral access in some species (e.g. hamsters, gerbils) • Increased vessel fragility due to small patient size • Requires increased levels of operator skill
Intraosseous	• Rapid support of central venous system • Useful in collapsed and very small patients where vascular access is difficult • May still be used for blood transfusions • Minimal risk of organ damage	• Not useful in fragile bones or metabolic bone disease • Not useful in cases of bone fractures or osteomyelitis • Increased risk of infection • Painful procedure requiring sedation/analgesia • Continuous perfusion required (syringe drivers) otherwise maximum boluses are 0.25–0.5 ml for rodents, 1–2 ml for hystricomorphs and 2–3 mls for rabbits and ferrets

one time. Guinea pigs and chinchillas are more likely to regurgitate than rabbits, especially when debilitated, so care is needed.

Ferret

Naso-oesophageal tubes are not so well tolerated in ferrets, but many will accept sweet-tasting oral electrolyte solutions from a syringe. Ferrets, especially when debilitated, can regurgitate, so care is needed.

Subcutaneous

The advantages and disadvantages of this method are given in Table 18.3.

Rabbit

The scruff or lateral thorax make ideal sites. This is a good technique for use as routine post-operative administration of fluids for minor surgical procedures such as speying or castration. It is possible to give a maximum of 30–60 ml split into two or more sites at one time depending on the size of rabbit.

Rat, mouse, gerbil and hamster

The scruff area is easily utilised for volumes of 3–4 ml of fluids for smaller rodents and up to 10 ml at any one time for rats. The use of a 25 gauge needle is recommended.

Guinea pig and chinchilla

This is an easily used route for post-operative fluids and mild dehydration in these species. The scruff area or lateral thorax are preferred sites (Fig. 18.4). The subcutaneous route may be painful for guinea pigs but doses of 25–30 ml may be given at one time, preferably at two or more sites. Fur slip is a problem in chinchillas.

Ferret

Volumes of 15–20 ml may be given in two or more sites over the scruff.

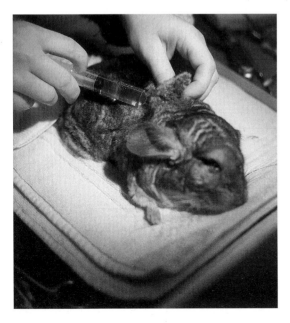

Fig. 18.4 Subcutaneous fluids being administered in the scruff region in a chinchilla post-operatively.

Intraperitoneal

The advantages and disadvantages of the intraperitoneal route in small mammals are given in Table 18.3.

Rabbit

The rabbit is placed in dorsal recumbancy to allow the gut contents to fall away from the injection zone. The needle is inserted in the lower right quadrant of the ventral abdomen, just through the abdominal wall and the syringe plunger drawn back to ensure that no puncture of the bladder or gut has occurred. A maximum volume of 20–30 ml may be given at one time depending on the size of the rabbit. Previous notes regarding concurrent respiratory or cardiovascular disease should be considered. If positioned correctly there should be no resistance to injection.

Rat, mouse, gerbil and hamster

The positioning and administration site for rodents is as for rabbits (Fig. 18.5). The needle should be 25 gauge or smaller and maximal volumes of 1–4 ml in smaller rodents, up to 10 ml in large rats, may be given.

Guinea pig and chinchilla

Similar principles apply for this route as for rabbits and rodents. Doses of 15–20 ml may be given. This is a good route for more serious cases, as intravenous fluids are not so well tolerated, particularly in chinchillas and guinea pigs.

Ferret

The technique is as for rabbits. Restraint may be difficult in the conscious patient, and maximum volumes are 20–25 ml.

Intravenous

The advantages and disadvantages of intravenous fluid therapy in small mammals are given in Table 18.3.

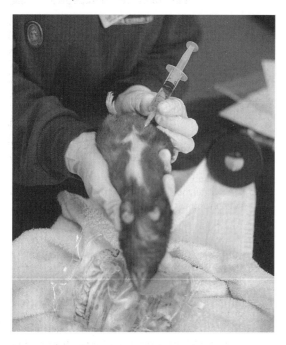

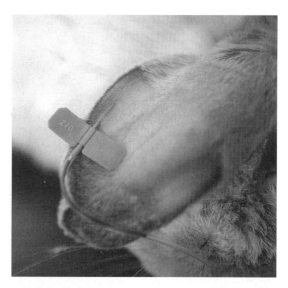

Fig. 18.6 Catheterisation of the lateral ear vein in a rabbit using a butterfly catheter.

Fig. 18.5 Intraperitoneal fluids administered to a rat showing positioning required for safe administration to avoid organ puncture.

Rabbit

The blood vessel that is best tolerated is the lateral ear vein. The technique for using it is described below.

Lateral ear vein catheterisation: the following technique should be used (Fig. 18.6):

(1) The area should be shaved and surgically prepared. Warm the ear under a lamp or hot water bottle or apply local anaesthetic cream to dilate the vessel. (NB If the rabbit is sedated, the ear veins will dilate anyway.)

(2) Use the lateral ear vein which runs along the curved most caudal/lateral margin of the pinna. Do not be tempted to use the apparently larger vessel that runs in the midline of the pinna as this is the central ear artery. Catheterisation of this vessel may lead to thrombosis followed by ear tip necrosis!

(3) Use a 25–27 gauge butterfly catheter, pre-flushed with heparinised saline. Once in place, tape it in securely and reflush. Attach the

intravenous drip tubing or catheter bung to the end of the butterfly catheter.

(4) Fit the rabbit with an Elizabethan collar or apply an intravenous drip guard to the intravenous tubing to prevent chewing, and attach this to the syringe driver. It is possible to tape the butterfly catheter to the back of the rabbit's head if using intermittent intravenous boluses, but it is important to ensure the catheter is regularly flushed with heparinised saline.

Cephalic vein: The cephalic vein may be used as for the cat and dog, although this vein may be split in some rabbits: A 25–27 gauge over-the-needle or butterfly catheter may be used for access and taped in as for cats and dogs.

Saphenous vein: for the saphenous vein it is best to use a 25–27 gauge butterfly catheter as it is relatively fragile. It runs over the lateral aspect of the hock (Fig. 18.7).

All of these routes can be used for intravenous boluses of up to 10 ml for larger rabbits and 5 ml for smaller dwarf breeds, but for continuous therapy a syringe driver is required.

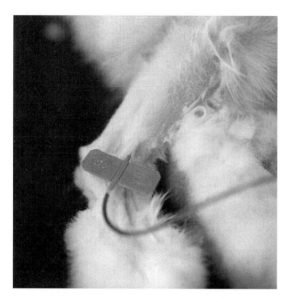

Fig. 18.7 Catheterisation of the saphenous vein in a rabbit using a butterfly catheter.

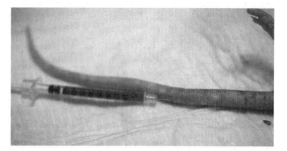

Fig. 18.8 Blood transfusion in a rat. Blood is administered to an anaesthetised patient via the tail vein, here in a pre-heparinised syringe.

Rat, mouse, gerbil and hamster

The intravenous route in hamsters and gerbils is extremely difficult to use, as they have few peripheral veins and the tail veins in gerbils are dangerous to use due to the risk of tail separation. In mice and rats, the lateral tail veins may be used. An intravenous bolus of fluids can be given using a 25–27 gauge insulin needle or by insertion of a butterfly catheter (Fig. 18.8). Warming the tail, applying local anaesthetic cream and sedation will help to dilate the vessels and make venipuncture easier. Volumes of 0.2 ml in mice up to 0.5 ml in rats as a bolus may be given. It is also possible to perform a cut-down jugular catheterisation but this requires anaesthesia.

Guinea pig and chinchilla

The cephalic and saphenous veins may be used – but generally these are very small and difficult to catheterise. A cut-down technique may be used to access the jugular veins in an emergency.

Jugular vein catheterisation: Sedation or anaesthesia is necessary for this procedure, which is as follows:

(1) The guinea pig or chinchilla is placed in dorsal recumbancy and the ventral neck is surgically prepared.
(2) An incision is made lateral to the midline and parallel to the trachea, through the skin, and the underlying tissues are bluntly dissected to expose the jugular vein.
(3) An over-the-needle catheter is preferred, preferably a 25 gauge with wings which can be sutured to the skin after insertion.
(4) The catheter is flushed with heparinised saline, a bung is placed over the port and the catheter bandaged in place.

Ferret

Ferrets are difficult to catheterise when fully conscious. The cephalic vein may be used, with 24–27 gauge over-the-needle catheters, however movement once consciousness has been regained frequently dislodges these catheters, and ferrets will often chew the dressings off. Bolus therapy when unconscious may be preferable with 5–10 ml given over several minutes.

Intraosseous

The advantages and disadvantages of this route in small mammals are given in Table 18.3.

Rabbit

The proximal femur is the easiest bone to use for intraosseous fluid administration. The landmark to aim for is the fossa between the hip joint and the greater trochanter. A 20–23 gauge hypodermic needle or spinal needle is used, and the procedure requires sedation. The area is surgically prepared and the needle is screwed into position in the same direction as the long axis of the femur. It may be necessary to cut down through the skin with a sterile scalpel blade in some rabbits. This method will require a syringe driver perfusion device.

It is possible to use the proximal tibia but this is less well tolerated due to interference with the stifle joint. There is frequently a need for tubing guards or Elizabethan collars for all intravenous or intraosseous techniques.

Rodents

The proximal femur may be tolerated as for rabbits in larger rats but smaller species often have too small a medullary cavity for needles to be safely inserted.

Hystricomorphs

This is the preferred route for severely dehydrated chinchillas and guinea-pigs with the proximal femur being the easiest site. Access is via the natural fossa created by the hip joint and the greater trochanter. Infusion devices such as syringe drivers are advised for this route of administration (Fig. 18.9).

Drug toxicities in small mammals

Lagomorpha

Drugs of the penicillin family, particularly the potentiated penicillins (e.g. potentiated amoxycillin), but also preparations containing ampicillin and amoxycillin should not be used due to their ability to cause an enterotoxaemia with *Clostridia* spp. gut overgrowth. The same is true of the cephalosporin and the macrolide family. Other antibiotic additives to avoid in rabbits include procaine which is often added to penicillin preparations.

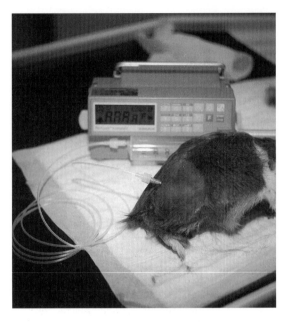

Fig. 18.9 Intraosseous catheter placement in a guinea pig using the proximal femur, showing attachment to drip set and infusion device, and prior to bandaging in place.

Muridae

Antibiotic treatment of rats and mice is less fraught with problems than is the case with many of the other rodents, as they are less susceptible to antibiotic side effects such as *Clostridia* spp. overgrowth and fatal diarrhoeas. It should be noted however that the following preparations should not be used: Medications containing procaine (such as procaine penicillin) and streptomycin have been reported as causing toxicity in mice and rats.

Gerbils (Cricetidae)

Gerbils are sensitive to streptomycin and dihydrostreptomycin containing antibiotics. They are mildly affected by potentiated penicillins, and these should be used with care. It is not advised to use any macrolides in gerbils (e.g. clindamycin, erythromycin, etc).

Hamsters (Cricetidae)

The following antibiotics should never be used in hamsters due to the ability to cause a fatal enterotoxaemic condition and in the case of the aminoglycosides because of the risks of renal damage and ototoxicity: these are all penicillins, all cephalosporins, all macrolides (clindamycin, erythromycin, etc.), the aminoglycosides streptomycin and dihydrostreptomycin, oral gentamicin.

Guinea pigs (Hystricomorpha)

The following antibiotics should not be used in guinea pigs for fear of causing a fatal enterotoxaemic condition: all penicillins, all cephalosporins and all macrolides.

Chinchillas (Hystricomorpha)

The following antibiotics should not be used in chinchillas for fear of inducing a fatal enterotoxaemia: all penicillins, all cephalosporins, and all macrolides. Metronidazole has been associated with liver failure in chinchillas.

Chipmunks (Sciuromorpha)

Chipmunks appear more resilient to antibiotics than many of the other animals mentioned here,

probably due to their slightly more omnivorous nature. However, avoid the macrolide family and the penicillins as both can cause diarrhoea, particularly the former.

Ferrets

Ferrets are generally unaffected by most antimicrobials.

Treatments for diseases in small mammals

The tables in this section are intended to give an overview of the therapies available and are by no means comprehensive. Readers are advised to consult one of the many excellent texts listed at the end of this chapter for further information.

Lagomorph disease therapies

Tables 18.4–18.7 discuss common treatments for diseases of lagomorphs on a system basis.

Table 18.4 Treatment of skin diseases in lagomorphs.

Diagnosis	Treatment
Mites, lice and fleas	Ivermectin is the drug of choice for mites and lice. In the UK, the drug imadocloprid (Advantage®, Bayer) is licensed for flea treatment in rabbits.
Blow-fly strike	Prevention is geared to removing risk of urine and faecal soiling, e.g. fine mesh used to cover outdoor hutch openings. The use of the topical growth inhibitor cyromazine (Rearguard®, Novartis) will prevent maggot maturation. Once infected, manually remove maggots, and use ivermectin, covering antibiotics and fluid therapy.
Bacterial diseases	Based on culture and sensitivity results. Blue fur disease requires enrofloxacin treatment, and rabbit syphilis requires penicillin (one dose given with care).
Dermatophytosis	Oral griseofulvin can be used, although not in pregnant does due to its terratogenic side-effects. Enilconazole washes may be used instead.
Myxomatosis	No treatment. Prevention is by vaccination with the Shope papilloma virus.

Table 18.5 Treatment of digestive system diseases in lagomorphs.

Diagnosis	Treatment
Dental disease	Prevention is better than cure. Access to good quality hay, dried grass or fresh grazing is essential. Homogenous pelleted grass-based foods are also useful. Once teeth are overgrown, regular burring to a normal shape must be performed every 6–8 weeks.
Hairballs	Digestive lubricants, liquid paraffin, fluid therapy and the enzyme papain (found in pineapple juice) are recommended. Surgery should be a last option.
Diarrhoea	Fluid therapy is very important. Cause must be determined before treatment. Loperamide may be used to symptomatically reduce diarrhoea. Coccidiosis may be treated with oral sulfadimidine at 1 g per litre of drinking water for 7 days. Repeat after 7 days. Nematode infections may be treated with an ivermectin injection at 0.2 mg/kg or oral fenbendazole at 20 mg/kg once daily for 4 days.
Mucoid enteropathy	Dietary management is important. Use of pro-kinetics such as metoclopramide and cisapride may be useful. Fluid therapy is also essential with oral probiotics therapy.

Table 18.6 Treatment of respiratory and urogenital diseases in lagomorphs.

Diagnosis	Treatment
Pasteurellosis	Fluid therapy is essential. Treatment with fluoroquinolone or sulphonamide antibiotic advised. Mucolytics, e.g. bromhexine hydrochloride, and manual cleaning of the nares is also useful.
Viral haemorrhagic disease	No treatment. Prevention with killed vaccine (UK Cylap®, Websters).
Urolithiasis	Flushing bladder of crystals and fluid therapy. Reduce dietary calcium and restrict dry food to maximum 25–30 g/day
Uterine adenocarcinoma	Treatment by surgical speying. Prevention is by surgical speying at 4–5 months of age.
Venereal spirochaetosis	Penicillin G, single dose, subcutaneously at 40,000 IU/kg. May need to repeat after 7 days. Care should be taken as it can be toxic.
Mastitis	Antibiosis based on culture and sensitivity. Analgesia with carprofen 5 mg/kg, meloxicam 0.2 mg/kg daily. Fluid therapy and supportive treatment is essential.

Table 18.7 Treatment of musculoskeletal and nervous system diseases in lagomorphs.

Diagnosis	Treatment
Fractures	Spinal dislocations and fractures with hind limb paresis carry a poor prognosis. Shock doses of short-acting corticosteroids, e.g. methyl prednisolone, should be considered if administered within 12 hours of injury. Limb fractures carry a better prognosis. Consider calcium and vitamin D3 supplementation in cases of metabolic bone disease.
Vestibular disease	Fluoroquinolone or sulphonamide antibiotics are useful in bacterial cases. Prognosis is guarded for full recovery, but generally not life-threatening if due to otitis media-interna.
Encephalitozoonosis	Fenbendazole may be used at 10–20 mg/kg orally once daily for 7–10 days. Prognosis is guarded.

Muridae disease therapies

Tables 18.8–18.10 discuss common treatments for diseases of Muridae (rats and mice, chiefly) on a system basis.

Table 18.8 Treatment of skin diseases in Muridae.

Diagnosis	Treatment
Mites	Ivermectin at 0.2 mg/kg is advised
Lice and fleas	Ivermectin or fipronil topically sprayed on a cloth and wiped lightly over fur.
Bacterial diseases	Based on culture and sensitivity results. Pododermatitis may require surgical debridement, analgesia (carprofen/meloxicam) and hydrating gels/dressings, as well as improving cage substrate to increase padding. Weight loss also advisable.
Dermatophytosis	Oral griseofulvin, but beware of terratogenicity in pregnant females. Alternatively, use topical enilconazole washes every 2–3 days.
Atopy	Topical soothing shampoos and oral essential fatty acids (oil of evening primrose) may help.

Table 18.9 Treatment of digestive and respiratory system diseases in Muridae.

Diagnosis	Treatment
Dental disease	Burring every 3–4 weeks with a low speed dental burr is advised for incisor malocclusion.
Parasitic diarrhoea	Ivermectin at 0.2 mg/kg once, or fenbendazole at 20 mg/kg orally once daily for 5 days for nematodes. For coccidiosis use sulfadimidine in water at 200 mg/litre for 7 days. Metronidazole is useful for other protozoa.
Bacterial diarrhoea	Oxytetracycline is used for Tyzzer's disease at 0.1 g per litre of drinking water. Other treatments are based on culture and sensitivity.
Respiratory disease	Culture and sensitivity selection of antibiosis is useful, otherwise oxytetracycline and enrofloxacin are useful against *Mycoplasma* spp. Consider mucolytics, e.g. bromhexine hydrochloride.

Table 18.10 Treatment of urinary tract, musculoskeletal, neurological and ocular diseases in Muridae.

Diagnosis	Treatment
Chronic nephrosis	Reduce dietary protein, but increase the biological value of that protein. Anabolic steroids and B vitamin supplementation are also useful.
Urolithiasis	Removal of blockages manually. Reduce calcium content of diet and increase bran levels. Use sulphonamide antibiotics for preputial gland abscess/cystitis.
Spondylosis	Meloxicam at 0.2 mg/kg orally once daily for pain relief.
Fractures	Splinting and strict confinement + analgesia (meloxicam/carprofen) allow rapid callus formation and repair (2–3 weeks).
Vestibular disease	If bacterial, use fluoroquinolone or sulphonamide antibiotics. If caused by a pituitary tumour surgery may be possible.
Keratoconjunctivitis sicca	Topical cyclopsporin may be used.

Cricetidae disease therapies

Tables 18.11–18.14 discuss common treatments for diseases of Cricetidae (gerbils and hamsters, chiefly) on a system basis.

Table 18.11   Treatment of skin diseases of gerbils.

Diagnosis	Treatment
Demodicosis	Amitraz washes (1 ml solution to 0.5 litres water) once every two weeks until negative scrapings. Beware toxicity. Storage mites are best treated by topical fipronil sprayed on a cloth and wiped lightly over infected area.
Bacterial diseases	Oral or parenteral antibiosis based on culture and sensitivity results. Enrofloxacin at 5 mg/kg once, twice daily or oxytetracycline at 0.8 mg/litre water may be useful.
Dermatophytosis	Oral griseofulvin, but beware terratogenic properties in pregnant females. Enilconazole washes every 2–3 days.
Skin tumours	Surgical excision of ventral scent gland adenocarcinomas advised.
Degloving tail injuries	Fluid therapy advised. Topical anticoagulants (calcium sprays) or pressure to stem bleeding. Topical/parenteral antibiotics advised. May need surgery to remove denuded coccygeal vertebrae.

Table 18.12   Treatment of digestive, respiratory and reproductive system diseases in gerbils.

Diagnosis	Treatment
Ileal hyperplasia (wet tail)	Extremely difficult, but the use of oxytetracyclines has been suggested.
Parasitic diarrhoea	Ivermectin at 0.2 mg/kg for nematode infestations. Praziquantel at 10 mg/kg orally once for *Hymenolepis nana* but may need to repeat after 2 weeks.
Respiratory diseases	As for rats and mice.
Cystic ovarian disease	Surgical speying is curative. Alternatively, human chorionic gonadotrophin at 100 IU/kg may remove the cysts for a time.

Table 18.13   Treatment of skin and digestive system diseases in hamsters.

Diagnosis	Treatment
Mites	Amitraz is the treatment of choice (see gerbils).
Bacterial skin disease	Enrofloxacin has a wide safety margin in hamsters at 5 mg/kg.
Dermatophytosis	As for gerbils.
Cushing's disease	This is often untreatable. Metapyrone has been used at 8 mg orally once daily, but this is potentially extremely toxic and may result in the death of the hamster.
Cheek pouch impactions	Scruffing the hamster and milking the contents manually cranially or with a dampened cotton bud is advised. Flushing the pouches with dilute chlorhexidine can remove any superficial infection.
Cheek pouch prolapses	Surgical replacement with a cotton bud under anaesthesia is advised. A suture may be placed through the skin into the cheek pouch behind the ear to keep in place.
Wet tail	As for gerbils.

Table 18.14 Treatment of cardiovascular, endocrine, reproductive and musculoskeletal diseases in hamsters.

Diagnosis	Treatment
Aortic thrombosis	Use of furosemide at 0.25–0.5 mg/kg may be useful, as may the ACE inhibitor enalapril at 0.25 mg/kg, orally once daily. Beware of hypotensive effects.
Cushing's disease	See skin diseases.
Diabetes mellitus	Protamine zinc insulin therapy may be attempted at 0.5–1 unit/kg (requires dilution in saline). Aim for 0.25–0.5% glucose in urine and water consumption 10–15 ml/day. Use glucose/saline intraperitoneally and human glucose oral gels on membranes if evidence of hypoglycaemic overdose.
Pyometra	Surgical neutering after fluid therapy and antibiotic stabilisation.
Cystic ovarian disease	See gerbils.
Fractures	Compound fractures of the tibia may require leg amputation. If closed they may heal conservatively with rest and analgesia. Intra-medullary pinning with 25–27 gauge needles is possible.

Hystricomorph disease therapies

Tables 18.15–18.19 discuss common treatments for diseases of hystricomorphs on a system basis (chiefly chinchillas and guinea pigs).

Table 18.15 Treatment of skin diseases in guinea pigs.

Diagnosis	Treatment
Mites	Ivermectin at 0.2 mg/kg is effective against *Trixicara caviae*. Analgesics such as carprofen and tranquilisers, such as diazepam, may be necessary in severe cases.
Lice	Fipronil sprayed on to a cloth and then wiped over the fur. Ivermectin may also be useful.
Cervical lymphadenitis	Surgical lancing of the abscess, and treatment with antibiotics such as enrofloxacin is advised.
Dermatophytosis	Griseofulvin and topical enilconazole may be used as for rats and mice.
Pododermatitis	Treatment is the same as for rats.

Table 18.16   Treatment of digestive, respiratory and urinary system diseases in guinea pigs.

Diagnosis	Treatment
Dental disease	This is similar to rabbits. Change the diet to increase abrasive, grass-based foods. Burr molar spikes every 6–8 weeks under sedation. Treat oral infections based on culture and sensitivity +/– information.
Bacterial digestive disease	As for hamsters and gerbils, based on culture and sensitivity. Enrofloxacin useful for *Salmonella* spp.
Parasitic digestive disease	Nematodes may be treated with 0.2 mg/kg ivermectin. Coccidiosis requires oral sulfadimidine at 40 mg/kg, once daily for 5 days. *B. coli* requires metronidazole orally but use with caution due to risk of liver damage.
Faecal impaction	Manual emptying of peri-anal skin folds daily and flushing with dilute chlorhexidine.
Respiratory disease	Enrofloxacin and sulphonamide drugs are useful. Mucolytics, e.g. bromhexine hydrochloride, are useful.
Chronic nephrosis	As for rats. Supplemental vitamin C is useful.
Urolithiasis	Restriction of dry food to 15–20 g per day to reduce dietary calcium levels is useful. Treat as for cystitis.

Table 18.17   Treatment of reproductive ocular and musculoskeletal diseases in guinea pigs.

Diagnosis	Treatment
Cystic ovarian disease	As for gerbils.
Pregnancy toxaemia	Oral glucose gel (Hypostop®), intravenous or intraperitoneal glucose-saline as a 5–7 ml bolus. Dexamethasone 0.2 mg/kg intramuscularly (but will cause abortion). To prevent, do not let sow become overweight or stressed.
Mastitis	Antibiosis such as enrofloxacin or sulphonamides with fluid therapy and NSAID analgesia. Surgery may be necessary.
Scurvy	Vitamin C parenterally at 50 mg/kg, and 200 mg/l drinking water.
Fractures	Splinting with hexalite materials may be possible. Otherwise cage restriction and analgesia or surgical fixation is required. Methyl-prednisolone may be needed if spinal trauma is involved.
Conjunctivitis	Chlortetracycline eye ointment for *Chlamydophila psittaci* conjunctivitis. See scurvy for vitamin C related problems

Table 18.18   Treatment of skin and digestive system diseases in chinchillas.

Diagnosis	Treatment
Dermatophytosis	Griseofulvin at 25 mg/kg orally once daily for 28 days. Avoid eniloconazole washes due to fur damage.
Dental disease	As for rabbits – dental burring under sedation every 6–8 weeks, dietary change to grass-based products. Analgesia for root pain using meloxicam orally.
Colic	Fluid therapy, analgesia (carprofen or meloxicam) and cisapride at 0.2–0.5 mg/kg orally.
Hepatic lipidosis	Reduce excess proteins in diet. Supplement with B vitamins, and use lactulose at 0.3 ml/kg orally daily to reduce bacterial toxins the liver has to remove.
Constipation	Lactulose is a mild laxative. Fluid therapy and dietary fibre useful. Once hydrated, oral cisapride may be helpful.
Bacterial diarrhoea	Based on culture and sensitivity results.
Parasitic diarrhoea	Treatment of giardiasis is with fenbendazole at 25 mg/kg orally once daily for 3 days (avoid metronidazole due to hepatotoxicity).

Table 18.19   Treatment of cardiovascular, musculoskeletal, nervous and ocular diseases in chinchillas.

Diagnosis	Treatment
Cardiomyopathies	Furosemide and ACE inhibitors, such as enalapril, may be of some use.
Fractures	Long bone fractures are best fixed with external fixation surgically. Smaller fractures may be splinted with human finger splints.
Fitting	Symptomatic treatment with 1–2 mg/kg diazepam intramuscularly. Heat-stroke can be treated with cooled intravenous/peritoneal fluids. Listeriosis may be treated with oxytetracycline 10 mg/kg twice daily intramuscularly.
Conjunctivitis	Use of chlortetracycline eye ointments is recommended for *Chlamydophila psittaci*. Always check for dental disease in any case of epiphora.

Sciuromorph disease therapies

Tables 18.20 and 18.21 discuss common treatments for diseases of sciuromorphs (chiefly the chipmunk) on a system basis.

Table 18.20   Treatment of skin, digestive and respiratory system diseases of chipmunks.

Diagnosis	Treatment
Mites	Ivermectin at 0.2 mg/kg is advised. In addition, for *Dermanyssus gallinae*, burn bedding and dust cage with bromcyclen powder.
Bacterial skin disease	Antibiosis based on culture and sensitivity. Generally, enrofloxacin, tetracycline and sulphonamides are safe and effective.
Dental disease	Burring of incisor malocclusion with a slow speed dental drill every 4–6 weeks.
Diarrhoea	As for rats and mice.
Respiratory disease	Oxytetracycline at 22 mg/kg once daily for 5–7 days is useful for *Mycoplasma* spp. Enrofloxacin may also be used.

Table 18.21   Treatment of urinary, reproductive, musculoskeletal and nervous system diseases of chipmunks.

Diagnosis	Treatment
Urolithiasis	Surgical or manual removal of obstructing uroliths. Give meat-based foods temporarily to acidify urine and dissolve crystals, or increase seeds and fruits and reduce biscuits.
Hypocalcaemic paralysis	100 mg/kg calcium gluconate intramuscularly. Prevention based on dietary supplementation.
Uterine infections	Based on culture and sensitivity results. Pyometra may require surgery after fluid stabilisation.
Mastitis	Enrofloxacin and oxytetracyclines may be useful with NSAID analgesia (carprofen).Surgery may be required.
Fractures	Spinal trauma has a poor prognosis, but methyl prednisolone may be used peracutely. Minor fractures may respond to cage rest and in-food analgesia (meloxicam).
Fitting	Removal from rooms with TV and computor screens. Use of 0.5–1 mg/kg diazepam intramuscularly may help.

Mustelid disease therapies

Tables 18.22–18.25 discuss common treatments for diseases of mustelids (chiefly the domestic ferret) on system basis.

Table 18.22   Treatment of skin diseases in mustelids.

Diagnosis	Treatment
Mites	Ivermectin at 0.2 mg/kg once, and repeated after 14 days.
Fleas and ticks	Use of fipronil at 7.5 mg/kg topically. (*Note:* this is not licensed for use in ferrets.)
Bacterial diseases	Based on culture and sensitivity with drugs such as enrofloxacin at 5–10 mg/kg, potentiated sulphonamides at 15–30 mg/kg twice daily and potentiated amoxicillin at 10–20 mg/kg twice daily.
Dermatophytosis	Oral griseofulvin as for rats chinchillas, or topical enilconazole washes every 3 days.
Tumours	Surgical excision.
Hormonal diseases	Testosterone-dependent alopecia requires surgical castration. Oestrogen-dependent alopecia requires surgical speying or castration if a seminoma. Hyperadrenocorticism treatment is given in Table 18.25.

Table 18.23   Treatment of digestive system diseases in mustelids.

Diagnosis	Treatment
Dental disease	Extraction of rotten teeth, antibiosis with clindamycin at 5.5 mg/kg twice daily or potentiated amoxicillin is recommended. Encourage dry foods to prevent recurrence.
Gastric ulcers	Use cytoprotectants: cimetidine (10 mg/kg twice daily), sucralfate (100 mg/kg daily orally) and bismuth subsalicylate (1 ml/kg three time daily, orally). If *Helicobacter mustelae* is present, combined amoxicillin and metronidazole is advised.
Proliferative ileitis	Chloramphenicol is the antibiotic of choice.
Lymphoma	Chemotherapy with drugs such as vincristine, cyclophosphamide and prednisolone has been tried but prognosis is guarded.
Bacterial disease	This is based on culture and sensitivity results of faeces samples.
Parasitic disease	Giardiasis treatment is with metronidazole. Coccidiosis is with sulfadimidine. Nematode infestations may be treated with 0.2 mg/kg ivermectin or with fenbendazole.
Liver disease	Lactulose at 1.5–3 mg/kg orally once daily may help. Supportive therapy with vitamin B supplements and reduced fat/high biological value proteins is advised.

Table 18.24   Treatment of respiratory, cardiovascular and urinary system diseases of mustelids.

Diagnosis	Treatment
Canine distemper virus	There is no treatment. Prevention is based on vaccination, but this has to be with one developed for a dogs. Care should be taken to choose a vaccine not raised in ferrets, and to use a reduced dose. Consultation with the vaccine manufacturer is advised. Ferrets may be dosed at 8 and 14 weeks, and then annually thereafter.
Bacterial pneumonia	This is based on culture and sensitivity results.
Dilated cardiomyopathy	Furosemide at 1–4 mg/kg in acute crisis is useful, intravenously or intramuscularly. ACE inhibitor enalapril may be used at 0.5 mg/kg every 48 hours but watch for hypotensive effects. Digoxin may also be used in heart failure.
Urolithiasis	Surgery may be required to remove obstructions and/or bladder stones. Feeding an all meat-based protein diet is essential to prevent formation. Treatment of any primary or secondary cystitis is based on culture and sensitivity results.

Table 18.25 Treatment of endocrine, reproductive and ocular diseases in mustelids.

Diagnosis	Treatment
Hyperadrenocorticism	Medical therapy is ineffective as the tumour is adrenal-based. Treatment is surgical excision of the tumour.
Diabetes mellitus	Based on protamine zinc insulin at 1–2 units per ferret, and increasing by 0.5 units until blood glucose falls to 15 mmol/l or urine glucose to 0.5%. Twice daily dosing may be required.
Pregnancy toxaemia	40% glucose at 0.5–1 ml/kg by slow intravenous bolus. Bicarbonate supplement to fluids is advised to counteract acidosis. Dexamethasone may be required in severe cases but abortion will occur.
Uterine infections	Surgical speying after fluid stabilisation and treatment with broad spectrum antibiotics until culture and sensitivity results are available.
Mastitis	Broad-spectrum antibiotics and NSAIDs with fluid therapy is advised. Surgical excision of abscesses may be needed.
Hyperoestrogenism	Prevention based on speying at 4–5 months or earlier, or mating with an entire or vasectomised hob, or regular proligesterone treatment at the start of the season (50 mg/jill). Treat with blood transfusion if PCV < 20%, or in early stages stop oestrus with proligesterone or human chorionic gonadotrophin.

Further reading

Beynon, P.H. and Cooper, J.E. (1991) *Manual of Exotic Pets*, 3*rd* edn. BSAVA Cheltenham.

Harkness. J.E. and Wagner, J.E. (1995) *The Biology and Medicine of Rabbits and Rodents*, 4*th* edn. Lea and Febiger, Philadelphia.

Meredith, A. and Redrobe, S. (2001) *Manual of Exotic Pets*, 4*th* edn. BSAVA Cheltenham.

Okerman, L. (1994) *Diseases of Domestic Rabbits*, 2*nd* edn. Blackwell Science, Oxford.

Quesenberry, K.E. and Hillyer, V.E. (1997) *Ferrets, Rabbits and Rodents: Clinical Medicine and Surgery*. W.B. Saunders, Philadelphia.

Appendix 1

Legislation Affecting Exotic Pet Species in the United Kingdom

Convention on the International Trade of Endangered Species (CITES)

Broadly this is the list of endangered species around the world, categorised into:

- Appendix 1, which contains those species highly endangered in which international trade is banned
- Appendix 2 contains those species considered seriously threatened in which trade is again banned or at least heavily controlled
- Appendix 3 contains those species which are at risk, and in which international trade is restricted.

In the United Kingdom these lists are enforced by European Union Control Of Trade in Endangered Species laws or COTES regulations (Council Regulation 339/97 and Commission Regulation 939/97) wherein the species are divided into four groups:

- Annex A includes species such as the Mediterranean tortoises, for example the Greek or spur-thighed tortoise (*Testudo graeca*). It also includes many endangered species of *native* bird, such as the red kite.
- Annex B includes all species under CITES Appendix 2 and some other species
- Annex C includes all species barring one or two under CITES Appendix 3
- Annex D includes non-CITES species which are considered as needing protection by the European Union.

It is important to note that any person selling a species listed in Annex A must have a licence, as well as having some form of permanent identification of that individual to prove its identity.

In the case of the Mediterranean tortoise species, the vendor must have a licence to prove that the mother of the hatchling is captive bred, or was obtained before the regulations came into force. The hatchling must be sold currently with a licence from the government and with an electronic identification chip which is to be implanted in a standard site. The British Veterinary Zoological Society currently recommends subcutaneously in the left thigh region. The chip is to be implanted as soon as the plastral length of the tortoise exceeds 100 mm.

Health and Safety at Work Act 1974

It is important to remember that many wildlife cases carry zoonotic diseases, such as *Salmonella* spp, rabies-related viruses in some wild bat populations, *Yersinia pseudotuberculosis* in many rodents and lagomorphs, chlamydiosis in many wild birds and psittacine species, etc. Many species of exotic pet may be aggressive when stressed or ill and will readily turn on the handler. Unpleasant bites, scratches or worse can result.

The veterinary nurse (and other members of staff) have an obligation to avoid hazards and prevent accidents and accidental cross infection in the workplace. In addition the employer has an obligation to ensure that facilities and training of staff are sufficient to minimise the risks of handling and treating these animals.

Protection of Animals Act 1911–1964

Under this legislation it is an offence to treat a captive animal cruelly or to cause it unnecessary suffering. This ensures that all cases receive proper care and attention, and that their accommodation is of the correct dimensions and provides suitable shelter from other animals as well as excessive noxious stimuli.

Abandonment of Animals Act 1960

Under this legislation it is an offence to release any wild animal which is not in a fit state to survive in the wild. Examples include release of birds of prey with foot injuries or beak injuries, release of mammals with fractures etc.

Wildlife and Countryside Act 1981

With regard to exotic pets, this legislation prohibits the release of non-native species into the wild in the United Kingdom (as listed in Schedule 9 of the Act).

Appendix 2
Useful Addresses

British Veterinary Zoological Society
(This society welcomes veterinary surgeons and veterinary nurses alike)
Mr D G Lyon BVSc MRCVS, Administrative Director
7 Bridgewater Mews,
Gresford Heath
Pandy,
Wrexham LL12 8EQ
Website www.bvzs.org

British Chelonia Group
PO Box 1176
Chippenham
Wiltshire
SN15 1XB
Website www.britishcheloniagroup.org.uk
Reg Charity 801818

Tortoise Trust
BM Tortoise
London
WC1N 3XX
Website www.tortoisetrust.org

The Rabbit Welfare Association Incorporating the British House-rabbit Association
RWF
PO Box 346
Newcastle-upon-Tyne
NE99 2YP
Reg Charity 1085689
Website www.rabbitwelfare.co.uk

The Association of Avian Veterinarians
(This association welcomes veterinary nurses/technicians)
PO Box 811720
Boca Raton
FL 33481
USA
Website www.aav.org

The Association of Reptilian and Amphibian Veterinarians
(This association welcomes veterinary nurses/technicians)
PO Box 605
Chester Heights
PA 19017
USA
Website www.arav.org

Index